Computational Theories and their Implementation in the Brain

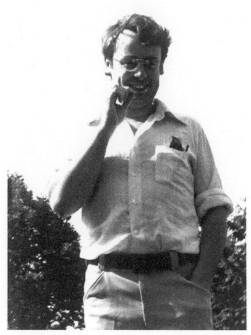

David Marr (taken in Cambridge, UK at the time that he was working on the papers featured in the book)

Computational Theories and their Implementation in the Brain
The legacy of David Marr

Edited by

Lucia M. Vaina and Richard E. Passingham

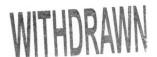

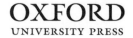

OXFORD
UNIVERSITY PRESS

OXFORD
UNIVERSITY PRESS

Great Clarendon Street, Oxford, OX2 6DP,
United Kingdom

Oxford University Press is a department of the University of Oxford.
It furthers the University's objective of excellence in research, scholarship,
and education by publishing worldwide. Oxford is a registered trade mark of
Oxford University Press in the UK and in certain other countries

First Edition published in 2017

Impression: 1

Published in the United States of America by Oxford University Press
198 Madison Avenue, New York, NY 10016, United States of America

British Library Cataloguing in Publication Data

Data available

Library of Congress Control Number: 2016937964

ISBN 978–0–19–874978–3

Printed and bound by
CPI Group (UK) Ltd, Croydon, CR0 4YY

Preface

David Marr would have been 70 in January 2015. Had he lived there would certainly have been a major Festschrift. In 2012 the journal *Perception* ran a special issue to mark 30 years since the publication of Marr's book *Vision* (1982). Marr was one of the early founders of the field of computational neuroscience (Marr and Poggio, 1976; Marr, 1982). He clearly distinguished between three levels of analysis: the computational level relates to the function of the system, the algorithmic level concerns its operations, and the implementational level concerns the details of hardware in which those operations are carried out. In his work on vision, Marr's stress on the computational and algorithmic levels has left a very substantial legacy.

However, to mark his 70th birthday, we decided to put together a volume to celebrate Marr's earlier legacy. This resulted from the publication of his pioneering early papers on the cerebellum (Marr, 1969), neocortex (Marr, 1970), and archicortex (Marr, 1971). In these papers Marr used mathematical tools to work out how these structures might perform their functions, given the details of their microstructure. The papers were an astonishing early attempt at the implementational level because they were models of simplicity and mathematical rigor and made clear predictions. They have also had a major influence that is still lasting, as this book demonstrates.

These papers were included in a book edited by Vaina (1991) that republished a selected set of Marr's papers together with commentaries. The aim of these commentaries was to expound the argument and bring the papers up to date. Thach did this in an experimental framework for the cerebellar paper (Marr, 1969) and McNaughton for the archicortex paper (Marr, 1971). Cowen compared the three papers, discussing how they were linked computationally while also emphasizing the neocortex paper in particular (Marr, 1970). Willshaw also commented on the archicortex paper (Marr, 1971) and examined how Marr used the constraints at three different levels to mould his theory. He had earlier presented small-scale simulations of the model (Willshaw and Buckingham, 1990).

The aim of the present book is different. We invited thirteen experts to reconsider one of the three papers. Their task was to discuss to what extent Marr's early papers can form the basis for convincing and detailed theories concerning implementation that take into account advances in knowledge in neuroanatomy, neurophysiology, and computational neuroscience.

We have divided the book into three sections, one for each of the three Marr papers. Dick Passingham contributes an introduction on Marr's views of the functions of the three structures and Lucia Vaina contributes a final one on David Marr's scientific work and its trajectory and his passions for the clarinet, flying, and life.

The contributors to each section have read and commented on the other chapters in the section. The book is a joint enterprise, a truly integrated account by all the authors. They read and commented on the other chapters in their section and discussed them in detail among themselves. It is a mark of the respect in which Marr is held that each of the contributors to this book has shown such dedication to the task.

We are indebted to David Willshaw and Peter Dayan for advice and encouragement throughout the preparation of this book. We are also grateful to Charlotte Green and Martin Baum, the editors of our book at Oxford University Press.

References

Marr D. (1969). A theory of cerebellar cortex. J Physiol. **202**:437–470.

Marr D. (1970). A theory for cerebral neocortex. Proc R Soc Lond B Biol Sci. **176**:161–234.

Marr D. (1971). Simple memory: a theory for archicortex. Philos Trans R Soc Lond B Biol Sci. **262**:23–81.

Marr D. (1982). Vision: A Computational Investigation into the Human Representation and Processing of Visual Information. San Francisco, CA: W. H. Freeman.

Marr D, Poggio T. (1976) Cooperative computation of stereo disparity. Science. **194**:283–287.

Vaina LM (ed.) (1991). From the Retina to the Neocortex: Selected Papers of David Marr. Boston: Birkhauser/Springer.

Willshaw DJ, Buckingham JT. (1990). An assessment of Marr's theory of the hippocampus as a temporary memory store. Philos Trans Roy Soc B Biol Sci. **329**:205–215.

Contents

Postlude

Contributors

Suzanna Becker
Department of Psychology,
Neuroscience and Behaviour,
Faculty of Science, McMaster University,
Hamilton, Canada

Egidio D'Angelo
Department of Brain and Behavioural
Sciences, University of Pavia and Brain
Connectivity Center, IRCCS Mondino
Neurological Institute, Pavia, Italy

Peter Dayan
Gatsby Computational Neuroscience Unit,
University College London, UK

Paul Dean
Department of Psychology,
University of Sheffield, UK

Rodney J. Douglas
Institute of Neuroinformatics,
University and ETH Zurich, Switzerland

Michael E. Hasselmo
Center for Systems Neuroscience,
Department of Psychological and Brain
Sciences, Center for Memory and Brain,
Graduate Program for Neuroscience,
Boston University, Massachusetts, USA

James R. Hinman
Center for Systems Neuroscience,
Boston University, Massachusetts, USA

Takeru Honda
Tokyo Metropolitan Institute of Medical
Science, Motor Disorders Project, Tokyo,
Japan; and RIKEN Brain Science Institute,
Japan

Masao Ito
Senior Advisor's Office,
RIKEN Brain Science Institute,
Japan

Kevan A. C. Martin
Institute of Neuroinformatics,
University and ETH Zurich,
Switzerland

Richard E. Passingham
Emeritus Professor of Cognitive
Neuroscience, Department of Experimental
Psychology, University of Oxford,
Oxford, UK

John Porrill
Sheffield Centre for Robotics,
University of Sheffield, UK

Alessandro Treves
SISSA, Cognitive Neuroscience,
Trieste, Italy and NTNU,
Centre for Neural Computation,
Trondheim, Norway

Lucia M. Vaina
Departments of Biomedical
Engineering, Neurology and the
Graduate Program for
Neuroscience, Boston University;
and Department of Neurology,
Harvard Medical School, Boston,
Massachusetts, USA

David Willshaw
Institute for Adaptive and Neural
Computation, School of Informatics,
University of Edinburgh, UK

Like the entomologist in pursuit of brightly coloured butterflies,
my attention hunted, in the flower garden of the gray matter, cells with
delicate and elegant forms, the mysterious butterflies of the soul, the beatings
of whose wings may someday—who knows?—clarify the secret of mental life.

Santiago Ramón y Cajal

Text extract from Santiago Ramón y Cajal, Recollections of My Life

Introduction

Chapter 1

Marr's views on the functions of the cerebellum, hippocampus, and neocortex

Richard E. Passingham

Introduction to Marr's early work

David Marr was a PhD student at the same time as me. Both our supervisors were working at the Institute of Psychiatry in London; his was Giles Brindley whereas mine was George Ettlinger. Marr and I used to meet at tea, and it was there that he once said to me that I "should read less and think more." And think he did.

It took him a year to read what he needed, and he then produced theories of how the cerebellar cortex, the neocortex, and the archicortex (hippocampus) operate. The papers were published in successive years: the theory of cerebellar cortex in 1969, the theory of neocortex in 1970, and the theory of archicortex in 1971. There can be few PhD theses in neuroscience that have had such an impact. The first paper (Marr, 1969) has been cited roughly 2500 times, the second (Marr, 1970) nearly 430 times. and the third (Marr, 1971) around 1800 times. And this measure surely understates the importance of these papers. So thorough and far-reaching was Marr's insight that much of what he had to say is simply accepted and repeated without attribution.

The attempt at such theories was courageous and greatly in advance of its time. Thus, it is worth recording that they were produced in a laboratory where experiments were being carried out that were also courageous and greatly in advance of their time. Brindley (1970) inserted an array of stimulating electrodes over the visual cortex of a person who was blind; the aim was to find out whether the phosphenes that were evoked could be used to form letters. And in the same laboratory Craggs (1974) recorded from the motor cortex in baboons to find out whether it was possible to read the signal; the hope was to use it to move a prosthesis or even to stimulate below the spinal cut so as to restore motor performance.

The problem with being ahead of your time is that the technical methods that are available may be inadequate for the task. It was a frustration to Marr that it was not practical to test even the most critical prediction of the cerebellar theory. In fact it was not until a decade later that it shown to be correct (Ito and Kano, 1982). So one can see why Marr was tempted to accept when he met Marvin Minsky in 1972 and was invited to work in the Artificial Intelligence Laboratory at the Massachusetts Institute of Technology (MIT). It was there that he went on to lay the foundations for computational neuroscience (Marr, 1982). The advantage is that theories of computational neuroscience can be proven to be sound even if it is not known how they are implemented in the brain.

It is now 45 years since Marr produced his three theories, and in that time computing has advanced beyond all recognition. In our laboratory at the Institute of Psychiatry, calculations were done on a large desktop calculator that could add, subtract, divide, and multiply; my supervisor had to pay significantly extra for the square root button. Computing was done on a PDP-8, a computer that was first marketed in 1965; its memory could store just over 4000 12-bit words.

Over the same 45 years neuroscience has also been transformed. Many techniques have been developed that have provided essential new information and that have also made it easier to test predictions. These techniques include the use of tracers to follow anatomical connections within cortical columns; recording from multiple cells while animals perform complex cognitive tasks; and imaging methods such as functional magnetic resonance imaging (fMRI) and magnetoencephalography (MEG), manipulations with optogenetics, and so on.

So it is time to reconsider whether it is now possible to produce theories of implementation that are both viable and testable. And there is no better way to see what form such theories should take than to look back at the abstract of Marr's (1969) first paper on the cerebellar cortex (Box 1.1).

Box 1.1 Abstract of Marr's 1969 paper on the cerebellar cortex

1 A detailed theory of cerebellar cortex is proposed whose consequence is that the cerebellum learns to perform motor skills. Two forms of input-output relations are described, both consistent with the cortical theory. One is suitable for learning movements (actions), and the other for learning to maintain posture and balance (maintenance reflexes).

2 It is known that the cells of the inferior olive and the cerebellar Purkinje cells have a special one-to-one relationship induced by the climbing fibre input. For learning actions it is assumed that:

(a) each olivary cell responds to a cerebral instruction for an elemental movement. Any action has a defining representation in terms of elemental movements, and this representation has a neural expression as a sequence of firing patterns in the inferior olive; and

(b) in the correct state of the nervous system, a Purkinje cells can initiate that elemental movement to which the corresponding olivary cell responds.

3 Whenever an olivary cell fires, it sends an impulse (via the climbing fibre input) to its corresponding Purkinje cell. This Purkinje cell is also exposed (via the mossy

fibre input) to information about the context in which its olivary cell fired, and it is shown how during rehearsal of an action, each Purkinje cell can learn to recognize such contexts. Later, when the action has been learnt, occurrence of the context alone is enough to fire the Purkinje cell, which then causes the next elemental movement. The action thus progresses as it did during rehearsal.

4   It is shown that an interpretation of cerebellar cortex as a structure which allows each Purkinje cell to learn a number of contexts is consistent with the distributions of the various types of cell, and with their known excitatory or inhibitory natures. It is demonstrated that the mossy-fibre granule cell arrangement provides the required pattern discrimination ability.

5   The following predictions are made:

   (a)   The synapses from parallel fibres to Purkinje cells are facilitated by the conjunction of presynaptic and climbing fibre (or post-synaptic) activity.

   (b)   No other cerebellar synapses are modifiable.

   (c)   Golgi cells are driven by the greater of the inputs from their upper and lower dendritic fields.

6   For learning maintenance reflexes, 2(a) and 2(b) are replaced by

   2′.   Each olivary cell is stimulated by one or more receptors, all of whose activities are usually reduced by the results of stimulating the corresponding Purkinje cell.

7   It is shown that if (2′) is satisfied, the circuit receptor–olivary cell–Purkinje cell–effector may be regarded as a stabilizing reflex circuit which is activated by learning mossy fibre inputs. This type of reflex has been called a learned conditional reflex, and it is shown how such reflexes can solve problems of maintain posture and balance.

8   5(a), and either (2) or (2′) are essential to the theory: 5(b) and 5(c) are not absolutely essential, and parts of the theory could survive the disproof of either.

Functions

This is an astonishing abstract It is of unrivaled precision and clarity. It says what the structure does, specifies the transformation from inputs to outputs, and states how the cells and their connections allow it to do what it does. These three proposals very roughly correspond to the three levels, computational, algorithmic, and implementation, distinctions that Marr was later to make (Marr and Poggio, 1977; Marr, 1982).

The abstract ends by making predictions and telling the reader how critical the different predictions are for the theory. In his later papers on the neocortex (Marr, 1970) and archicortex (Marr, 1971) he introduced a starring system for his predictions. If a three-starred prediction is falsified, the theory falls; but if a one-starred prediction is falsified, the theory can be maintained, though with modification.

In the cerebellar abstract shown in Box 1.1 Marr makes several predictions. Predictions 5(a), 5(b), and 5(c) relate to the level of implementation. Predictions 2(a) and 2(b) relate to the transformation between inputs and outputs. But no predictions are made as to function, though the implementation is predicated on the assumption that the cerebellum is involved in learning motor skills, as indeed it is.

In conversations at the time, it was clear that Marr took it to be essential to be sure what a structure did before proposing a detailed theory on how it did it. In suggesting functions for the three structures, Marr depended heavily on what was known at the time about their microstructure. It is the internal wiring that makes possible the transformation from inputs to outputs, and this transformation relates to the algorithmic level.

However, what the internal wiring can do is constrained by the nature of the extrinsic inputs and outputs. The reason is that it is these that provide the information and that determine its range of influence (Passingham et al., 2002). At the time that Marr wrote, detailed information was not available on the exact sites of origin and termination of long-range connections. This has been provided since then by the use of tracing techniques.

This introduction therefore considers two issues. The first is what the inputs and outputs of the cerebellum, hippocampus, and neocortex tell us about their functions. Here the aim is to compare what we now know about the functions of these structures with the functions as proposed or assumed by Marr. The second issue is whether theories concerning implementation can be shown to be false if the function assumed for the structure is incorrect. Here the aim is to see to what extent the implementations suggested by Marr do or do not depend on assumptions concerning function.

The term "function" will be used to describe what the structure does for the animal's behavioral repertoire. It is in this sense that Marr (1969) used the term "motor skills" when proposing his cerebellar theory. The term can equally be used to describe computations, as in Marr's (1982) example of a cash register, but it is not so used here.

Cerebellum

In taking the functions of the cerebellum to include the learning of motor skills, Marr was drawing on an inspired guess by his supervisor. Brindley (1964) had suggested that the cerebellar cortex might be involved in learning motor tasks through Hebbian learning. The suggestion that it learns motor skills was based on clinical experience with patients.

The essence of skill is precision in accuracy, force, and timing. That the cerebellum is critical for skilled performance can be illustrated by three studies on patients with cerebellar pathology. The first concerns accuracy: patients with lesions in the inferior olive are inaccurate when learning to throw while wearing distorting prisms (Martin et al., 1996). The second study concerns force: patients with cerebellar cortical lesions are poor at learning to adjust their reaches in the face of predictable but opposing forces (Gibo et al., 2013). And the third study concerns timing: patients with cerebellar lesions are poor at learning to produce rhythms (Keele and Ivry, 1990).

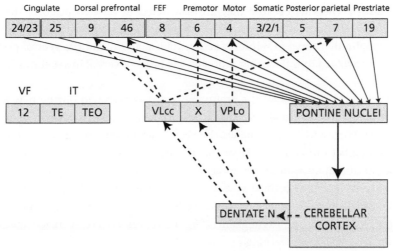

Cingulate		Dorsal prefrontal		FEF	Premotor	Motor	Somatic	Posterior parietal		Prestriate
24/23	25	9	46	8	6	4	3/2/1	5	7	19

VF	IT						
12	TE	TEO		VLcc	X	VPLo	PONTINE NUCLEI

DENTATE N ◄ - - CEREBELLAR CORTEX

Figure 1.1 Simplified diagram of the neocortical inputs and outputs of the cerebellum. References in text.

Marr (1969) suggested that the cerebellum learns skills by associating the context with the subsequent action and so learning to produce the action on the basis of that context alone. The context is provided by the inputs, and there are extensive inputs from the neocortex. However, at the time that Marr produced his theory, very little was known of the pattern of interconnections. These have been worked out in detail for the macaque brain as shown in Figure 1.1.

The neocortex projects indirectly to the cerebellum via the pons (Glickstein et al., 1985; Glickstein et al., 1994). However, the connections do not come from all areas. There are projections from the motor cortex and somatosensory cortex including the proprioceptive area 3a, as well as from the parietal association cortex, the premotor cortex, the supplementary motor cortex (not shown), the dorsal prefrontal cortex, and the cingulate cortex (Glickstein et al., 1985; Schmahmann and Pandya, 1997). There are also some projections from the superior temporal cortex (not shown) and from the posterior part of the orbitofrontal cortex (not shown). However, there are few if any projections from the inferotemporal cortex or the ventral prefrontal cortex.

The return projections via the dentate and interpositus nucleus are described by Dum and Strick (2003). They include projections to parietal area 7b, and the dorsal prefrontal areas 9 and 46. Middleton and Strick (2000) have argued that the outputs to the different cortical areas are relatively independent, and that the same is true for the outputs from the basal ganglia. However, we now know that there is overlap between the projections from neighboring cortical areas to the striatum (Averbeck et al., 2014), and the same appears to be true for the cortical projections to the pons. Thus, there can be an interaction between cortical areas not only at the cortical level but also at the subcortical level through projections to the cerebellum.

The pattern of connections is critical for understanding the role of the cerebellum. Animals learn skills because they pay in terms of obtaining food or other resources.

Children also learn skills because they are instructed in how to perform them. The inputs to the cerebellum do not provide the information needed for initial learning. It is the basal ganglia that serve to reinforce action (Doya, 1999) and the ventral prefrontal cortex that is involved in influencing action on the basis of verbal instructions (Hartstra et al., 2012).

Studies using fMRI show that the prefrontal cortex is activated during new learning of a motor task, whether visual cues specify the relevant sequence of finger movements (Toni et al., 1998), the force to be applied (Floyer-Lea and Matthews, 2004), or the timing of the movements (Ramnani and Passingham, 2001). However, in each of these experiments the prefrontal activations decreased to near baseline as the task was overlearned while there were cerebellar activations that increased with automaticity. Furthermore, as the task became automatic the subjects became less dependent on the visual cues; in the experiment by Ramnani and Passingham (2001) there was a decrease in activation in the inferotemporal cortex with learning.

The critical finding is that, as the subjects learned, they became more dependent on proprioceptive cues. In the study by Floyer-Lea and Matthews (2005) there was an increase in activation in the primary somatosensory cortex with learning. As shown in Figure 1.1 this area, including the proprioceptive area 3a, projects via the pons to the cerebellum. Thus, the results of the fMRI study are consistent with the suggestion that, with learning, one movement provides the context for the next one and that the cerebellum learns the association. The cerebellum can then influence movement via projections via the thalamus to the motor cortex. In the study by Floyer-Lea and Matthews (2005) there was an increase in activation in the motor cortex with automaticity.

If this interpretation is correct, lesions of the cerebellum should impair automatic performance but spare initial learning. If the dentate nucleus is temporarily inactivated, monkeys make many errors when performing sequences that they have previously learned (Lu et al., 1998). But the same animals can learn new sequences. However, though they can learn a new sequence, monkeys with lesions in the dentate are no longer able to learn it to automaticity as measured in terms of response times (Nixon and Passingham, 2000).

Conclusions

Marr's (1969) theory of the cerebellar cortex concerned the microstructure. It was produced before the inputs and outputs were fully described and before the functional experiments had been performed that could compare new learning with automation. It is the essence of automaticity that the subject no longer has to attend to what is done, and this can be demonstrated by the relative lack of costs during dual-task performance (Grol et al., 2006). The reason for the lack of costs is that the action now depends on a relatively simple circuit, and this no longer includes the prefrontal cortex. As Marr (1969) suggested, the sequence depends on a simple chain in which one element provides the context for the next.

Hippocampus

The hippocampus is similar to the cerebellum in having a linear array of cells: pyramidal cells in lamellae in the hippocampus, Purkinje cells in the case of the cerebellum. But, as Marr (1971) noted, there is an absence of climbing fibers in the hippocampus, though these are found both in the cerebellum (Marr, 1969) and in the neocortex (Marr, 1970). Marr (1971) argued that the existence of climbing fibers in the neocortex meant that classificatory units could be formed as well as memories, and that their absence in the hippocampus meant that its role was restricted to "simple memory." That the archicortex was involved in simple memory was a three-starred prediction.

Marr pointed out that there was a severe restraint on the capacity of the hippocampus, given the number of pyramidal cells. For this reason he suggested that memories were coded sparsely in relatively few cells. However, they were coded in such a way as to be distinct, thus involving pattern separation. Finally, he proposed that a memory could be retrieved via a mechanism of pattern completion. Pattern completion relates to the algorithmic level, that is to the input/output transformations. Pattern separation can be regarded in the same way. However, it also has implications for function: it implies the ability to discriminate between two representations.

In suggesting that the hippocampus was involved in memory, Marr (1971) was drawing on the earlier work of Milner (1959). She had reported that bilateral removal of the hippocampus produced a dense amnesia in patients. The syndrome was first described in patient HM (Scoville and Milner, 1957), but similar findings were reported later in other patients. Not only could these patients not remember recent experiences, they were unable to remember short strings of digits if their attention was briefly interrupted and they were unable to learn verbal paired associates.

We now know that the surgical lesion in patient HM was not confined to the hippocampus. It also involved the entorhinal cortex and the perirhinal cortex. The latter finding matters because we now know from experiments on macaque monkeys that it is the perirhinal cortex that is involved in recognizing items such as objects (Buckley and Gaffan, 1998b) and the associations between them (Buckley and Gaffan, 1998a; Hirabayashi et al., 2013a). Lesions that are confined to the hippocampus do not disturb either object recognition or object associations (Murray et al., 1993; Baxter and Murray, 2001).

While his paper was in press, Marr (1971) added a footnote mentioning the recent demonstration by Lomo (1971) that tetanic stimulation of the perforant path led to potentiation in the granule cells in the dentate gyrus. This provided a potential mechanism via which memories might be stored by synaptic change.

However, it was in the same year that O'Keefe and Dostrovsky (1971) reported the equally seminal finding that there are place cells in the hippocampus. Ten years later it was shown that rats with hippocampal lesions are severely impaired at finding the location of the underwater platform on the Morris water maze task (Morris et al., 1982). Since the start position of the animal is varied from trial to trial, it must use its position with respect to the surroundings to work out the location of the platform.

Inputs and outputs

As in the case of the cerebellum, charting the inputs and outputs is critical for understanding function. Figure 1.2 shows these as established for the hippocampus by tracer experiments on macaque monkeys. The key finding is that there are direct projections to the hippocampus from the inferior parietal area 7a (Zhong and Rockland, 2004). The parietal cortex also sends indirect projections via the retrosplenial cortex (Kobayashi and Amaral, 2003) and the parahippocampal cortex (Lavenex et al., 2002).

The significance of these results is that the inferior parietal area 7a forms part of the dorsal visual system for spatial processing (Kravitz et al., 2011); and importantly its inputs are mainly for peripheral vision (Baizer et al., 1991). This is in contrast to the inferotemporal cortex where the inputs from V4 are mainly for foveal vision.

There is thus a functional distinction between a system that specifies the surroundings and a system that specifies the nature of objects. However, there is also a functional division in the object system, since V4 also sends a projection for the peripheral field to the parahippocampal cortex (Ungerleider et al., 2008). The inferotemporal cortex is concerned with objects that are relatively small, such as manipulable objects. The parahippocampal cortex is concerned with larger objects such as occur within scenes (Levy et al., 2001). If monkeys or human subjects are scanned with fMRI, the parahippocampal cortex is activated when they view scenes (Nasr et al., 2011).

The importance of scenes is that they form the context for action. When rats are tested in the water maze, they judge their location by their view of the surroundings. The pool

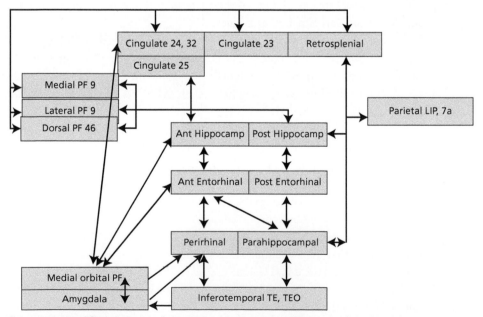

Figure 1.2 Simplified diagram of the neocortical inputs and outputs of the hippocampus. References in text.

is in a room full of objects, large and small, and the surroundings include not only the spatial organization of those objects but also the walls or boundaries. The term "scene" can be used to refer to the room as the animals view it.

There is evidence both from brain imaging and from the effects of lesions that the hippocampus is critical for distinguishing between scenes. If healthy human subjects are scanned, the pattern of activation across voxels has been shown to discriminate between scenes that are highly similar (Bonnici et al., 2012). This discrimination is made on the basis of the overall global strength of the relational match (Aly et al., 2013), and this is a test of the effectiveness of pattern separation. Monkeys (Baxter and Murray, 2001) and patients (Lee et al., 2005) with selective hippocampal lesions are impaired at discriminating between scenes. And knockout mice that are unable to express long-term potentiation (LTP) are able to find a single platform on the basis of the scene, but impaired when required to distinguish between two hidden platforms only one of which will support them (Bannerman et al., 2014).

From navigation to episodic memory

Given the fundamental role of the hippocampus in navigation it has been a problem to explain how it has been adapted to support episodic memory in people. There are two phenomena to be explained. The first is that if the lesion is confined to the hippocampus, it impairs the ability of patients to remember personal events in their life, that is it has a selective effect on episodic memory and not the ability to retrieve factual information (Vargha-Khadem et al., 1997). The second is that the patients report that they are unable to "re-experience" the event.

Activations during recall of episodic memories are found most often in the posterior hippocampus (Hassabis et al., 2007). This is the part of the hippocampus that corresponds in a rodent to the dorsal hippocampus (Moser and Moser, 1998), and it is lesions of the dorsal hippocampus that impair performance on the water maze in rats (Bannerman et al., 1999). As already mentioned, place cells in this region can code for where the animal is on an elevated maze. However, the human posterior hippocampus can also represent the place of the person in the environment; this has been shown by analyzing the pattern of activation across voxels when subject navigate in a virtual reality environment (Hassabis et al., 2009).

There is a further similarity. In rats the patterns of activity in place cells can also reflect the path that animal is *going* to take so as to reach a goal it has visited in the past (Pfeiffer and Foster, 2013). And when human subjects navigate in a virtual reality environment, the posterior hippocampus is activated specifically when they plan a future route from their current position (Spiers and Maguire, 2006).

There is, however, a critical difference and this is that human beings, unlike rats, can plan for the distant future. This is the consequence of the fact that like other primates, but unlike other mammals, they possess a granular prefrontal cortex (Passingham and Wise, 2012).; and furthermore it is greatly expanded as a proportion of the neocortex compared with the brain of a chimpanzee (Avants et al., 2006).

The significance of this development can be illustrated by experiments that use brain imaging. The lateral prefrontal cortex is activated when subjects imagine moving their fingers, but not when they actually move them (Ehrsson et al., 2003). Similarly it is activated when subjects imagine viewing a face or house, but not when they actually see them (Ishai et al., 2000). But the critical finding is that during imagination the prefrontal cortex activates the appropriate motor (Ehrsson et al., 2003) or sensory representations (Mechelli et al., 2004). One possibility is that it is this that leads to the subjective experience.

When subjects imagine a series of future steps toward some personal life goal it the medial prefrontal cortex that is activated (Spreng et al., 2010). This area is connected to the hippocampus via the retrosplenial cortex (Kobayashi and Amaral, 2003) and presubiculum (Morris et al., 1999). There is activation in all three areas whether subjects imagine future events or retrieve past ones from their life (Addis et al., 2007; Hassabis et al., 2007).

So the first suggestion is that the reason why episodic memory involves personal events is that the fundamental role of the hippocampus is to represent the current location of individual in space and to use it to determine the route of travel. There is a relation between the distance traveled and the time taken. To use the metaphor suggested by Tulving (2005), whether the person imagines the future or the past it is as if they are traveling in time.

The second suggestion is that the reason why retrieving memories is like "re-experiencing" them is that the prefrontal cortex is activated whether the subjects are imagining the future or remembering the past. One possibility is that the link is that imagining the future necessarily involves reference to events in the past. But an alternative is that we acquired our ability to re-experience the distant past because it paid to be able to imagine the distant future. There is a clear evolutionary advantage of foresight in that one can take precautions in advance.

Conclusions

It will be clear that, when Marr (1971) produced his theory of the hippocampus and simple memory, many important things were not known. It had not been established that in people the hippocampus is specifically involved in retrieving personal events and in "re-experiencing" them. Nevertheless, Marr was correct that the hippocampus is involved in recall and not in recognition (Aggleton and Brown, 2006).

Marr was also correct that the hippocampus provides a mechanism for the retrieval memories on the basis of partial cues. He made this suggestion because he was concerned about the problem of constraints, given the limited number of pyramidal cells. On the basis of what we now know, it is possible to suggest a solution to this problem. This assumes that the fundamental role of the hippocampus is to represent the location of the individual in the three-dimensional scene. If so, the partial cues are the locations or scenes in which events occurred, the assumption being that the representations of those events are stored in the neocortex.

Neocortex

The account given in the previous section on the hippocampus assumes that, as Marr (1970) suggested, it is the neocortex that classifies inputs and so forms and stores novel representations. In proposing that the fundamental function of the neocortex is to form classificatory units, he was drawing on the work of Hubel and Wiesel on the striate cortex in cats (Hubel and Wiesel, 1962) and monkeys (Hubel and Wiesel, 1968). Hubel and Wiesel had found cell types that they referred to as simple, complex, and hypercomplex. They had further suggested that the more complex cells might derive their properties from several inputs from cells with simpler properties

The term "classification" can be used in several ways. For example, it can be used to refer to the identification of an object where the animal has to learn that view A is of the same object as view A′. It can be used for the formation of concrete classes of objects, such as balls or cups. And it can be used to refer to abstract classes, such as the numbers 10 or 12. The findings that are relevant to Marr's notion of classificatory units concern cells that fire similarly to different inputs.

Structure of the neocortex

At the outset Marr took it to be a problem that "The mammalian cortex can learn to perform a wide variety of tasks, yet its structure is strikingly uniform (Ramón y Cajal, 1911)". Later studies have confirmed that there are similarities between the structure of cortical columns across the neocortex, even if they are not identical (da Costa and Martin, 2010). The explanation for the apparent paradox is that the neocortex is divided into many different areas, and each of these has a different *overall* pattern of inputs and outputs. This has been shown by using multidimensional scaling that uses a high-dimensional metric representation: each area has a unique place in the two-dimensional space (Passingham et al., 2002). As mentioned in the introduction, it is the extrinsic connections that constrain what each area does.

The basic way in which the different cortical areas are connected was worked out by Jones and Powell (1970). These authors documented the pattern of cortico-cortical connections in the macaque brain, with both feedforward and feedback connections. Figure 1.3 shows a very simplified diagram.

The work of Jones and Powell was published in the same year as Marr's (1970) neocortical theory. He does not cite it, presumably because he was not aware of it when he wrote the paper. Yet, it is the cortico-cortical organization of the connections that explains what the neocortex can do. And it is the lack of such an organization that limits what the basal ganglia can do.

As brains enlarge, there is a tendency for the number of neocortical areas to increase (Changizi and Shimojo, 2005). The reason is that there is a need to maintain efficient connectivity and this leads to the differentiation of areas into interconnected subareas (Krubitzer and Huffman, 2000). However, these subareas are not simply organized randomly: a hierarchical organization also develops such that when area A differentiates, the outputs from area A′ become the inputs to the new area A″.

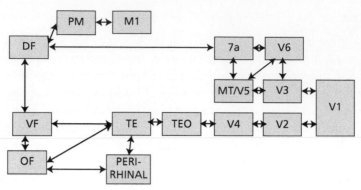

Figure 1.3 Simplified diagram of the ventral and dorsal visual system and their extensions in the prefrontal cortex. The diagram omits the system for controlling eye movements and spatial attention as well as the system for reaching for and grasping objects. Connections from Young (1993).

The consequence of such a hierarchical organization is that the cells in area A″ can combine inputs from different cells in area A′. That this combination occurs is suggested by comparing the size of the receptive fields in V1, V2, and V4. The fields in V4 are larger than those in V2 (Desimone and Schein, 1987). A plausible explanation is that the larger receptive fields are achieved by combining inputs from many cells with smaller receptive fields.

At the same time, the optimal stimulus for the cell becomes more complex. Whereas it may be a line in V1, it may be a stopped line in V4 (Desimone et al., 1985) or a simple shape in the inferotemporal cortex (Tanaka, 1997). Again a plausible explanation is that the property of invariance is achieved by combining inputs in a hierarchical fashion (Cadieu et al., 2007). In this way a cell could fire to—and thus "recognize"—shape X irrespective of size or location.

The functional progression in the ventral visual system is accompanied by an anatomical progression. Elston (2007) has counted the spines on the basal dendrites of layer III pyramidal cells. The number of spines increases from V1 through to the perirhinal cortex, stage by stage. It is at its greatest in ventral prefrontal cortex, area 12, to which the inferotemporal cortex projects (Webster et al., 1994). This points to a high degree of integration onto each cell, and the prefrontal cortex is notable for the proportion of cells that have conjunctive properties (Passingham and Wise, 2012).

This is a consequence of the hierarchical progression. Whereas early in the hierarchy one cell might fire to A or A′ and another to B or B′, later in the hierarchy a conjunctive cell might fire to A, A′, B and B′. Such a cell could, for example, code for an abstract category in which both A and B and their variants are included.

Training cells

The suggestion is that the properties of such cells would be trained up during development. It was critical to Marr's (1970) theory that classificatory units could learn to recognize patterns of inputs as being the same. We now know that this is indeed the case.

It has been shown, for example, for the shape selectivity of cells in the inferotemporal cortex (Freedman et al., 2006). The selectivity of cells in this area is influenced by the visual stimuli the animal is presented with so that it can learn to categorize them (Sigala and Logothetis, 2002).

A worked example of the trainability of cells is provided by the work of Sakai and Miyashita (1991) on pair-coding cells in the perirhinal and inferotemporal cortex. Even though the pairs of fractals that the monkeys learn to associate do not look alike, pair-coding cells fire when either one of the two fractals is presented. In other words, they learn to fire similarly to disparate inputs.

The functional properties of the cells in the perirhinal cortex can be predicted on the basis of the properties of the cells in the inferotemporal cortex. This is interconnected with the perirhinal cortex (Hirabayashi et al., 2013b), and the pair-coding cells in the inferotemporal cortex can be shown to be dependent on top-down projections from the perirhinal and entorhinal cortex (Hirabayashi et al., 2013a).

The fact that cells can be trained to associate A with X provides a mechanism for learning categories. There are cells in the ventral prefrontal cortex, as well as the inferotemporal cortex, that respond to object categories such as cats and dogs (Meyers et al., 2008). Furthermore, the prefrontal cells are flexible in their properties in that, having learned to associate morphs of cats or dogs to the prototype, they can then learn to associate a morph of a cat with a morph of a dog (Freedman et al., 2002).

These are effectively pair-coding neurones. However, though the recordings are taken from individual cells, it should not be thought the categorization is achieved via individual cells. The classification of an item such as a cat or dog depends on subpopulations of cells (Meyers et al., 2008).

The examples provided so far concern the ventral visual system and its extension into the ventral prefrontal cortex. But there are also classificatory cells in the dorsal visual system, for example cells in the parietal and dorsal prefrontal cortex (Tudusciuc and Nieder, 2009) that respond to specific numbers, irrespective of the actual items in the array. And there are also cells in prefrontal cortex with conjunctive properties such that they respond both to form and spatial location (Rao et al., 1997). The inputs for form come from the ventral visual system and for location from the dorsal visual system.

Conclusions

Marr's (1970) theory of the cerebral cortex concerns both the algorithm and the implementation. He did not put forward a theory as to the function of the neocortex as a whole. However, he did ask how a relatively uniform structure could perform so many different functions. There are two possible answers, and they are not mutually exclusive. The first is that the structure is not totally uniform: the microstructure of the frontal eye fields (Heinzle et al., 2007) or the dorsal prefrontal cortex (Kritzer and Goldman-Rakic, 1995) is not exactly the same as that of the visual cortex. The differences in microstructure seem to be shaped in part by the anatomical inputs that are available during development (Sur and Leamey, 2001).

The second answer is that the areas differ in their extrinsic inputs and outputs. For example, whereas the visual cortex has visual outputs, the frontal eye fields have both visual inputs and motor outputs.

Marr's (1970) theory of neocortex was based on the microstructure. However, his suggestion that the neocortex can form classificatory units is consistent with the fact the neocortex can learn to recognize categories. Unlike the neocortex, the basal ganglia lack a hierarchical structure, and it for this reason that categories are first learned at the neocortical level (Antzoulatos and Miller, 2011).

The relation between function and mechanism

It will be apparent that Marr's suggestions as to the function of the three structures, whether explicit or implied, were prescient. However, this leaves the question as to whether the algorithms and implementations proposed could be proved to be wrong if the functions assumed were wrong.

Cerebellum

In the case of the cerebellum it was not known when Marr (1969) produced his theory that there were indirect interconnections with the dorsal prefrontal cortex (Middleton and Strick, 2001), and this has led to speculation that the role of the cerebellum might be involved in higher cognition. If correct, this would prove a challenge to Marr's theory.

The reason is that the theory (Marr, 1969) proposed a simple associative structure for automating motor skills. The same mechanism was used to explain the maintenance of postural reflexes. And the theory can also be extended to account for the more recent evidence that the cerebellum is involved in associating a conditioned stimulus with an eyeblink (Ramnani et al., 2000) or with changes in skin conductance and heart rate (Maschke et al., 2002).

Yet there have been claims that the cerebellum is involved in verbal working memory (Desmond and Fiez, 1998), verb generation (Desmond and Fiez, 1998), set shifting (Lie et al., 2006), and problem solving (Kim et al., 1994b). These findings pose a challenge for Marr's (1969) theory. It is not clear, for example, how a mechanism for associating a context with a response can account for the generation of *novel* responses during problem solving. This is not, of course, to say that other theories, such as those that depend on internal models, might not be flexible enough to do so (Ito, 2008).

However, given the challenge to Marr's (1969) theory, it is important to assess the potency of the challenge. It is based on anatomical and functional evidence. To take the anatomy first, the fact that there are interconnections between the dorsal prefrontal cortex and the cerebellum (Schmahmann and Pandya, 2008) does not prove that the cerebellum is itself involved in higher cognition.

The point can be made by work on macaque monkeys. The role of the dorsal prefrontal cortex in cognition has often been assessed by training the animals on delayed response tasks. Yet, though monkeys with dorsal prefrontal lesions fail to relearn the delayed alternation task after surgery, monkeys with lesions in the dentate nucleus can relearn the task normally (Nixon and Passingham, 1999). Though the areas are connected, the evidence is that, unlike the dorsal prefrontal cortex (Passingham and Wise, 2012), the cerebellum is not involved in generating novel responses or in maintaining them in prospective memory.

It could be argued that the situation may be different for the human brain. In experiments using delayed response tasks the responses are manual or oculomotor, but humans can speak. However, there is no reason why Marr's theory cannot be extended to accommodate articulatory responses. There is activation in the cerebellum when subjects engage in verbal working memory (Desmond and Fiez, 1998) and patients with cerebellar lesions can show poor verbal memory (Ravizza et al., 2006). But verbal working memory involves subvocal articulation (Baddeley, 1986) and this is true even if the words or letters are read (Conrad, 1973). The pronunciation of words, whether heard or read, is a skill that has been learned and automated, and the disruption of the mechanism might well affect verbal working memory.

A similar explanation could be given for other findings that have been taken to involve semantic processing. There is activation in the cerebellum when subjects generate verbs that are appropriate for nouns (Desmond and Fiez, 1998) and a cerebellar lesion can lead to inappropriate responses (Fiez et al., 1992). However, Marr could accommodate these findings on the grounds that the associations have been learned over a lifetime and each noun forms the context for the articulation of the appropriate verb. The cerebellum is also activated when subjects learn to predict the end of a sentence on the basis of the way it starts (Moberget et al., 2014). Here the initial part of the sentence serves as a context for the subvocal articulation of the last word.

The same explanation will not, however, account for the claims that the cerebellum is involved in performance of the Wisconsin Card Sorting task (Schmahmann and Sherman, 1998). Lie et al. (2006) used fMRI to scan subjects while they engaged in set shifting on this task, and a comparison was made between shifts that were instructed and shifts that were not. The cerebellar activation was associated with shifts that were not instructed, that is that were made on the basis of negative feedback alone. Given the fact that the amygdala is connected with the pons (Price and Amaral, 1981), one possibility is that the cerebellum is activated during shifts of this sort because successful performance depends on generating a galvanic skin response to prompt shifts, as on the Iowa gambling task (Wagar and Dixon, 2006).

So none of the examples cited so far are incompatible with a simple associative theory. However, this is not true of claims that the cerebellum is involved in problem solving since this would require the cerebellum to be equipped for the generation of *novel* responses. Yet, Kim et al. (1994a) scanned human subjects while they planned moves in a pegboard maze, and there was an activation in the dentate nucleus. The contrast was with a control condition in which the subjects simply moved the pegs.

The problem is that the two conditions differ in several ways, for example in preparatory activity and in the eye movements that are involved (Glickstein and Doron, 2008).

So there is a confound in the contrast. It seems unlikely that the cerebellar activation genuinely involved planning and response selection since patients with lesions that are confined to the cerebellum can solve problems that require planning moves, as on the Tower of Hanoi (Daum et al., 1993).

It will be clear that there is a danger of using the term "cognition" loosely, and then assuming that a theory of implementation by the cerebellum has to accommodate "cognitive" functions. There are, as yet, no data that could not be explained by a simple mechanism for the automation of associations between context and response. To falsify Marr's (1969) implementation it would be necessary to prove that the cerebellum is equipped to generate novel responses as is required on tasks of problem solving or reasoning.

Hippocampus

In his theory of archicortex Marr (1971) used the term "events" for the inputs to the codons rather than the conventional term "stimuli." The term "event" has the advantage of referring to inputs over time as well as space. An example of such an event is an action. And it has indeed turned out that the hippocampus is involved in remembering events rather than objects.

The term "events" can be used to refer not only to actions but also to the consequences of those actions. If selective lesions are placed in the hippocampus, macaque monkeys are not only impaired on the recognition of scenes but also, though less severely, on the object reversal task (Murray et al., 1998). The reason is probably that the lesion included the anterior sector and this is interconnected with the medial orbital cortex (Cavada et al., 2000). There are activations in the medial orbital cortex when human subjects modify their actions as the result of a change in the consequences (Glascher et al., 2009).

As already mentioned, that the hippocampus is a simple memory store was a three-starred prediction. This can survive the evidence that the hippocampus either stores scenes or the links between locations or scenes and events. Given that Marr (1971) did not specify what events were stored in the hippocampus, the theory is not falsified by findings such as these.

The theory would only be shown to be false if it turned out that the hippocampus was not a storage device at all or if it could classify in the same way as the neocortex. It is true that at the time that Marr (1971) wrote it was not known that the hippocampus is involved in imagining new events (Addis et al., 2007; Hassabis et al., 2007). However, this is easily accommodated if we suppose that the common factor is the ability to "experience" the event, whether imagining the future or re-experiencing the past.

Neocortex

Marr (1970) proposed that the neocortex could form classificatory units. But this is not the same as saying that the function of the neocortex is to classify. Clearly this is one function, but the neocortex performs other functions as well. For example, because the connections run both ways, information in early sensory streams can be modulated by top-down effects, providing mechanisms for voluntary attention and control (Shulman et al., 1997). Furthermore, the neocortex also evaluates actions in the light of current needs and guides actions according to the appropriate context (Passingham and Wise, 2012).

However, the theory of classificatory units refers to a basic operation and this could be as much involved in learning rules or the appropriate action as in learning to recognize visual inputs. In macaque monkeys there are cells in the prefrontal cortex that code for the rules of "matching" and " non-matching" (Wallis et al., 2001) and others that code for abstract sequences of responses (Shima et al., 2007). It is not possible to disprove Marr's (1970) neocortical theory by evidence concerning overall function because his theory involves the algorithms and implementation alone.

It should, however, still be possible to disprove a theory concerning implementation in neocortex that purports to explain how a particular area does what it does. For example, Deco and Rolls (2003) suggested how prefrontal cortex might provide a mechanism for short-term memory. However, recent results have suggested that it may not act in this way (Passingham and Wise, 2012). Monkeys with dorsal prefrontal lesions appear to know where the remembered location is, even if this is sometimes not the first location that they look to (Tsujimoto and Postle, 2012).

Whether a theory of implementation can be disproved because the function that is assumed is incorrect depends on the level of detail with which the implementation is specified. It has turned out, for example, that Deco and Rolls (2005) have been able to adapt their theory so as to explain action selection. The theory is specified at a general level.

Current theories concerning implementation are most convincing where the function of the structure is well established. For example, it is clear that the frontal eye fields are involved in visual search (Schall, 2002). As expected, there are visual, visuomotor and motor cells in the area (Schall, 2002). Inactivation of the frontal eye fields leads to saccades that are in the wrong direction given the visual cue (Keller et al., 2008). Thus, there is now a firm basis for suggesting how the cell populations and their interconnections might perform the appropriate transformations (Heinzle et al., 2007).

Conclusions

The challenge is now to produce theories at Marr's algorithmic and implementation level that are of sufficient detail that they can only be true if the function of the structure is indeed as assumed. Furthermore, it would be helpful if future implementations adopted the starring system, as devised by Marr. This will make it clear what a particular theory predicts that no other theory predicts. It is one thing to propose that an implementation that is consistent with the data, another to show that it and no other theory is the correct one.

Marr clarified what needs to be done and the levels that need to be addressed. The remaining chapters in this book show where, given advances in neuroscience, his insights have now led.

Acknowledgments

I am grateful to Steve Wise, Tim Behrens, Eleanor Maguire, and Lucia Vaina for comments on a draft of this chapter.

References

Addis DR, Wong AT, Schacter DL. (2007). Remembering the past and imagining the future: common and distinct neural substrates during event construction and elaboration. Neuropsychology. 45:1363–1377.

Aggleton JP, Brown MW. (2006). Interleaving brain systems for episodic and recognition memory. Trends Cogn Sci. 10:455–463.

Aly M, Ranganath C, Yonelinas AP. (2013). Detecting changes in scenes: the hippocampus is critical for strength-based perception. Neuron. 78:1127–1137.

Antzoulatos EG, Miller EK. (2011). Differences between neural activity in prefrontal cortex and striatum during learning of novel abstract categories. Neuron. 71:243–249.

Avants BB, Schoenemann PT, Gee JC. (2006). Lagrangian frame diffeomorphic image registration: Morphometric comparison of human and chimpanzee cortex. Med Image Anal. 10:397–412.

Averbeck BB, Lehman J, Jacobson M, Haber SN. (2014). Estimates of projection overlap and zones of convergence within frontal-striatal circuits. J Neurosci. 34:9497–9505.

Baddeley A. (1986). Working Memory. Oxford: Oxford University Press.

Baizer JS, Ungerleider LG, Desimone R. (1991). Organization of visual inputs to the inferior temporal and posterior parietal cortex in macaques. J Neurosci. 11:168–190.

Bannerman DM, Sprengel R, Sanderson DJ, McHugh SB, Rawlins JN, Monyer H, Seeburg PH. (2014). Hippocampal synaptic plasticity, spatial memory and anxiety. Nat Rev Neurosci. 15:181–192.

Bannerman DM, Yee BK, Good MA, Heupel MJ, Iversen SD, Rawlins JN. (1999). Double dissociation of function within the hippocampus: a comparison of dorsal, ventral, and complete hippocampal cytotoxic lesions. Behav Neurosci. 113:1170–1188.

Baxter MG, Murray EA. (2001). Opposite relationship of hippocampal and rhinal cortex damage to delayed nonmatching-to-sample deficits in monkeys. Hippocampus. 11:61–71.

Bonnici HM, Kumaran D, Chadwick MJ, Weiskopf N, Hassabis D, Maguire EA. (2012). Decoding representations of scenes in the medial temporal lobes. Hippocampus. 22:1143–1153.

Brindley GS. (1964). The use made by the cerebellum of the information that it receives from sense organs. IBRO Bull. 3:80.

Brindley GS. (1970). Sensations produced by electrical stimulation of the occipital poles of the cerebral hemispheres, and their use in constructing visual prostheses. Ann Roy Coll Surg Engl. 47:106–108.

Buckley MJ, Gaffan D (1998a) Perirhinal cortex ablation impairs configural learning and paired-associate learning equally. Neuropsychology. 36:535–546.

Buckley MJ, Gaffan D (1998b) Perirhinal cortex ablation impairs visual object identification. J Neurosci. 18:2268–2275.

Cadieu C, Kouh M, Pasupathy A, Connor CE, Riesenhuber M, Poggio T. (2007). A model of V4 shape selectivity and invariance. J Neurophysiol. 98:1733–1750.

Ramón y Cajal S. (1911/1955). Histologie du système nerveux de l'homme et des vertébrés. Paris: A. Maloine/Madrid: Consejo Superior De Investigation Cientificas.

Cavada C, Company T, Tejedor J, Cruz-Rizzolo RJ, Reinoso-Suarez F. (2000). The anatomical connections of the macaque monkey orbitofrontal cortex. A review. Cereb Cortex. 10:243–251.

Changizi MA, Shimojo S. (2005). Parcellation and area-area connectivity as a function of neocortex size. Brain Behav Evol. 66:88–98.

Conrad R. (1973). Some correlates of speech coding in the short-term memory of the deaf. J Speech Hear Res. **16**:375–384.

Craggs MD. (1974). Electrical activity of the motor cortex associated with voluntary movements in the baboon. J Physiol. **237**:12P–13P.

da Costa NM, Martin KA. (2010). Whose cortical column would that be? Front Neuroanat. **4**:16.

Daum I, Ackermann H, Schugens MM, Reimold C, Dichgans J, Birbaumer N. (1993). The cerebellum and cognitive functions in humans. Behav Neurosci. **107**:411–419.

Deco G, Rolls ET. (2003). Attention and working memory: a dynamical model of neuronal activity in the prefrontal cortex. Eur J Neurosci. **18**:2374–2390.

Deco G, Rolls ET. (2005). Attention, short-term memory, and action selection: a unifying theory. Prog Neurobiol. **76**:236–256.

Desimone R, Schein SJ. (1987). Visual properties of neurons in area V4 of the macaque: sensitivity to stimulus form. J Neurophysiol. **57**:835–868.

Desimone R, Schein SJ, Moran J, Ungerleider LG. (1985). Contour, color and shape analysis beyond the striate cortex. Vision Res. **25**:441–452.

Desmond JE, Fiez J. (1998). Neuroimaging studies of the cerebellum: language, learning and memory. Trends Cogn Sci. **2**:355–361.

Doya K. (1999). What are the computations of the cerebellum, the basal ganglia and the cerebral cortex? Neural Netw. **12**:961–974.

Dum RP, Strick PL. (2003). An unfolded map of the cerebellar dentate nucleus and its projections to the cerebral cortex. J Neurophysiol. **89**:634–639.

Ehrsson HH, Geyer S, Naito E. (2003). Imagery of voluntary movement of fingers, toes, and tongue activates corresponding body-part-specific motor representations. J Neurophysiol. **90**:3304–3316.

Elston GN (2007). Specialization of the neocortical pyramidal cell during primate evolution. In: Evolution of Nervous Systems: A Comprehensive Reference (Kaas J, Preuss TM, eds) vol. **4**, pp. 191–242. New York: Elsevier.

Fiez JA, Petersen SE, Cheney MK, Raichle ME. (1992). Impaired non-motor learning and error detection associated with cerebellar damage. Brain. **115**:155–178.

Floyer-Lea A, Matthews PM. (2004). Changing brain networks for visuomotor control with increased movement automaticity. J Neurophysiol. **92**:2405–2412.

Floyer-Lea A, Matthews PM. (2005). Distinguishable brain activation networks for short- and long-term motor skill learning. J Neurophysiol. **94**:512–518.

Freedman DJ, Riesenhuber M, Poggio T, Miller EK. (2002). Visual categorization and the primate prefrontal cortex: neurophysiology and behavior. J Neurophysiol. **88**:929–941.

Freedman DJ, Riesenhuber M, Poggio T, Miller EK. (2006). Experience-dependent sharpening of visual shape selectivity in inferior temporal cortex. Cereb Cortex. **16**:1631–1644.

Gibo TL, Criscimagna-Hemminger SE, Okamura AM, Bastian AJ. (2013). Cerebellar motor learning: are environment dynamics more important than error size? J Neurophysiol. **110**:322–333.

Glascher J, Hampton AN, O'Doherty JP. (2009). Determining a role for ventromedial prefrontal cortex in encoding action-based value signals during reward-related decision making. Cereb Cortex. **19**:483–495.

Glickstein M, Doron K. (2008). Cerebellum: connections and functions. Cerebellum. **7**:589–594.

Glickstein M, Gerrits N, Kralj I, Mercier B, Stein J, Voogd J. (1994). Visual pontocerebellar projections in the macaque. J Comp Neurol. **349**:51–72.

Glickstein M, May JG, Mercier RE. (1985). Corticopontine projections in the macaque: the distribution of labelled cortical cells after large injections of horseradish peroxidase in the pontine nuclei. J Comp Neurol. **235**:343–359.

Grol MJ, de Lange FP, Verstraten FA, Passingham RE, Toni I. (2006). Cerebral changes during performance of overlearned arbitrary visuomotor associations. J Neurosci. 26:117–125.

Hartstra E, Waszak F, Brass M. (2012). The implementation of verbal instructions: dissociating motor preparation from the formation of stimulus-response associations. Neuroimage. 63:1143–1153.

Hassabis D, Chu C, Rees G, Weiskopf N, Molyneux PD, Maguire EA. (2009). Decoding neuronal ensembles in the human hippocampus. Curr Biol. 19:546–554.

Hassabis D, Kumaran D, Maguire EA. (2007). Using imagination to understand the neural basis of episodic memory. J Neurosci. 27:14365–14374.

Heinzle J, Hepp K, Martin KA. (2007). A microcircuit model of the frontal eye fields. J Neurosci. 27:9341–9353.

Hirabayashi T, Takeuchi D, Tamura K, Miyashita Y. (2013a). Functional microcircuit recruited during retrieval of object association memory in monkey perirhinal cortex. Neuron. 77:192–203.

Hirabayashi T, Takeuchi D, Tamura K, Miyashita Y. (2013b). Microcircuits for hierarchical elaboration of object coding across primate temporal areas. Science. 341:191–195.

Hubel DH, Wiesel TN. (1962). Receptive fields, binocular interaction and functional architecture in the cat's visual cortex. J Physiol. 160:106–154.

Hubel DH, Wiesel TN. (1968). Receptive fields and functional architecture of monkey striate cortex. J Physiol. 195:215–243.

Ishai A, Ungerleider LG, Haxby JV. (2000). Distributed neural systems for the generation of visual images. Neuron. 28:979–990.

Ito M. (2008). Control of mental activities by internal models in the cerebellum. Nat Rev Neurosci. 9:304–313.

Ito M, Kano M. (1982). Long-lasting depression of parallel fiber-Purkinje cell transmission induced by conjunctive stimulation of parallel fibers and climbing fibers in the cerebellar cortex. Neurosci Lett. 33:253–258.

Jones EG, Powell TP. (1970). An anatomical study of converging sensory pathways within the cerebral cortex of the monkey. Brain. 93:793–820.

Keele SW, Ivry R. (1990). Does the cerebellum provide a common computation for diverse tasks? A timing hypothesis. Ann N Y Acad Sci. 608:179–207; discussion 207–111.

Keller EL, Lee KM, Park SW, Hill JA. (2008). Effect of inactivation of the cortical frontal eye field on saccades generated in a choice response paradigm. J Neurophysiol. 100:2726–2737.

Kim S-G, Ugurbil S, Strick PL. (1994a). Activation of cerebellar output nucleus during cognitive processing. Science. 265:949–961.

Kim SG, Ugurbil K, Strick PL. (1994b). Activation of a cerebellar output nucleus during cognitive processing. Science. 265:949–951.

Kobayashi Y, Amaral DG. (2003). Macaque monkey retrosplenial cortex: II. Cortical afferents. J Comp Neurol. 466:48–79.

Kravitz DJ, Saleem KS, Baker CI, Mishkin M. (2011). A new neural framework for visuospatial processing. Nat Rev Neurosci. 12:217–230.

Kritzer MF, Goldman-Rakic PS. (1995). Intrinsic circuit organization of the major layers and sublayers of the dorsolateral prefrontal cortex in the rhesus monkey. J Comp Neurol. 359:131–143.

Krubitzer L, Huffman KJ. (2000). Arealization of the neocortex in mammals: genetic and epigenetic contributions to the phenotype. Brain Behav Evol. 55:322–335.

Lavenex P, Suzuki WA, Amaral DG. (2002). Perirhinal and parahippocampal cortices of the macaque monkey: projections to the neocortex. J Comp Neurol. 447:394–420.

Lee AC, Bussey TJ, Murray EA, Saksida LM, Epstein RA, Kapur N, et al. (2005). Perceptual deficits in amnesia: challenging the medial temporal lobe "mnemonic" view. Neuropsychol. 43:1–11.

Levy I, Hasson U, Avidan G, Hendler T, Malach R. (2001). Center-periphery organization of human object areas. Nat Neurosci. **4**:533–539.

Lie CH, Specht K, Marshall JC, Fink GR. (2006). Using fMRI to decompose the neural processes underlying the Wisconsin Card Sorting Test. Neuroimage. **30**:1038–1049.

Lomo T. (1971). Potentiation of monosynaptic EPSPs in the perforant path-dentate granule cell synapse. Exp Brain Res. **12**:46–63.

Lu X, Hikosaka O, Miyachi S. (1998). Role of monkey cerebellar nuclei in skill for sequential movement. J Neurophysiol. **79**:2245–2254.

Marr D. (1969). A theory of cerebellar cortex. J Physiol. **202**:437–470.

Marr D. (1970). A theory for cerebral neocortex. Proc R Soc Lond B Biol Sci. **176**:161–234.

Marr D. (1971). Simple memory: a theory for archicortex. Philos Trans R Soc Lond B Biol Sci. **262**:23–81.

Marr D. (1982). Vision. Cambridge, MA: MIT Press.

Marr D, Poggio T. (1977). From understanding computation to understanding neural circuitry. Neurosci Res Progr Bull. **15**:470–488.

Martin TA, Keating JG, Goodkin HP, Bastian AJ, Thach WT. (1996). Throwing while looking through prisms. I. Focal olivocerebellar lesions impair adaptation. Brain **119** (Pt 4):1183–1198.

Maschke M, Schugens M, Kindsvater K, Drepper J, Kolb FP, Diener HC, et al. (2002). Fear conditioned changes of heart rate in patients with medial cerebellar lesions. J Neurol Neurosurg Psychiatr. **72**:116–118.

Mechelli A, Price CJ, Friston KJ, Ishai A. (2004). Where bottom-up meets top-down: neuronal interactions during perception and imagery. Cereb Cortex. **14**:1256–1265.

Meyers EM, Freedman DJ, Kreiman G, Miller EK, Poggio T. (2008). Dynamic population coding of category information in inferior temporal and prefrontal cortex. J Neurophysiol. **100**:1407–1419.

Middleton FA, Strick PL. (2000). Basal ganglia and cerebellar loops: motor and cognitive circuits. Brain Res Brain Res Rev. **31**:236–250.

Middleton FA, Strick PL. (2001). Cerebellar projections to the prefrontal cortex of the primate. J Neurosci. **21**:700–712.

Milner B. (1959). The memory defect in bilateral hippocampal lesions. Psychiatric Res Rep **11**:43–58.

Moberget T, Gullesen EH, Andersson S, Ivry RB, Endestad T. (2014). Generalized role for the cerebellum in encoding internal models: evidence from semantic processing. J Neurosci. **34**:2871–2878.

Morris R, Pandya DN, Petrides M. (1999). Fiber system linking the mid-dorsolateral frontal cortex with the retrosplenial/presubicular region in the rhesus monkey. J Comp Neurol. **407**:183–192.

Morris RG, Garrud P, Rawlins JN, O'Keefe J. (1982). Place navigation impaired in rats with hippocampal lesions. Nature. **297**:681–683.

Moser MB, Moser EI. (1998). Functional differentiation in the hippocampus. Hippocampus. **8**:608–619.

Murray EA, Baxter MG, Gaffan D. (1998). Monkeys with rhinal cortex damage or neurotoxic hippocampal lesions are impaired on spatial scene learning and object reversals. Behav Neurosci. **112**:1291–1303.

Murray EA, Gaffan D, Mishkin M. (1993). Neural substrates of visual stimulus-stimulus association in rhesus monkeys. J Neurosci. **13**:4549–4561.

Nasr S, Liu N, Devaney KJ, Yue X, Rajimehr R, Ungerleider LG, Tootell RB. (2011). Scene-selective cortical regions in human and nonhuman primates. J Neurosci. **31**:13771–13785.

Nixon PD, Passingham RE. (1999). The cerebellum and cognition: cerebellar lesions do not impair spatial working memory or visual associative learning in monkeys. Eur J Neurosci. **11**:4070–4080.

Nixon PD, Passingham RE. (2000). The cerebellum and cognition: cerebellar lesions impair sequence learning but not conditional visuomotor learning in monkeys. Neuropsychol. **38**:1054–1072.

O'Keefe J, Dostrovsky J. (1971). The hippocampus as a spatial map. Preliminary evidence from unit activity in the freely-moving rat. Brain Res. **34**:171–175.

Passingham RE, Stephan KE, Kotter R. (2002). The anatomical basis of functional localization in the cortex. Nat Rev Neurosci. **3**:606–616.

Passingham RE, Wise SP. (2012). The Neurobiology of Prefrontal Cortex. Oxford: Oxford University Press.

Pfeiffer BE, Foster DJ. (2013). Hippocampal place-cell sequences depict future paths to remembered goals. Nature. **497**:74–79.

Price JL, Amaral DG. (1981). An autoradiographic study of the projections of the central nucleus of the monkey amygdala. J Neurosci. **1**:1242–1259.

Ramnani N, Passingham RE. (2001). Changes in the human brain during rhythm learning. J Cogn Neurosci. **13**:952–966.

Ramnani N, Toni I, Josephs O, Ashburner J, Passingham RE. (2000). Learning- and expectation-related changes in the human brain during motor learning. J Neurophysiol. **84**:3026–3035.

Rao SC, Rainer G, Miller EK. (1997). Integration of what and where in the primate prefrontal cortex. Science. **276**:821–824.

Ravizza SM, McCormick CA, Schlerf JE, Justus T, Ivry RB, Fiez JA. (2006). Cerebellar damage produces selective deficits in verbal working memory. Brain. **129**:306–320.

Sakai K, Miyashita Y. (1991). Neural organization for the long-term memory of paired associates. Nature. **354**:152–155.

Schall JD. (2002). The neural selection and control of saccades by the frontal eye field. Philos Trans R Soc Lond B Biol Sci. **357**:1073–1082.

Schmahmann JD, Pandya DN. (1997). The cerebrocerellar system. In: The Cerebellum and Cognition (Schmahmann JD, ed.), pp. 31–60. San Diego, CA: Academic Press.

Schmahmann JD, Pandya DN. (2008). Disconnection syndromes of basal ganglia, thalamus, and cerebrocerebellar systems. Cortex. **44**:1037–1066.

Schmahmann JD, Sherman JC. (1998). The cerebellar cognitive affective syndrome. Brain. **121** (Pt 4):561–579.

Scoville WB, Milner B. (1957). Loss of recent memory after bilateral hippocampal lesions. J Neurol Neurosurg Psychiatr. **20**:11–21.

Shima K, Isoda M, Mushiake H, Tanji J. (2007). Categorization of behavioural sequences in the prefrontal cortex. Nature. **445**:315–318.

Shulman GL, Corbetta M, Buckner RL, Raichle ME, Fiez JA, Miezin FM, Petersen SE. (1997). Top-down modulation of early sensory cortex. Cereb Cortex. **7**:193–206.

Sigala N, Logothetis NK. (2002). Visual categorization shapes feature selectivity in the primate temporal cortex. Nature. **415**:318–320.

Spiers HJ, Maguire EA. (2006). Thoughts, behaviour, and brain dynamics during navigation in the real world. Neuroimage. **31**:1826–1840.

Spreng RN, Stevens WD, Chamberlain JP, Gilmore AW, Schacter DL. (2010). Default network activity, coupled with the frontoparietal control network, supports goal-directed cognition. Neuroimage. **53**:303–317.

Sur M, Leamey CA. (2001). Development and plasticity of cortical areas and networks. Nat Rev Neurosci. **2**:251–262.

Tanaka K. (1997). Mechanisms of visual object recognition. Curr Opin Neurobiol. **7**:523–529.

Toni I, Krams M, Turner R, Passingham RE. (1998). The time-course of changes during motor sequence learning: a whole-brain fMRI study. Neuroimage. **8**:50–61.

Tsujimoto S, Postle BR. (2012). The prefrontal cortex and oculomotor delayed response: a reconsideration of the "mnemonic scotoma." J Cogn Neurosci. **24**:627–635.

Tudusciuc O, Nieder A. (2009). Contributions of primate prefrontal and posterior parietal cortices to length and numerosity representation. J Neurophysiol. **101**:2984–2994.

Tulving E. (2005). Episodic memory and autonoesis: uniquely human? In: The Missing Link in Cognition (Terrace HS, Metcalfe J, eds), pp. 3–56. Oxford: Oxford University Press.

Ungerleider LG, Galkin TW, Desimone R, Gattass R. (2008). Cortical connections of area V4 in the macaque. Cereb Cortex. **18**:477–499.

Vargha-Khadem F, Gadian DG, Watkins KE, Connelly A, van Paesschen W, Mishkin M. (1997). Differential effects of early hippocampal pathology on episodic and semantic memory. Science. **277**:330–331 (comment); 376–380.

Wagar BM, Dixon M. (2006). Affective guidance in the Iowa gambling task. Cogn Affect Behav Neurosci. **6**:277–290.

Wallis JD, Anderson KC, Miller EK. (2001). Single neurons in prefrontal cortex encode abstract rules. Nature. **411**:953–956.

Webster MJ, Bachevalier J, Ungerleider LG. (1994). Connections of inferior temporal areas TEO and TE with parietal and frontal cortex in macaque monkeys. Cereb Cortex. **4**:471–483.

Young MP. (1993). The organization of neural systems in the primate cerebral cortex. Proc R Soc Lond B Biol Sci. **252**:13–18.

Zhong YM, Rockland KS. (2004). Connections between the anterior inferotemporal cortex (area TE) and CA1 of the hippocampus in monkey. Exp Brain Res. **155**:311–319.

A theory of cerebellar cortex

Chapter 2

Development from Marr's theory of the cerebellum

Takeru Honda and Masao Ito

Forty-five years ago—Marr's 1969 paper and its background

In the early 1960s, analyses of neuronal circuit connections in the cerebellum advanced markedly. The results were summarized in the monograph entitled *The Cerebellum as a Neuronal Machine* (Eccles et al., 1967). In this book, neuronal circuits of the cerebellum are described in detail in terms of convergence/divergence and excitation/inhibition, but there is not much about the functions that such a neuronal circuit could produce. It merely states that these circuits are involved in "certain essential information processing."

Many researchers tried to decipher the excellent diagrams of neuronal circuits illustrated in the book. In particular, the characteristic dual innervation of Purkinje cells (PCs: the sole output neurons of the cerebellar cortex) by two excitatory pathways was the focus of heated discussions: a mossy fiber (MF)–granule cell (GC)–parallel fiber (PF) pathway and an inferior olive cell–climbing fiber (CF) pathway converge to the same PC (Figure 2.1). In the international symposium on "Information Processing in the Cerebellum" held in 1967 at Salishan Lodge on the Oregon coast of the USA, several possible functions of these connections were raised, but none of them appeared to get to the crux of the arguments (Ito, 2006). Marr did not join that symposium, but two years later his 1969 paper appeared in the *Journal of Physiology*. It clearly defined the role of the dual innervation as a memory device, which is vital to any computer. This paper transformed the cerebellar neuronal circuit from just an elegant diagram to a blueprint of a functional learning machine.

Marr (1969) agreed with Brindley's (1964) suggestion that, when both PFs and a CF impinging on one and the same PC are activated synchronously, PF–PC synapses are activated both presynaptically and postsynaptically, which in turn induces a Hebbian form of plasticity (Hebb, 1949), i.e., long-term potentiation (LTP). With this LTP mechanism, MFs, GCs, and PCs constitute a three-layered associative learning network. Marr (1969) assumed that each CF conveys a cerebral (or peripheral) instruction for an elemental movement, and the receiving PC is also exposed via the MF inputs to information about the context in which the CF fires. During rehearsal of an action, each PC learns

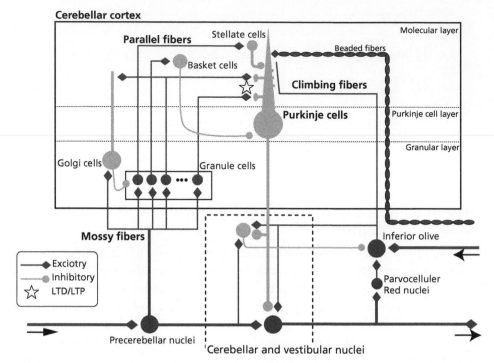

Figure 2.1 Neuronal circuit of the cerebellum. Explanation is in the text.

to recognize such contexts, and later, after the action has been learned, the occurrence of the context alone is sufficient to fire the PC, which then initiates the next elemental movement.

Two years later, Albus (1971) proposed another model based on a close analogy to the simple perceptron (Rosenblatt, 1958). In this model, the inferior olive acts as an outside teacher that generates CF signals. These CF signals change the transmission efficacy of the conjunctively activated PF–PC synapses. When the performance of the cerebellum is erroneous, relevant CFs send error signals, which generate long-term depression (LTD, see section "Synaptic plasticity as memory"). LTD depresses concurrently activated PF–PC synapses that are responsible for the erroneous performance of the cerebellum. Around 1970, CF-dependent LTD at PF–PC synapses was only a theoretical possibility, but it is now substantiated experimentally as a type of synaptic plasticity.

Marr's 1969 paper presented a highly novel theory, yet the reaction of experimental neuroscientists at that time was disappointingly negative. Only a few seemed to recognize its importance, and a majority criticized it as being based on an unrealistic or even an illusory assumption of synaptic plasticity. Indeed, there was no experimental evidence before Bliss and Lomo (1973) reported on LTP in the hippocampus. On our side, there was a specific reason to support the Marr–Albus model; it was known that adaptation of the vestibulo-ocular reflex (VOR) occurs in a neuronal circuit within the

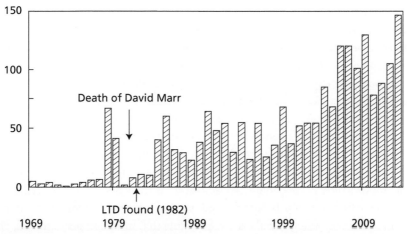

Figure 2.2 Citation pattern for Marr (1969), "A theory of the cerebellar cortex". Ordinate, total citations per year. Abscissa, year.
Estimated by Google Scholar.

cerebellar flocculus (Ito, 1972, 1982), but supporters of Marr's theory were still hardly found. This lack of support is reflected in the fact that Marr's model initially had a low impact, as indicated by the modest number of citations during the decade following its publication (Figure 2.2). The number of citations has since then increased markedly over three decades up to the present. This is a typical example showing the difficulty in evaluating a highly creative work from its early citation patterns. In general, paradigm-changing discoveries have a notoriously limited early impact, because the more a discovery deviates from the current paradigm, the longer it takes to be appreciated by the community (Wang et al., 2013).

Synaptic plasticity as memory

Marr's theory of the cerebellar cortex is built on a number of assumptions and makes a number of predictions. Since its proposal, these assumptions and predictions have been the subjects of fruitful experimental examinations. In this subsection, we review the current knowledge of synaptic plasticity of PCs, which is one of the major cores of Marr's theory of the cerebellum.

LTP and LTD

Marr (1969) assumed that the CF-dependent plasticity of PF–PC synapses is LTP, in accordance with Brindley's (1964) suggestion, whereas Albus (1971) considered it to be LTD on the basis of the better stability of the simple perceptron operating with LTD. In the simple perceptron, an outside teacher intensifies the transmission across PF–PC synapses (by LTP) operating when the machine responds correctly, as Marr (1969) assumed, whereas the transmission across wrongly responding PF–PC synapses are suppressed (by

LTD), as Albus (1971) proposed. Therefore, both the Marr and the Albus models are consistent with the learning mechanism adopted in the simple perceptron. The essential difference between the two models is in the assumptions that CF signals represent errorless responses of the machine in Marr's model but erroneous responses in Albus's model. Decade-long experimental efforts yielded substantial evidence for LTD to occur after conjunctive stimulation of a CF and PFs impinging on the same PC (Ito and Kano, 1982; Ito et al., 1982; Ekerot and Kano, 1985; Sakurai, 1987; Ito, 1989).

Among a number of predictions Marr made is the following: "5. (a) The synapses from parallel fibres to PCs are facilitated by the conjunction of presynaptic and climbing fibre (or post-synaptic) activity." This is often taken as being wrong in the sense that the actual event that follows the PF–CF conjunctive activation is LTD, but is not the predicted LTP. However, the actual situation is complicated, so that a simple statement of the prediction being "correct or wrong" would not apply. Note that in a perceptron model, an outside teacher intensifies the PF–PC synaptic transmission (by LTP) when the machine's response is error-free, whereas the teacher weakens the PF–PC synaptic transmission (by LTD) when the machine responds incorrectly. However, it is not possible in a real synapse that only one CF acts to induce both LTP and LTD by conjunction. Then, Marr chose LTP, whereas Albus preferred LTD. What actually happens is that LTD is induced by conjunction whereas LTP is induced by the lack of conjunction.

Error representation by CFs

This has been conceived and experimentally verified in studies of various motor systems (for review, see Ito, 2013). Although error-representing CF signals induce LTD, the absence of such signals leads to LTP (Sakurai, 1987; Shibuki and Okada, 1992; Lev-Ram et al., 2002). This bilateral synaptic plasticity contributes to a unique type of learning from errors (error learning, Doya, 1999, 2000; Dean et al., 2002). The rule for this error learning has been formulated; PFs carrying signals that positively correlate with an error signal have their synaptic weights reduced (LTD), whereas those carrying signals that negatively correlate with the error signal have their weights increased (LTP) (see Dean and Porril, Chapter 4, this volume).

Soon after the synaptic-plasticity-based learning mechanism was formulated in the 1980s, many laboratories joined the exploration of the molecular mechanisms of LTD. Various pathways of signal transduction and receptor trafficking have been identified (for review, see Ito et al., 2014). LTD can now be blocked effectively using various inhibitors and gene manipulation techniques (for review, see Yuzaki, 2013; Ito et al., 2014).

LTD–motor learning linkage

The marked advance we have witnessed since the 1970s and 1980s is that several types of elementary motor control, reflexive or voluntary, have been identified as specifically connected to a cerebellar circuit and thereby adaptively controlled. These are VOR, optokinetic eye movement response (OKR), saccade, eyeblink conditioning, hand reaching, and cursor tracking. These types of motor learning provided a way to examine whether LTD is critically involved in motor learning. A pharmacological inhibitor or genetic manipulation that blocks LTD induction in slices or tissue cultures should impair motor learning in animal behavior. This LTD–motor learning linkage has been the basis for the Marr–Albus–Ito hypothesis that LTD plays a key role in cerebellar motor learning (Ito, 2000).

Recent experimental evidence further supports the LTD–motor learning linkage concept (Yuzaki, 2013). A cyclooxygenase (COX)-2 inhibitor (nimesulide) blocked LTD in acute slices, while its intraperitoneal administration impaired OKR adaptation in mice in vivo (Le et al., 2010). Concomitant impairment of LTD induction and motor learning has been observed in mGluR1 knockout (KO) mice (Ichise et al., 2000), GluD2 KO mice (Kakegawa et al., 2009), and GluD2-mutated mice (Kakegawa et al., 2011). KO of C1ql1 in CF, which binds to the brain-specific angiogenesis inhibitor 3 (Bai3) at CF–PC synapses, also impaired both LTD and cerebellar motor learning (Kakegawa et al., 2015). A recent electron microscopy study also supports the LTD–motor learning linkage concept because the decrease in the expression level of AMPA-type glutamate receptors (AMPARs) in PF–PC synapses is associated with OKR adaptation (Wang et al., 2014).

LTD–motor learning mismatch

The hypothesis has, however, been challenged on the basis of three lines of recent evidence. First, LTD–motor learning coincidence is lacking in the mice carrying the mutated GluA2-C terminus (Steinberg et al., 2004; Schonewille et al., 2011). Although these mutant mice exhibited normal motor learning, LTD was not induced in cerebellar slices obtained from them. Nevertheless, it has recently been found that LTD occurs in these mutants under certain stimulation conditions (Yamaguchi et al., 2015); hence, the possibility that LTD occurs in vivo cannot be excluded. Second, the inhibitor T-588, which blocks LTD in slices, did not interfere with motor learning when administered orally to rats (Welsh et al., 2005) or intraperitoneally to mice (Schonewille et al., 2011). However, in a recent study of marmosets, the intraperitoneal injection of T-588 depressed OKR adaptation dose-dependently (Anzai and Nagao, 2014). The reason for this species difference is yet to be explored, but a possible reason is the difference in the ease with which T-588 reaches PCs across the gastrointestinal or peritoneal membrane and blood–brain barrier. Third, in protein phosphatase-2B KO PCs, in which LTP is absent, motor learning was impaired whereas LTD occurred normally. This observation may lead to the suspicion that LTP, but not LTD, is essential for motor learning (Schonewille et al., 2011). However, the observation can also be interpreted on the basis of the Marr–Albus–Ito hypothesis, as suggested in a recent modeling study (Yamazaki et al., 2015). That is, when LTP is absent in protein phosphatase-2B KO PCs, spontaneous LTD may fail to be balanced by spontaneous LTP and hence accumulate to the extent that these PCs become unable to function normally; consequently, motor learning might be impaired. For these reasons, we consider that the LTD–motor learning mismatch should be resolved so that the Marr–Albus–Ito hypothesis remains acceptable.

The LTD–motor learning mismatch has also been raised in connection with the eyeblink conditioning (Hesslow et al., 2013). This is based on four lines of experimental evidence, all of which are, however, explicable and consistent with LTD (see the section "Solving controversies on LTD mechanism of eyeblink conditioning").

Silent synapses

A recent surprising discovery is that the vast majority (up to 97%) of PF–PC synapses are silent (Wang et al., 2000; Isope and Barbour, 2002; Ekerot and Jörntell, 2003). How PF–PC synapses become silent is as yet unknown, but it is speculated that repeated LTD inductions in PF–PC synapses involved in an erroneous behavior render these synapses silent, whereas repeated LTP inductions in PF–PC synapses involved in an error-free behavior may keep these synapses functional. However, in in-vitro cerebellar slices, an LTD causes only a 30–40% reduction in PF-excitatory postsynaptic currents (EPSCs) (e.g., Le et al. 2010), and how repeatedly evoked LTD accumulates to nullify PF-EPSCs has been unclear. The rate of occurrence of silent synapses (up to 97%) may seem very high, but taking the total number of PF–PC synapses as 150 000, there will still be 4500 functional synapses in each PC, which is sufficient to form a neurocomputing circuit for specific information. It is likely that neuronal circuits in the cerebellar cortex, which are originally randomly connected at birth, are specialized by silencing redundant PF–PC synapses during repeated learning from errors.

Memory capacity of a PC

Using the classic perceptron model and assuming the binary operation (0 or 1 action potential) of PF–PC synapses, it is estimated that a PC could learn up to 5 kB of information in the form of 40 000 input–output associations (Brunel et al., 2004). The pattern recognition capacity of a PC was calculated using a multicompartmental model, in which all spines were activated independently by a random sequence of PF inputs, firing at an average rate of 0.3 Hz. This background excitation was balanced by tonic background inhibition, so that the PC model fired simple spikes at an average frequency of 48 Hz, similarly to real PCs (De Schutter and Bower, 1994a, 1994b). The PC model was elaborated by adding experimentally determined response variability and pattern size on the basis of a linear algorithm (Walter and Khodakhah, 2006, 2009). In this model, each pattern was generated by 650 different randomly selected inputs from the entire pool of 150 000 inputs. This model's response showed a linear function of the strength of its inputs, with the 650 inputs increasing the model's firing rate by 200 spikes per second. Learning occurred in this PC model by LTD at PF–PC synapses, halving the strength of all the inputs that comprised the learned pattern. The capacity of a PC to participate in pattern recognition was estimated by altering the number of patterns the model had to learn and by quantifying its ability to distinguish between learned and novel patterns. To quantify the latter, the resulting signal-to-noise ratio of the maximum firing rate of the model is calculated in response to learned novel patterns (Walter and Khodakhah, 2009).

Yet another unique PC model was proposed, assuming that PCs encode information using pauses in their discharge rather than acceleration (Steuber et al., 2007). Such pauses were observed in computer-simulated or experimentally recorded PCs after applying a strong shock to GCs. The applicability of this model to real cerebellar tissues under natural conditions has been questioned, however, because a relatively milder and temporally dispersed (i.e., more natural) GC activation fails to cause such pauses (Walter and Khodakhah, 2009). Compared with this pause coding, the linear encoding of information enables cerebellar nuclear neurons to use a simple averaging mechanism. In contrast to the pause encoding, a linear algorithm enables PCs to recognize a large number of both synchronous and asynchronous input patterns in the presence or absence of inhibitory synaptic transmission. In any case, the number of patterns recognized by PCs, as determined using a linear algorithm, could be greater than that achieved by PCs encoding information in pauses (Walter and Khodakhah, 2009).

Actual cellular/molecular mechanisms controlling PC activities involve multiple ion channels that are distributed along dendrites and axons (e.g., Masoli et al., 2015) and complex molecular signal transduction processes (e.g., Ito et al., 2014). These new lines of evidence may further help with improved neuronal circuit modeling of the cerebellum.

Multiple sites of synaptic plasticity

Marr's prediction 5(b) in the abstract of his 1969 paper (see Chapter 1) denotes that no cerebellar synapses (other than PF–PC synapses) are modifiable. Apparently, in constructing his model of the cerebellar cortex, Marr (1969) avoided unnecessary complications by assuming that other synapses are all nonmodifiable. This was a good strategy at the time Marr was writing, but since then various types of synaptic plasticity have been found at many sites not only within the cerebellar cortex, but also in cerebellar and vestibular nuclei (for review, see Hansel et al., 2001; Ito, 2011; Gao et al., 2012; Mapelli et al. 2015). We are, therefore, required to analyze the characteristic features of these types of synaptic plasticity and their specific functional roles in the cerebellum.

PFs form excitatory synapses on not only PCs but also stellate cells (SCs) and basket cells in the superficial and deep molecular layer (see Figure 2.1). Recording of field potentials from SCs revealed that the conjunctive stimulation of PFs and CFs induces LTP, opposite to the LTD that appears in PCs (Jörntell and Ekerot, 2002; Ekerot and Jörntell 2003). In in-vitro cerebellar slices, the conjunction of PF-EPSCs and depolarization, the latter replacing CF stimuli, also induced LTP (Rancillac and Crépel, 2004). Because SCs form inhibitory synapses on PCs, LTD in PF–PC synapses and LTP in PF–SC synapses should have synergistic depressant action on PCs. Very recently, triple mutants have been generated in which both LTD and the molecular layer interneuron output were impaired, and they showed highly significantly more reduced eyeblink conditioning than when either of them alone was blocked (Henk-Jan Boele and Chris De Zeeuw, personal communication). This suggests that PF–SC LTP may compensate for part of PF–PC LTD. Another example of synaptic plasticity involving SCs is rebound depolarization (RD) (Kano et al., 1992). CF- or current-evoked membrane depolarization induces a long-lasting enhancement of inhibitory postsynaptic potentials in a PC. In RD-impaired transgenic mice, VOR adaptation was subnormal, suggesting that RD is involved in motor learning (Hirano and Kawaguchi, 2014).

MF–GC synapses have been found to generate LTP following high-frequency stimulation (D'Angelo et al., 1999). This LTP is associated with an increase in GC input resistance and a decrease in spike threshold (Armano et al., 2000). These changes depend on postsynaptic depolarization and NMDA receptor activation and were prevented in the presence of inhibitory synaptic activity.

Plasticity at synapses from MF collaterals to vestibular nuclear (VN) neurons has been postulated as a mechanism of cerebellar learning (Miles and Lisberger, 1981; Medina and Mauk, 1999), and indeed, LTP has actually been found to occur (Kassardjian et al., 2005; Pugh and Raman, 2006; Shutoh et al., 2006; Zhang and Linden, 2006; Anzai et al., 2010; McElvain et al., 2010). Nagao's group revealed that PF–PC plasticity underlies the fast adaptation of OKR (lasting for a day), whereas MF–VN plasticity accounts for its slow adaptation (lasting for a week; Shutoh et al., 2006). The relationship between these two types of synaptic plasticity has been shown to be as follows. Normally, the shutdown of the flocculus cortex impairs not only the fast adaptation, but also the slow adaptation; however, after adaptation has been performed, the flocculus shutdown impairs only the fast adaptation, leaving the slow adaptation virtually intact. These findings have been interpreted to indicate that a memory trace of OKR adaptation experienced by mice is initially acquired in PF–PC synapses by LTD as a short-term memory (for fast adaptation). After repetition of training, the memory trace is transferred to MF–VN synapses and consolidated as a long-term memory (for slow adaptation; Shutoh et al., 2006; Okamoto et al., 2011). These observations suggest an important role of nuclear LTP in cerebellar memory, at least in the vestibulocerebellar system. Miles and Lisberger (1981) and Medina and Mauk (1999) assumed that PCs act as a teacher for nuclear synaptic plasticity, but Yamazaki et al. (2015) reproduced the memory transfer simply by applying the bidirectional Hebbian rule to MF–VN synapses.

Thus, the cerebellar circuit contains more than 15 different types of synaptic plasticity (Hansel et al., 2001; Ito, 2011; D'Angelo, 2014; Mapelli et al., 2015). Each type has its own mechanism and is devoted conjointly to improving the learning capability of cerebellar neuronal circuits. These are important additional aspects of Marr's theory of the cerebellum. To determine the possible roles of various types of synaptic plasticity, D'Angelo's group analyzed the cerebellar model-controlled manipulation of a robotic arm. Notably, they found that the incorporation of LTP/LTD in the synapses that CF collaterals supply to CN neurons accelerated the otherwise slow PF–PC LTP/LTD-based learning by an order or two (Luque et al., 2014). Introduction of both LTD and LTP at MF–CN and PC–CN synapses, in addition to PF–PC synapses, improved the quality of control by learning (Garrido et al., 2013). A realistic model of the cerebellum with synaptic plasticity at these three sites reproduced robustly humanlike effective learning properties in acquisition, extinction, and re-extinction, dealing with different external and noisy stimuli in the real world (Casellato et al., 2015).

From codon theory to liquid-state machine (LSM)

Beside the memory at PF–PC networks already dealt with in the section "Memory capacity of a PC," information representation in MF–GC networks is another major focus of Marr's theory of the cerebellar cortex. In this section, we explain Marr's codon theory and follow its development to the random projection model to the LSM.

Spatial representation in the codon model

Considering the MF–GC arrangement characterized by a small convergence and a large divergence, Marr (1969) introduced the term "codon" as a subset of a collection of active MFs, and "codon representation" as the representation of a MF input by a sample of such subsets. A codon then activates a combination of GCs. Because the number of GCs is much larger than that of MFs, the GC representation may amplify differences between input patterns represented by active MFs (Albus, 1971).

To visualize a possible behavior of the MF–GC arrangement, we used a network model composed of 4 MFs connected to 6 GCs (Figure 2.3A). When a combination of 3 active MFs constitutes a codon, there will be 4-codon representations. We calculate the number of GCs to be activated according to Marr's (1969) codon theory. As a result, each of these 4 codons activates 3 of the 6 GCs in different combinations, and 20 different patterns of distribution of activated GCs are possible (Figure 2.3B and the equation in its legend). Because 4 activity patterns conveyed by MFs generate 4 activity patterns each involving 6 GCs, the total number of combinations of GC activity patterns is calculated (20 choose 4) to be 4845. In this model, we estimated the similarity between the 4 MF or GC activity patterns (4 choose 2 = 6 ways) by calculating the factor N, which denotes the average number of active MFs or GCs common to 2 patterns (e.g., GC2 at p_2 and p_3 in the left box of Figure 2.3B). Note that in contrast to $N = 2.0$ in all of the 4 patterns of active MFs, only 30 of the 4845 patterns of GC activity showed $N = 2.0$ and lower than 2.0 in the remaining 4815 patterns. It indicates that in this MF–GC arrangement, the similarity between GC activity patterns decreases as the number of GCs increases; hence, it becomes easier to distinguish their activity patterns. The anatomically determined ratio of the number of GCs to that of MFs is approximately 300 in cats (see Ito, 1984). The number of GC activity patterns will then be as large as 287 280 400 (4 × 300 choose 3).

Golgi cell (GO) inhibition of GCs decreases codon size and consequently improves pattern discriminations (Marr, 1969; Pellionisz and Szentagothai, 1973). In our model, if we assume that GO inhibition decreases the number of active GCs involved in each GC activity pattern from 3 to 2, N would decrease from 1.0–2.0 to 0.33–0.66 (Figures 2.3B and 2.3C).

Therefore, the large number of GCs and the GO inhibition are two important factors that determine codon discriminability. Possible pattern discrimination capability was calculated previously by computer simulation with a model of the cerebellum consisting of 13 000 MFs, 200 000 GCs, and 100 GOs (Tyrrell and Willshaw, 1992). This simulation discriminated about 70 MF activity patterns, a number that is, however, less than those

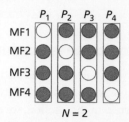

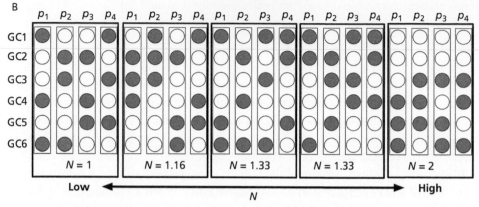

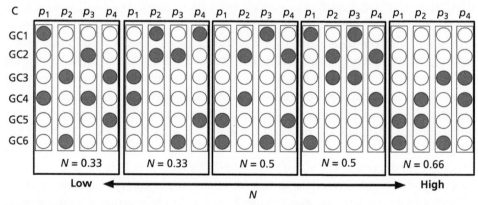

Figure 2.3 Example of codon representation. (A) The postulated MF–GC network contains four MFs, three of which are active (●) and one is inactive (○) at a time. These MFs generate four MF activity patterns: P1, P2, P3, and P4. (B) At the succeeding GC stage, there are six GCs, three of which are activated (●) and the other three are inactivated (○) at a time. Twenty possible GC activity patterns occur: p1,..., p20. Using equation (2) in Marr's theory of the cerebellar cortex (Marr, 1969), the number of active GCs per PC [#(active GCs)] can be calculated as a function of the number of GCs [#(GCs)], that of active MFs (L), that of MFs [#(MFs)], and threshold for GC spiking (R) by binomial statistical analysis.

$$\#(active\ GCs) = \#(GCs) \times \binom{L}{R} \bigg/ \binom{\#(MFs)}{R}$$

As shown in (A) and (B), #(active GCs) is 3 when #(GCs) = 6, L = 3, R = 2, and #(MFs) = 4. Four patterns having the same values of N are grouped. (C) GC activity patterns to be generated when MF patterns in (A) activate 2 (instead of 3) GCs at a time under Golgi cell inhibition. Indicated values of N are calculated for MFs as $N = (P_1P_2 + P_1P_3 + P_1P_4 + P_2P_3 + P_2P_4 + P_3P_4)/6$, where $P_1 = (0, 1, 1, 1)^T$, $P_2 = (1, 0, 1, 1)^T$, $P_3 = (1, 1, 0, 1)^T$, and $P_4 = (1, 1, 1, 0)^T$ and the inner product of their patterns (e.g. P_1P_2). Values of N in (B) and (C) were calculated similarly as $N = (p_1p_2 + p_1p_3 + p_1p_4 + p_2p_3 + p_2p_4 + p_3p_4)/6$. Lower values of N in a group of 4 imply relative ease in discriminating the 4 patterns.

calculated using the present model. A third factor that potentially affects the sensitivity of discrimination of MF input patterns is LTP in MF–GC synapses (D'Angelo, 2014 and Chapter 4 of this volume; Mapelli et al., 2015).

Extension toward temporal representation

Whereas the codon model processes spatial information, MFs, in general, also convey temporal information. Two types of models have been developed to deal with temporally coded MF information. One is the "adaptive filter" model in which GCs behave as oscillators with different frequencies and phases (Fujita, 1982; Dean et al., 2010). GCs are activated with various phase lags originating from random MF–GC connections and GO inhibition. As a result, the integrated GC activity represents a certain function of time. In this model, GC activity represents more information by focusing on amplitude and frequency rather than the number of discriminated patterns in the codon model. Details of the adaptive filter model of the cerebellum are introduced by Dean and Porril (see Chapter 4).

Another is the "random projection model" composed of a realistic network structure and parameters (Buonomano and Mauk, 1994). Yamazai and Tanaka's (2005) analysis of Buonomano and Mauk's (1994) simulation importantly revealed that the same population of GCs becomes active only once during the lifetime of the model unless reset by strong stimulation of MFs. In a simple network model involving MFs, GCs, and GOs, for example, a population of active GCs is converted step by step to a different population with time (Figure 2.4B) even when MF activity continues to represent only one pattern (Figure 2.4A). The correlation coefficient $C_{t1}(t)$ between the population of active GCs at $t1$ and each population of active GCs at $t1$, $t2$, $t3$, and $t4$ linearly decreases (Figure 2.4C and its legend). Therefore, one population of active GCs represents one time (passage-of-time representation, for example, $t2$, $t3$, and $t4$ in Figure 2.4B). Analysis of this model revealed that the passage-of-time representation is induced by a long-decay constant of NMDA receptor-mediated excitatory postsynaptic potentials (EPSP) at GOs and the random inhibitory recurrent GC–GO–GC connections (Yamazaki and Tanaka, 2005).

LSM model of the cerebellum

The simple perceptron proposed by Rosenblatt (1962) consists of three layers of neurons connected in one direction, from the sensory cell layer to the association cell layer and the response cell layer. In the simple perceptron model of the cerebellar cortex, Albus (1971) placed the cells of origin of MFs in the sensory cell layer, GCs in the association cell layer, and PCs in the response cell layer. CFs function as the outside teacher that modifies GC–PC connectivity according to errors in the machine's performance. The simple perceptron is the first manufactured learning machine, but its capability to learn is limited (Minsky and Papert, 1969, 1988).

The LSM proposed by Maass et al. (2002) provides a computational basis for Buonomano–Mauk's random projection model of the cerebellum introduced above (Yamazaki and Tanaka, 2007a). Its name comes from an analogy to the spatiotemporal

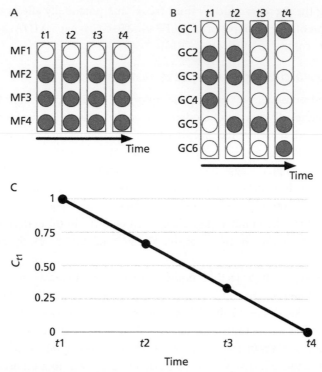

Figure 2.4 GC activity patterns in LSM. (A) Activity patterns in four MFs remain unchanged with time. (B) Corresponding GC activity patterns, which, with time ($t1$, $t2$, $t3$, and $t4$), gradually change to different patterns. (C) Monotonic decrease in correlation coefficient C of GC activity patterns with time. Ordinate: $C_{t1}(t)$ (C as function of time) calculated using $C_{t1}(t) = t_1 t / |t_1||t|$ where $t_1 = (0,1,1,1,0,0)^T$, t is t_1, $t_2 = (0,1,1,0,1,0)^T$, $t_3 = (1,0,1,0,1,0)^T$, or $t_4 = (1,0,0,0,1,1)^T$, and the inner product of their patterns (e.g. $t_1 t$). Abscissa: time.

pattern of ripples produced by a stone falling into a still water surface. Corresponding to the association cell layer of the simple perceptron (Figure 2.5A), the LSM also consists of a network called the "reservoir," in which a number of neurons corresponding to GCs constitute a random recurrent network (Figure 2.5B). Being fed with external contextual information, the recurrent network generates a spatiotemporal activity pattern. The signals mapped in the reservoir are then fed to "readout neurons" corresponding to PCs. The readout neurons can learn to choose desired spatiotemporal activity patterns by modifying the reservoir neuron-to-readout neuron connectivity using external error signals. In the three-layered structures, the simple perceptron and LSM appear similar except for the recurrent inhibition by GOs incorporated in the LSM, but not in the simple perceptron (compare Figures 2.5A and 2.5B). Note that the direct projection of MFs to GOs forms a MF–GO–GC feedforward inhibition pathway in addition to the GC–GO–GC feedback inhibition pathway (Eccles et al., 1967). The feedforward inhibition may function in the sharp timing of MF-evoked spiking in GCs (e.g., Brunel et al.,

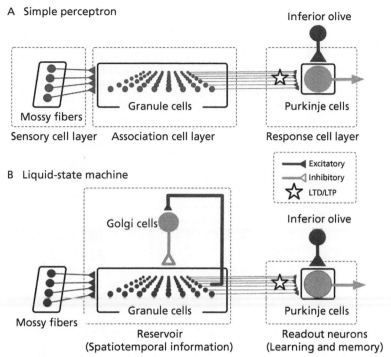

Figure 2.5 Computational neural network model for the cerebellum. (A) Simple perceptron model, consisting of three layers: sensory cell layer (containing MFs), association cell layer (GCs), and response cell layer (PCs). (B) LSM model consisting of reservoir (GCs and GOs) and readout (PCs). CFs function as an external teacher in both of these models.

2004) whereas the feedback inhibition generates broad spatiotemporal patterns of LSM. The simulations by Honda et al. (2011) demonstrated that as long as the MF–GO connection is relatively weak, this connection does not interfere with the feedback inhibition.

To show the operation of the MF–GC–PC arrangement in the LSM manner, we examined a model composed of 15 GCs projecting their axons to one and the same PC and mapped the spatiotemporal pattern that emerged in it in response to MF inputs with a constant spatial pattern, as shown in Figure 2.6A. This model behaved in such a way that after resetting at $t1$, MF inputs activate 7 of the 15 GCs whose spatial pattern of distribution changed similarly to that adopted in the previous simulation studies (Yamazaki and Tanaka, 2005, 2007a, 2007b; Honda et al., 2011). This characteristic behavior of MF–GC–GO arrangement can be observed in the simulation platform (http://sim.neuroinf.jp). The model presented in Figure 2.6A is designed in such a way that with time, one of the seven spiking GCs becomes silent, and at the same time another GC that has been silent becomes spiking. Owing to this status rotation among the 15 GCs, the total number of spiking GCs remains constant. In this situation, some GCs may continue to spike monotonously for a while and then are silenced, whereas other GCs may continue to be silent and after a while they continuously spike. This status rotation among GCs changes the spatial distribution pattern of spiking GCs, but the total number of spiking GCs within

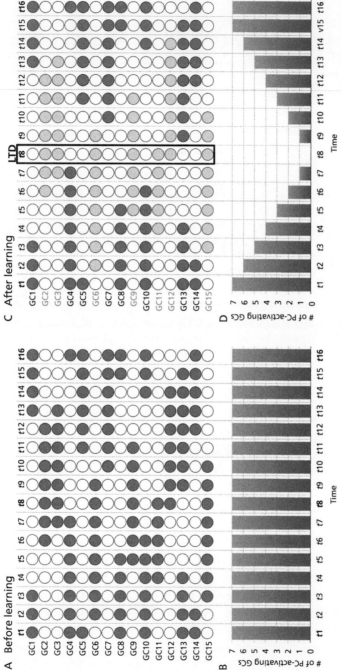

Figure 2.6 GC activities in an LSM model of the cerebellum. (A) Spatiotemporal patterns of distribution of spiking GCs. ●, spiking GC, ○ silent GC. (B) Time-dependent changes in the number of spiking GCs in (A). (C) Similar to (A), but after training by CF signals at $t8$. those GCs spiking but not activating the target PC because of LTD. (D) Similar to (B), but for PC-activating GCs in (C).

the group of 15 GCs remains unchanged (Figure 2.6B). The target PC reads out the spatiotemporal pattern of GC activities.

To examine how LTD is represented in the LSM model, we trained the model by applying a CF stimulus to the target PC at $t8$ and thereby induced LTD in the synapses supplied by the GCs that spiked at $t8$ (that is, GC2, GC3, GC6, GC9, GC11, GC12, and GC15 in Figure 2.6C). After the training, these GCs (○ within the boxed column in Figure 2.6) no longer activate the target PC even when they are spiking. Hence, they are functionally removed from the 15 GCs. Thus, the number of GCs that activate the target PC (●) gradually decreases to zero with time from $t1$ to $t8$ and then gradually increases again from $t8$ to $t16$ (Figure 2.6D). The time-varying pattern of spatial distribution of GCs acting on the target PC (Figure 2.6A) and its changes after the induction of LTD (Figure 2.6C) are essential features of the LSM model, but we must realize that, to experimentally observe such features in the real cerebellum, more than 1000 GCs must be monitored simultaneously (Yamazaki and Tanaka, 2005).

LSM modeling of eyeblink conditioning

In delayed eyeblink conditioning, repeated combined stimulations of MFs as the conditioned stimulus (CS) and CFs as the unconditioned stimulus (US) induce changes in the effectiveness of CS so that CS alone causes eye blinking (Figure 2.7A; for review, see Yeo and Hesslow, 1998; Thompson and Steinmetz, 2009). It has been reported that around the time of the onset of US, PCs firing in the cerebellum exhibit a pause, which causes eyeblinking, as shown in Figure 2.7B (Jirenhed and Hesslow, 2011a). The mechanism of the delayed eyeblink conditioning has been explained on the basis of the classic delay line hypothesis; that is, GCs converging onto a PC fire with systematically varied delay time (Hesslow et al., 2013). When CF signals representing US are presented, a conjunctively activated PF as CS will generate LTD and thus block transmission from the PF to the PC. Thence, the PC will stop firing at the time of CF signaling and consequently an eyeblink will occur. However, the actually observed firing of PCs does not conform to the delay line hypothesis (Hesslow et al., 2013), which therefore has to be discarded. On the other hand, conditioned eyeblink conditioning was reproduced by computer simulation using a random projection model (Buonomano and Mauk, 1994; Medina et al., 2000) or the LSM model of the cerebellum (Yamazaki and Tanaka, 2007b, Honda et al., 2011). The characteristic inverted-triangle-like pause of PC discharges observed in the cerebellum (Figure 2.7B) is well reproduced by simulation using the LSM model, as illustrated in Figure 2.7C (compare with Figure 2.7B).

An LSM model of the cerebellum also reproduces the gain adaptation of OKR (Yamazaki and Nagao, 2012). The LSM model of the cerebellum also calculates exclusive OR (XOR) (Yamazaki and Tanaka, 2007a), which the simple perceptron cannot (Minsky and Papert, 1969, 1988). However, because an adaptive filter model can also calculate XOR (Mapelli et al., 2010), this is not a proof of a uniquely powerful information processing capability of the LSM model of the cerebellum. A computer-simulated LSM has successfully simulated force-field adaptation (Casellato et al., 2014) and weight manipulation (Garrido et al.,

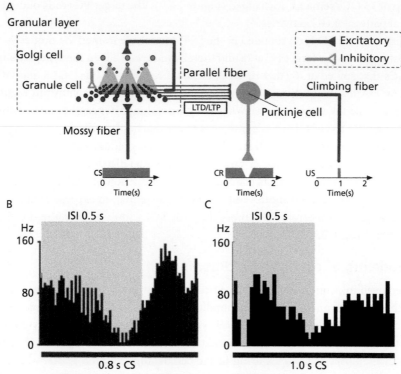

Figure 2.7 PC activities in eyeblink conditioning: experimental recording and LSM simulation. (A) Cerebellar circuit operating in eyeblink conditioning. (B) Simple spike frequency extracellarly recorded from a PC in response to conditioned stimulation (CS) after training with US. Note that CS alone induced a decrease in simple spike activity. The horizontal bar indicates 0.8 s time period during which CS was presented. The gray window shows the interstimulus interval (ISI) between CS and US, which was 0.5 s. (C) LSM simulation of the experimental situation described in (B). Calculated using the cerebellar model of Honda et al., (2011). The horizontal bar indicates CS that continued for 1.0 s. ISI is shown similarly to that in (B).

B, C: Learning stimulus intervals—adaptive timing of conditioned Purkinje cell responses, Cerebellum, 10, 2011, pp. 523–535 Jirenhed and Hesslow © Springer Science+Business Media Dordrecht. With permission of Springer.

2013; Luque et al., 2014), and real-time control of a robotic arm (Yamazaki and Igarashi, 2013). The LSM model will show its merit when applied to solving more complex control problems.

Solving controversies on LTD mechanism of eyeblink conditioning

Whereas the LSM incorporating LTD excellently reproduces PC behavior in eyeblink conditioning (Figure 2.7C), the following four major experimental observations have been claimed not to be explicable by LTD (Hesslow et al., 2013) and are thus the focus of debate.

1 During CR, the simple spike firing of PCs observed before training is completely suppressed by CS, too severely to be ascribed to LTD. This finding can, however, be explained by the possibility that CS activates also inhibitory interneurons and that this inhibition critically cancels PF-evoked EPSP, as reported by Brunel et al. (2004). LTD that attenuates PF-EPSP would make the inhibitory postsynaptic potential (IPSP) dominant over the EPSP and consequently suppress PC simple spike discharges.

2 Whereas simultaneous PF–CF conjunction is most efficient in inducing LTD in slices, paired CS–US presentations at intervals of 150 ms or longer lead to the development of typical pause responses in PCs. This delay in CS–US presentation can, however, be ascribed to the latent time for IP3-mediated intracellular release of Ca^{2+} after PF stimulation as CS. In in-vitro slices, PF-evoked IPSPs are blocked pharmacologically to render PF-EPSPs prominent. Hence, the concentration of Ca^{2+} entering through voltage-dependent Ca^{2+} channels would be sufficiently high for the Ca^{2+} to interact supralinearly with the Ca^{2+} entering during CF-evoked complex spikes to cause a considerable Ca^{2+} surge that triggers LTD. Under in-vivo conditions for testing eyeblink conditioning, CS-evoked EPSPs could be curtailed by IPSPs and would not induce entry of sufficient Ca^{2+}. Instead, IP3-mediated Ca^{2+} release from intracellular stores will be a dominant factor for inducing the Ca^{2+} surge with a delay of 50–400 ms (Doi et al., 2005) after the onset of CS.

3 It is not easy to explain on the basis of LTD how the trained PCs take a specific learned time course with a long delay, a maximum immediately before the US, and terminating 300–500 ms after the US (see Figure 2.7C). Examination of poststimulus time histograms of PC responses to each of the repetitive MF stimuli by Jirenhed and Hesslow (2011b) also revealed only temporary depression around the time of US presentation (compare Figures. 2.8B and 2.8D, with special attention to b). This is, however, what is reproduced in the LSM model of the cerebellum, in which PC-activating GCs decrease gradually and after US, increase back gradually (see Figure 2.6C and 2.6D). This induces simple spike activities of PCs that modulate with a temporal pattern of a characteristic inverted triangle (see Figure 2.7C).

4 There seems to be no evidence of LTD because no persistent depression of MF–GC–PC transmission was observed in conditioned PCs (see Figure 2.7B). In the learned LSM model, the number of GCs activating the target PC decreases only temporarily, but not persistently (see Figures 2.7 and 2.8). This is because in the LSM model, GCs that have been involved in LTD rotate their status with other PC-activating GCs (see Figures 2.6C and 2.8C). One possible way to reveal LTD, therefore, is to eliminate (perhaps pharmacologically or genetically) the GO-mediated inhibition of GCs, thus stopping the status rotation of GCs. Another possible way to reveal LTD is to induce LTD in all GC–PC synapses, so that no PC-activating GCs remain to be status-rotated with those undergoing LTD.

Thus, the results of rigorous experimental testing performed by Jirenhed and Hesslow (2011b) and reviewed by Hesslow et al. (2013) can be reconciled with the LSM model of

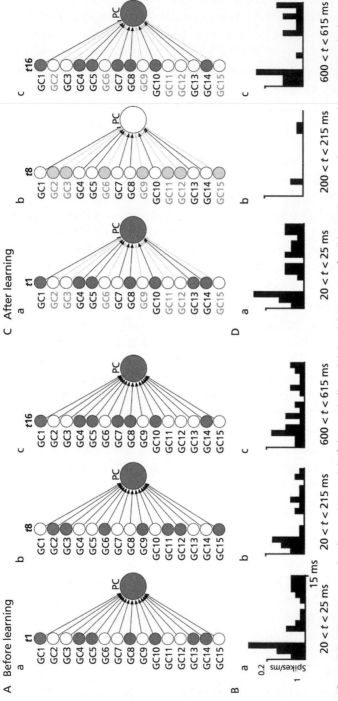

Figure 2.8 LTD representation in an LSM model of the cerebellum. (A) Spatial patterns of spiking GCs converging onto the target PC, (Aa) at $t1$ (before a CS-evoked PC pause); (Ab) at $t8$ (throughout the PC pause), and (Ac) at $t16$ (after the PC pause). (B) Poststimulation time histograms of PC responses to MF stimulation. Ba, Bb, and Bc approximately correspond in time to Aa, Ab, and Ac. (C) Similar to (A), but showing the effect of LTD induction at $t18$ (A). The GC axons undergoing LTD at GC–PC synapses are shown in light gray. (D) Similar to (B) but for (C). Histograms in (B) and (D) are reproduced from Jirenhed and Hesslow, 2011b. Time course of classically conditioned Purkinje cell response is determined by initial part of conditioned stimulus. ●, ○, and ● indicate similarly to those in Figures. 2.6A and C. B, D: Reprinted with permission of The Journal of Neuroscience, 31:9070–9074, 2011.

the cerebellum with LTD as its memory element. Because the LSM model is presently the only model that can defend against the four challenges listed here, it must be the most plausible model of the cerebellum.

Roles of NMDA receptor channels in the LSM model

A network model connecting GCs and GOs was constructed by Maex and De Schutter (1998) on the basis of the Hodgkin–Huxley theory. This model generated synchronized firing of GCs and GOs and reproduced an oscillatory local field potential observed in the granular layer at 7–8 Hz in rats (Hartmann and Bower, 1998) and 13–14 Hz in monkeys (Pellerin and Lamarre, 1997; Courtemanche et al., 2009) at rest without any external stimuli. Simulation studies suggest that adding weak gap junctions to GOs (Dugué et al., 2005) or weak connections between MFs and GOs (Solinas et al., 2010; Honda et al., 2011) makes these oscillations more marked than in the case without the weak connections. The spontaneous firing rate of MFs is as low as 5 Hz, but it increases to 30 Hz when an animal is simulated with a tone (e.g., CS) (Freeman and Muckler, 2003). Honda et al. (2011) added NMDA receptor channels to dendrites of GOs and randomly connected GCs and GOs, and demonstrated that Maex and De Schutter's (1998) model can reproduce spatiotemporal patterns in the LSM. Furthermore, the density of Mg^{2+} ions in NMDA channels on the dendrites of GOs is a key factor for the stimulus-dependent state transition between the synchronized oscillation of GCs in oscillatory local field potential and the passage-of-time representation of GCs in eyeblink conditioning.

Internal model in the cerebellum

Marr's (1969) theory of the cerebellum provided a reliable basis for assuming that the cerebellum is an enormous assembly of similarly structured small modules having learning capability (i.e., nucleocortical microcomplex or microcomplex, Ito, 1984, 2014). The question of what functional role each microcomplex plays in neural control functions led to the idea that the cerebellum provides an internal model of the controlled object.

The first clue was the unique structure called the "cerebrocerebellar communication loop," which links a cerebellar hemispheric area to the primary motor cortex (Dum and Strick, 2003; Kelly and Strick, 2003). Considering the function of this loop, Ito (1970) suggested that it serves as the internal feedback via the cerebellum toward the primary motor cortex that functions as the controller of voluntary movements (Figure 2.9A). One may suppose that at the beginning of a movement exercise, the primary motor cortex closely refers to the external feedback through sensory systems. As the exercise proceeds, this external feedback is gradually replaced by an internal feedback through the cerebellum, in which an internal model could be formed to simulate the physical properties of the controlled object, that is, a moving arm, leg, or body. Then, the primary motor cortex will execute a precise movement using the internal feedback through the forward model instead of the external feedback from the real control object. In developing a computational theory for the control of a robot arm, Kawato et al. (1987) defined a *forward model*

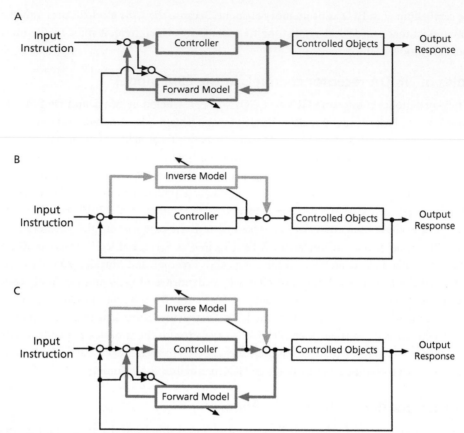

Figure 2.9 Control systems with internal models. (A) Forward model mediating internal feedback. (B) Inverse model mediating feedback-error-dependent learning. (C) Hybrid system with forward and inverse models.
(Honda et al., 2015).

as a representation mimicking the input–output relationship of a controlled object. The forward model represents a description of motion of the body or its various parts in space in terms of position, velocity, acceleration, and direction (termed "kinematics"). Another group expanded the meaning of the forward model in that the cerebellum estimates the current state of the motor system (Miall et al., 2007). To this end, the cerebellum may "state estimate" by collecting sensory information about the last known position of the arm and predict its future responses to the most recent movement commands. One can then plan and control an intended movement accurately.

Another type of internal model, the *inverse model*, represents a reciprocal of the input–output relationship of a controlled object (Figure 2.9B). This concept emerged from Kawato et al.'s (1987) unique idea of the two-degrees-of-freedom adaptive control. In this system, a voluntary movement is controlled by a combination of the primary motor cortex equipped with a classic feedback and a module of the cerebellar circuit (microcomplex,

Ito, 2014), the latter representing an inverse model of the controlled object and acting as a feedforward controller without feedback. Before learning, feedback control by the primary motor cortex is predominant, but as learning proceeds in the cerebellum, feedforward control becomes predominant. Neuronal connections required in incorporating an inverse model for a voluntary movement (Figure 2.9B) have been revealed anatomically or physiologically. Neurons in the supplementary motor cortex and premotor cortex project to both the primary motor cortex (Fang et al., 2005) and cerebellum via the pontine nucleus (Wiesendanger et al., 1979). Furthermore, the outputs of the primary motor cortex and the cerebellar interpositus nucleus converge on some descending tract neurons: for example, rubrospinal tract neurons receive input from the anterior interpositus nucleus (Toyama et al., 1970) and also from the primary motor cortex (Tsukahara and Kosaka, 1968).

The two types of internal model are dedicated to different functions: a forward model predicts for the controller where to move a limb in space (Miall et al., 1993; Wolpert and Miall, 1996; Izawa et al., 2012), whereas an inverse model represents motor command information about how to move the limb (Gomi and Kawato, 1996). Which of the two internal models is operating in the real cerebellum has been a subject of debate (Kobayashi et al., 1998; Winkelman and Frens, 2006; Ebner and Pasalar, 2008; Ebner et al., 2011). However, there is no reason to assume that forward and inverse models should work exclusively; they may work jointly. Honda et al. (2015) proposed a hybrid system of forward and inverse models, which accounts for the prism adaptation of reaching movements in humans (Figure 2.9C). We therefore suggest that both the inverse and forward models play their important respective roles in voluntary movements. Indeed, cerebellar diseases impair inverse and forward models differentially (Hashimoto et al., 2015; Honda et al., 2015).

The control system structure of spinal and brainstem reflexes is identical to that of voluntary movements except that reflexes are driven by peripheral stimuli instead of central instruction signals that drive voluntary movements (see Ito, 2011). The presence of long spinocerebellar communication loops connecting reflex centers with the cerebellum via dorsal and ventral spinocerebellar tracts, and rubrospinal, vestibulospinal, and reticulospinal descending tracts would suggest a forward model. On the other hand, the pathway for the limb withdrawal reflex in response to nociceptive stimuli is connected to the cerebellum in the manner of an inverse model (see Apps and Garwicz, 2005). Whether the two forms of internal model work in combination in some reflexes has yet to be investigated.

Role of the cerebellum in cognition

In Marr's time (i.e., around the 1970s), evidence to suggest that the cerebellum is involved in cognitive functions was scarce. Two decades later, clinical observations revealed that lesions in the cerebellum are often associated with mental disorders with characteristic symptoms, which Schmahmann and Sherman (1998) called mental dysmetria. The role of the cerebellum in language acquisition was also suggested on the basis of the considerable expansion of the most lateral part of the cerebellar hemispheres in humans (Leiner et al., 1993). From the aspect of internal model-assisted control, it is important that a cerebrocerebellar communication loop, which is particularly prominent in humans, connects the cerebellar hemisphere to the prefrontal and temporoparietal association cortices, which constitute the centers of cognitive function (Ramnani, 2006). Recently, much brain imaging data has been accumulated that reveals cerebellar activities associated with certain cognitive tasks, typically the Wisconsin Card Sorting test (Lie et al., 2006; see Passingham, Chapter 1 of this volume). While the question on what mechanisms the cerebellum contributes to cognition was eagerly addressed, Ito (1990, 1993, 2005, 2008) pointed out that there is a formalistic analogy between movements and certain cognitive functions. For example, as we move a limb, we manipulate an idea in our mind. When we practice a movement repeatedly, we become able to conduct it unconsciously. Analogously, we become able to conduct a repeatedly exerted thought unconsciously. This analogy of thought to voluntary motor control is a basis for assuming that the cerebellum contributes to the thought mechanism (Ito, 2006, 2008; Ramnani, 2006). In the thought mechanism, the prefrontal cortex should play the role of a controller, which manipulates a controlled object, such as an image, idea, or concept, represented in the temporoparietal cortex. When an object is repeatedly manipulated in the mind, an internal model of the controlled object will be formed or reformed in the cerebellum. As the object manipulation in mind is further repeated, the internal model will be refined by learning to closely mimic the controlled object. The thought may then proceed implicitly without conscious concern of what the thought is. This view of the cognitive internal model is supported by the presence of a well-developed cerebrocerebellar communication loop in humans connecting the prefrontal cortex to the temporoparietal cortex. Further considering anatomical evidence for large-scale cerebrocerebellar connections, D'Angelo and Casali (2012) proposed that the cerebellum operates as a general-purpose coprocessor, whose effects depend on the specific brain centers to which individual modules are connected.

In cognition, we use language, evaluate, and come to decisions, these being the major components of human intelligence. Brain imaging studies of humans by functional magnetic resonance imaging (fMRI) and positron emission tomography (PET) have demonstrated the involvement of the cerebellum in language. Both the right and left cerebellar hemispheres and cerebellar vermis are activated in language tasks (Ackermann, 2008; Stoodley and Schmahmann, 2010). After learning the relationship between a noun and a verb, subjects can automatically think out a verb for a noun. In this learning, a loop including the right cerebellar hemisphere is mainly related to this language task (Raichle et al., 1994). The right cerebellum might present an internal model for language as working memory for priming effects (Durisko and Fiez, 2010; Marvel and Desmond, 2010). A clear role of the cerebellar in silent numerical counting has recently been reported; that is, greater activation is induced in the right cerebellum in the task of counting forward (from 1 to 30) than in counting backward (from 30 to 1). For counting backward, greater activation was found in the prefrontal cortex, supplementary motor area, and anterior cingulate of both hemispheres (Šveljo et al., 2014).

In common thoughts, however, counterparts of control objects are much more complex. Indeed, there is the term "mental model," which Craik (1943) and Johnson-Laird (1983) defined as a psychological substrate for a mental representation of real or imaginary situations. It is a small-scale model of reality that the mind constructs and uses to reason, underlie explanations, and anticipate a future event. Another term is "schema," which Jean Piaget (1896–1980) defined as being formed in a growing child learning to interpret and understand the surrounding world (Piaget, 1951). Piaget's schema includes both a category of knowledge and the process of obtaining that knowledge. Currently, these two concepts are not mechanistic, and they lack a computational basis. The question on how to apply neural circuit models developed for movements in the physical domain to cognitive function in the psychological domain remains unanswered as yet.

Involvement of the cerebellum in emotion

The cerebellum is connected also to the hypothalamus, the center of emotion and innate behavior (Haines et al., 1984). This connection includes the third type of afferent fiber (Haines and Dietrichs, 1984; King et al., 1992). This third type of afferent fiber characteristically has beaded structures (Figure 2.1), which contain amines or neuropeptides as neurotransmitters or neuromodulators (Schweighofer et al., 2004; Ito, 2009). For example, histamine-containing fibers originate from the tuberomamillary nucleus of the hypothalamus and broadly extend in the cerebellum (King et al., 1992). In contrast, orexin-containing fibers originate solely from the perifornical regions of the hypothalamus and innervate almost exclusively the flocculus, that is, the phylogenetically old part of the cerebellum (Nambu et al., 1999). Beaded fibers containing angiotensin II arise from the paraventricular and supraoptic nuclei of the hypothalamus (Lind et al., 1985) and impinge globally on the cerebellum. Four different amines (serotonin, histamine, acetylcholine, and dopamine) (Schweighofer et al., 2004) and 24 different neuropeptides have so far been located in the cerebellum (Ito, 2009).

Aminergic and peptidergic fibers are distributed broadly in the brainstem, spinal cord, and cerebellum in a characteristically sparse and diffuse manner. For example, through the granular layers, Purkinje cell layers, and molecular layers of the rabbit flocculus, the spatial density of orexinergic fibers is at the maximum 3.33 pieces per mm^2 coronal cross-sectional area of the flocculus (Nisimaru et al., 2013). It appears that, whereas MFs and CFs form neuron-to-neuron-specific connections, aminergic and peptidergic fibers convey information diffusely to determine the general activity or the mode of operation of their target neurons in terms of neuromodulation (Marder and Thirumalai, 2002). Each peptide or amine may assemble a unique set of neuronal circuits through the spinal cord, brainstem, and cerebellum, which jointly express a specific emotion and behavior. A number of neuropeptides and amines of hypothalamic origin may thus provide a selection mechanism for different types of emotion and behavior.

A specific role of orexinergic fibers in rabbits is to mediate the cardiovascular component of defense reactions to harmful stimuli (Nisimaru et al., 2013) and thereby contribute, at least in part, to the expressions of anger and anxiety that lead to emergence of fight and flight behaviors respectively. Another important clue for linking the cerebellum to emotion is the intracerebellar presence of dopaminergic fibers (Giompres and Delis, 2005), which is generally related to emotion.

Perspectives

In Marr's well-known three levels of understanding of a complex information processing machine (Table 2.1; Marr, 1982), the computational theory that determines the goal of the computation is at the first level. At the second level is the question of with what representation and algorithm this computational theory is implemented in the machine. At the third level is the question of how the representation and algorithm are implemented with hardware. To understand the problems regarding the cerebellum, one may ask similar questions in reverse order (Ito, 1984):

(a) how is the cerebellum constructed? (structure);

(b) how does the neuronal circuitry operate? (circuit operation); and

(c) what does the cerebellum do? (functional principle) (Table 2.1).

Over the past four decades, owing to the advancement of a variety of research technologies, an enormous amount of hardware knowledge about the brain has been accumulated (neurons, synapses, genes, connections; e.g., Shepherd and Grillner, 2010). Theoretical models such as the Marr–Albus model of the cerebellar cortex, an adaptive filter model, and an LSM model are advancements at the representation and algorithm level (Yamazaki and Tanaka, 2007a; Casellato et al., 2014; Casellato et al., 2015). The idea of internal models now applies broadly to problems at the level of computational principle. Owing to Marr's initiative, the cerebellum is the best analyzed region of the brain at all three levels (see also Dean and Porril, Chapter 4 of this volume).

So far, research of the cerebellum has yielded three types of computational model with unique representations and algorithms: the simple perceptron, LSM, and adaptive filter. The overall purposes of operation of these cerebellar neuronal machine models have been defined in terms of adaptive control of reflexes and internal model-assisted control of voluntary limb movements. Figuratively speaking, the cerebellum may act as an all-purpose simulator. However, the roles of the cerebellum in cognition have only been conceptually defined; it is not yet possible to reproduce cognitive functions using computational models. Presently, no distinct difference is found at the hardware level between the cerebellar areas related to movement and cognition. A crucial element in cognition might still be missing from the hardware of the cerebellum. However, it is also possible that the cerebellum utilizes similar local circuits for both movement and cognition. Whether the cerebellum serves movements or cognition might depend on the overall system structures involving the cerebral association cortex.

How the brain shifts from the physical domain for movements to the psychological domain for cognition is a question raised in the effort to develop an artificial intelligence that could reproduce human capabilities of using language and forming abstraction and concepts (McCarthy et al., 1955). Despite the great efforts so far devoted to it, this attempt

Table 2.1 Marr's three levels of understanding and their applications to the cerebellum

	1st level	2nd level	3rd level
Levels of understanding complex information processing machine (from Marr, 1982)	**Computational theory** What is the goal of computation, why is it appropriate, and what is the logic of the strategy by which it can be carried out?	**Representation and algorithm** How can this computational theory be implemented? In particular, what is the representation for the input and output, and what is the algorithm for the transformation?	**Hardware implementation** How can the representation and algorithm be realized physically?
	Level c	Level b	Level a
Levels of questions to be asked to the cerebellum (modified from Ito, 1984)	**Functional principle** What does the cerebellum or a part of the cerebellum do?	**Circuitry operation** How does the neuronal circuitry of the cerebellum operate?	**Structure** How is the cerebellum constructed?
Examples in the cerebellum	Internal models that assist motor, sensory, cognitive, and emotional systems	Marr–Albus model, adaptive filter model, LSM	Neurons, synapses, genes, neuronal circuits

Data from Marr (1982) and Ito (1984).

has not been successful. Note, however, that the human brain does express and process both movements and cognition. We still do not know yet how ideas, abstraction, or concepts are expressed and processed in neuronal circuits. The gap that we face in studies of the cerebellum appears to imply one of the most profound challenges in science.

If we gain sufficient knowledge at all three levels of understanding, a neuronal circuit can be reproduced by manufactured hardware, which will closely mimic the behavior of real brain tissues. One may hope that this approach, in the long run, leads us to the development of an artificial brain. Nowadays, technology has advanced to the extent of a brain chip consisting of 4096 neurosynaptic cores, each core including 5.4 billion transistors, 1 million neurons, and 256 million synapses interconnected with each other via an intrachip network (Merolla et al., 2014). This brain chip exhibits a superb pattern recognition capability. Moreover, the palm-sized graphical processing unit can achieve high-performance computing and has successfully controlled a robotic arm with real-time LSM (Yamazaki and Igarashi, 2013). At the level of principle, whether the brain contains a Turing machine mechanism remains an as-yet-unanswered critical question in science. If not, what type of new computing principle could we find in the brain? The cerebellum should be at the highest level of brain hierarchy where such a final question could be addressed.

References

Ackermann H. (2008). Cerebellar contributions to speech production and speech perception: psycholinguistic and neurobiological perspectives. Trends Neurosci. **31**:265–272.

Albus JS. (1971). A theory of cerebellar function. Math Biosci. **10**:25–61.

Anzai M, Kitazawa H, Nagao S. (2010). Effects of reversible pharmacological shutdown of cerebellar flocculus on the memory of long-term horizontal vestibulo-ocular reflex adaptation in monkeys. Neuroscience Res. **68**:191–198.

Anzai M, Nagao S. (2014). Motor learning in common marmosets: Vestibulo-ocular reflex adaptation and its sensitivity to inhibitors of Purkinje cell long-term depression. Neuroscience Res. **83**:33–42.

Apps R, Garwicz M. (2005). Anatomical and physiological foundations of cerebellar information processing. Nat Rev Neurosci. **6**:297–311.

Armano S, Rossi P, Taglietti V, D'Angelo E. (2000). Long-term potentiation of intrinsic excitability at the mossy fiber-granule cell synapse of rat cerebellum. J Neurosci. **20**:5208–5216.

Bliss TV, Lomo T. (1973). Long-lasting potentiation of synaptic transmission in the dentate area of the anaesthetized rabbit following stimulation of the perforant path. J Physiol. **232**:331–356.

Brindley G. (1964). The use made by the cerebellum of the information that it receives from sense organs. IBRO Bull. **3**:80.

Brunel N, Hakim V, Isope P, Nadal J-P, Barbour B. (2004). Optimal information storage and the distribution of synaptic weights: perceptron versus Purkinje cell. Neuron. **43**:745–757.

Buonomano DV, Mauk MD. (1994). Neural network model of the cerebellum: temporal discrimination and the timing of motor responses. Neural Comput. **6**:38–55.

Casellato C, Antonietti A, Garrido JA, Carrillo RR, Luque NR, Ros E, et al. (2014). Adaptive robotic control driven by a versatile spiking cerebellar network. PloS ONE **9**:e112265.

Casellato C, Antonietti A, Garrido JA, Ferrigno G, D'Angelo E, Pedrocchi A. (2015). Distributed cerebellar plasticity implements generalized multiple-scale memory components in real-robot sensorimotor tasks. Front Comput Neurosci. **9**:24.

Courtemanche R, Chabaud P, Lamarre Y. (2009). Synchronization in primate cerebellar granule cell layer local field potentials: basic anisotropy and dynamic changes during active expectancy. Front Cell Neurosci. 3:6.

Craik H. (1943). The Nature of Explanation. Cambridge: Cambridge University Press.

D'Angelo E. (2014). The organization of plasticity in the cerebellar cortex: from synapses to control. Prog Brain Res. 210:31–58.

D'Angelo E, Casali S. (2012). Seeking a unified framework for cerebellar function and dysfunction: from circuit operations to cognition. Front Neural Circuits. 6:116.

D'Angelo E, Rossi P, Armano S, Taglietti V. (1999). Evidence for NMDA and mGlu receptor-dependent long-term potentiation of mossy fiber-granule cell transmission in rat cerebellum. J Neurophysiol. 81:277–287.

De Schutter E, Bower JM (1994a) An active membrane model of the cerebellar Purkinje cell II. Simulation of synaptic responses. J Neurophysiol. 71:401–419.

De Schutter E, Bower JM (1994b) An active membrane model of the cerebellar Purkinje cell. I. Simulation of current clamps in slice. J Neurophysiol. 71:375–400.

Dean P, Porrill J, Ekerot CF, Jörntell H. (2010). The cerebellar microcircuit as an adaptive filter: experimental and computational evidence. Nat Rev Neurosci. 11:30–43.

Dean P, Porrill J, Stone JV. (2002). Decorrelation control by the cerebellum achieves oculomotor plant compensation in simulated vestibulo-ocular reflex. Proc Biol Sci. 269:1895–1904.

Doi T, Kuroda S, Michikawa T, Kawato M. (2005). Inositol 1,4,5-trisphosphate-dependent Ca^{2+} threshold dynamics detect spike timing in cerebellar Purkinje cells. J Neurosci. 25:950–961.

Doya K. (1999). What are the computations of the cerebellum, the basal ganglia and the cerebral cortex? Neural Netw. 12:961–974.

Doya K. (2000). Complementary roles of basal ganglia and cerebellum in learning and motor control. Curr Opin Neurobiol. 10:732–739.

Dugué GP, Dumoulin A, Triller A, Dieudonne S. (2005). Target-dependent use of co-released inhibitory transmitters at central synapses. J Neurosci. 25:6490–6498.

Dum RP, Strick PL. (2003). An unfolded map of the cerebellar dentate nucleus and its projections to the cerebral cortex. J Neurophysiol. 89:634–639.

Durisko C, Fiez JA. (2010). Functional activation in the cerebellum during working memory and simple speech tasks. Cortex. 46:896–906.

Ebner TJ, Hewitt AL, Popa LS. (2011). What features of limb movements are encoded in the discharge of cerebellar neurons? Cerebellum. 10:683–693.

Ebner TJ, Pasalar S. (2008). Cerebellum predicts the future motor state. Cerebellum. 7:583–588.

Eccles J, Ito M, Szentagothai J. (1967). The Cerebellum as a Neuronal Machine. Berlin: Springer-Verlag.

Ekerot C-F, Kano M. (1985). Long-term depression of parallel fibre synapses following stimulation of climbing fibres. Brain Res. 342:357–360.

Ekerot CF, Jörntell H. (2003). Parallel fiber receptive fields: a key to understanding cerebellar operation and learning. Cerebellum. 2:101–109.

Fang PC, Stepniewska I, Kaas JH. (2005). Ipsilateral cortical connections of motor, premotor, frontal eye, and posterior parietal fields in a prosimian primate, *Otolemur garnetti*. J Comp Neurol. 490:305–333.

Freeman JH, Jr., Muckler AS. (2003). Developmental changes in eyeblink conditioning and neuronal activity in the pontine nuclei. Learn Mem. 10:337–345.

Fujita M. (1982). Adaptive filter model of the cerebellum. Biol Cybernet. 45:195–206.

Gao Z, van Beugen BJ, De Zeeuw CI. (2012). Distributed synergistic plasticity and cerebellar learning. Nat Rev Neurosci. 13:619–635.

Garrido JA, Luque NR, D'Angelo E, Ros E. (2013). Distributed cerebellar plasticity implements adaptable gain control in a manipulation task: a closed-loop robotic simulation. Front Neural Circuits. **7**:159.

Giompres P, Delis F. (2005). Dopamine transporters in the cerebellum of mutant mice. Cerebellum. **4**:105–111.

Gomi H, Kawato M. (1996). Equilibrium-point control hypothesis examined by measured arm stiffness during multijoint movement. Science. **272**:117–120.

Haines D, Dietrichs E. (1984). An HRP study of hypothalamo-cerebellar and cerebello-hypothalamic connections in squirrel monkey (*Saimiri sciureus*). J Comp Neurol. **229**:559–575.

Haines D, Dietrichs E, Sowa T. (1984). Hypothalamo-cerebellar and cerebello-hypothalamic pathways: a review and hypothesis concerning cerebellar circuits which may influence autonomic centers and affective behavior (part 2 of 2). Brain Behav Evol. **24**:210–220.

Hansel C, Linden DJ, D'Angelo E. (2001). Beyond parallel fiber LTD: the diversity of synaptic and non-synaptic plasticity in the cerebellum. Nat Neurosci. **4**:467–475.

Hartmann MJ, Bower JM. (1998). Oscillatory activity in the cerebellar hemispheres of unrestrained rats. J Neurophysiol. **80**:1598–1604.

Hashimoto Y, Honda T, Matsumura K, Nakao M, Soga K, Katano K, et al. (2015). Quantitative evaluation of human cerebellum-dependent motor learning through prism adaptation of hand-reaching movement. PloS ONE. **10**:e0119376.

Hebb DO. (1949). The Organization of Behavior: A Neuropsychological Theory. New York: Wiley.

Hesslow G, Jirenhed D-A, Rasmussen A, Johansson F. (2013). Classical conditioning of motor responses: what is the learning mechanism? Neural Netw. **47**:81–87.

Hirano T, Kawaguchi SY. (2014). Regulation and functional roles of rebound potentiation at cerebellar stellate cell-Purkinje cell synapses. Front Cell Neurosci. **8**:42.

Honda T, Matsumura K, Hashimoto Y, Ishikawa K, Mizusawa H, Nagao S, Ito M. (2015). Dynamics of cerebellar internal models during prism adaptation of human hand-reaching task. Neuroscience 2015: Japan Neuroscience Society, 38th Annual Meeting, Kobe, Japan.

Honda T, Yamazaki T, Tanaka S, Nagao S, Nishino T. (2011). Stimulus-dependent state transition between synchronized oscillation and randomly repetitive burst in a model cerebellar granular layer. PLoS Comput Biol. **7**:e1002087.

Ichise T, Kano M, Hashimoto K, Yanagihara D, Nakao K, Shigemoto R, Katsuki M, Aiba A. (2000). mGluR1 in cerebellar Purkinje cells essential for long-term depression, synapse elimination, and motor coordination. Science. **288**:1832–1835.

Isope P, Barbour B. (2002). Properties of unitary granule cell→Purkinje cell synapses in adult rat cerebellar slices. J Neurosci. **22**:9668–9678.

Ito M. (1970). Neurophysiological aspects of the cerebellar motor control system. Int J Neurol. **7**:162–176.

Ito M. (1972). Neural design of the cerebellar motor control system. Brain Res. **40**:81–84.

Ito M. (1982). Cerebellar control of the vestibulo-ocular reflex—around the flocculus hypothesis. Annu Rev Neurosci. **5**:275–297.

Ito M. (1984). The Cerebellum and Neural Control. New York: Raven Press.

Ito M. (1989). Long-term depression. Annu Rev Neurosci. **12**:85–102.

Ito M. (1990). Neural control as a major aspect of high-order brain function. In: The Principles of Design and Operation of the Brain, pp. 281–301. Berlin: Springer.

Ito M. (1993). Movement and thought: identical control mechanisms by the cerebellum. Trends Neurosci. **16**:448–450; discussion 453–444.

Ito M. (2000). Mechanisms of motor learning in the cerebellum. Brain Res. **886**:237–245.

Ito M. (2005). Bases and implications of learning in the cerebellum—adaptive control and internal model mechanism. Prog Brain Res. **148**:95–109.

Ito M. (2006). Cerebellar circuitry as a neuronal machine. Prog Neurobiol. **78**:272–303.

Ito M. (2008). Control of mental activities by internal models in the cerebellum. Nat Rev Neurosci. **9**:304–313.

Ito M. (2009). Functional roles of neuropeptides in cerebellar circuits. Neuroscience. **162**:666–672.

Ito M. (2011). The Cerebellum: Brain for an Implicit Self. Upper Saddle River, NJ: FT Press.

Ito M. (2013). Error detection and representation in the olivo-cerebellar system. Front Neural Circuits. **7**:1.

Ito M. (2014). Cerebellar microcircuitry? In: Reference Module in Biomedical Sciences, Elsevier, http://dx.doi.org/10.1016/B978-0-12-801238-3.04544-X. (http://www.sciencedirect.com/science/article/pii/B978012801238304544X)

Ito M, Kano M. (1982). Long-lasting depression of parallel fiber-Purkinje cell transmission induced by conjunctive stimulation of parallel fibers and climbing fibers in the cerebellar cortex. Neurosci Lett. **33**:253–258.

Ito M, Sakurai M, Tongroach P. (1982). Climbing fibre induced depression of both mossy fibre responsiveness and glutamate sensitivity of cerebellar Purkinje cells. J Physiol. **324**:113–134.

Ito M, Yamaguchi K, Nagao S, Yamazaki T. (2014). Long-term depression as a model of cerebellar plasticity. Prog Brain Res. **210**:1–30.

Izawa J, Criscimagna-Hemminger SE, Shadmehr R. (2012). Cerebellar contributions to reach adaptation and learning sensory consequences of action. J Neurosci. **32**:4230–4239.

Jirenhed D-A, Hesslow G (2011b) Time course of classically conditioned Purkinje cell response is determined by initial part of conditioned stimulus. J Neurosci. **31**:9070–9074.

Jirenhed DA, Hesslow G (2011a) Learning stimulus intervals—adaptive timing of conditioned purkinje cell responses. Cerebellum **10**:523–535.

Johnson-Laird P. (1983). Mental Models: Towards a Cognitive Science of Language, Inference, and Conciousness. Cambridge: Cambridge University Press.

Jörntell H, Ekerot CF. (2002). Reciprocal bidirectional plasticity of parallel fiber receptive fields in cerebellar Purkinje cells and their afferent interneurons. Neuron. **34**:797–806.

Jörntell H, Ekerot CF. (2003). Receptive field plasticity profoundly alters the cutaneous parallel fiber synaptic input to cerebellar interneurons in vivo. J Neurosci. **23**:9620–9631.

Kakegawa W, Mitakidis N, Miura E, Abe M, Matsuda K, Takeo YH, et al. (2015). Anterograde C1ql1 signaling is required in order to determine and maintain a single-winner climbing fiber in the mouse cerebellum. Neuron. **85**:316–329.

Kakegawa W, Miyazaki T, Kohda K, Matsuda K, Emi K, Motohashi J, et al. (2009). The N-terminal domain of GluD2 (GluRdelta2) recruits presynaptic terminals and regulates synaptogenesis in the cerebellum in vivo. J Neurosci. **29**:5738–5748.

Kakegawa W, Miyoshi Y, Hamase K, Matsuda S, Matsuda K, Kohda K, et al. (2011). D-serine regulates cerebellar LTD and motor coordination through the delta2 glutamate receptor. Nat Neurosci. **14**:603–611.

Kano M, Rexhausen U, Dreessen J, Konnerth A. (1992). Synaptic excitation produces a long-lasting rebound potentiation of inhibitory synaptic signals in cerebellar Purkinje cells. Nature. **356**:601–604.

Kassardjian CD, Tan Y-F, Chung J-YJ, Heskin R, Peterson MJ, Broussard DM. (2005). The site of a motor memory shifts with consolidation. J Neurosci. **25**:7979–7985.

Kawato M, Furukawa K, Suzuki R. (1987). A hierarchical neural-network model for control and learning of voluntary movement. Biol Cybernet. **57**:169–185.

Kelly RM, Strick PL. (2003). Cerebellar loops with motor cortex and prefrontal cortex of a nonhuman primate. J Neurosci. **23**:8432–8444.

King JS, Cummings SL, Bishop GA. (1992). Peptides in cerebellar circuits. Prog Neurobiol. **39**:423–442.

Kobayashi Y, Kawano K, Takemura A, Inoue Y, Kitama T, Gomi H, Kawato M. (1998). Temporal firing patterns of Purkinje cells in the cerebellar ventral paraflocculus during ocular following responses in monkeys II. Complex spikes. J Neurophysiol. **80**:832–848.

Le TD, Shirai Y, Okamoto T, Tatsukawa T, Nagao S, Shimizu T, Ito M. (2010). Lipid signaling in cytosolic phospholipase A2α–cyclooxygenase-2 cascade mediates cerebellar long-term depression and motor learning. Proc Natl Acad Sci U S A. **107**:3198–3203.

Leiner HC, Leiner AL, Dow RS. (1993). Cognitive and language functions of the human cerebellum. Trends Neurosci. **16**:444–447.

Lev-Ram V, Wong ST, Storm DR, Tsien RY. (2002). A new form of cerebellar long-term potentiation is postsynaptic and depends on nitric oxide but not cAMP. Proc Natl Acad Sci U S A. **99**:8389–8393.

Lie CH, Specht K, Marshall JC, Fink GR. (2006). Using fMRI to decompose the neural processes underlying the Wisconsin Card Sorting Test. NeuroImage. **30**:1038–1049.

Lind RW, Swanson LW, Ganten D. (1985). Organization of angiotensin II immunoreactive cells and fibers in the rat central nervous system. An immunohistochemical study. Neuroendocrinology. **40**:2–24.

Luque NR, Garrido JA, Carrillo RR, D'Angelo E, Ros E. (2014). Fast convergence of learning requires plasticity between inferior olive and deep cerebellar nuclei in a manipulation task: a closed-loop robotic simulation. Front Comput Neurosci. **8**:97.

Maass W, Natschläger T, Markram H. (2002). Real-time computing without stable states: A new framework for neural computation based on perturbations. Neural Comput. **14**:2531–2560.

Maex R, De Schutter E. (1998). Synchronization of golgi and granule cell firing in a detailed network model of the cerebellar granule cell layer. J Neurophysiol. **80**:2521–2537.

Mapelli J, Gandolfi D, D'Angelo E. (2010). Combinatorial responses controlled by synaptic inhibition in the cerebellum granular layer. J Neurophysiol. **103**:250–261.

Mapelli L, Pagani M, Garrido JA, D'Angelo E. (2015). Integrated plasticity at inhibitory and excitatory synapses in the cerebellar circuit. Front Cell Neurosci. **9**:169.

Marder E, Thirumalai V. (2002). Cellular, synaptic and network effects of neuromodulation. Neural Netw. **15**:479–493.

Marr D. (1969). A theory of cerebellar cortex. J Physiol. **202**:437–470.

Marr D. (1982). Vision. Cambridge, MA: MIT Press.

Marvel CL, Desmond JE. (2010). Functional topography of the cerebellum in verbal working memory. Neuropsychol Rev. **20**:271–279.

Masoli S, Solinas S, D'Angelo E. (2015). Action potential processing in a detailed Purkinje cell model reveals a critical role for axonal compartmentalization. Front Cell Neurosci. **9**:47.

McCarthy J, Minsky ML, Rochester N, Shannon CE. (1955). A proposal for the Dartmouth Summer Research Project on artificial intelligence. http://www-formal.stanford.edu/jmc/history/dartmouth/dartmouth.html.

McElvain LE, Bagnall MW, Sakatos A, du Lac S. (2010). Bidirectional plasticity gated by hyperpolarization controls the gain of postsynaptic firing responses at central vestibular nerve synapses. Neuron. **68**:763–775.

Medina JF, Garcia KS, Nores WL, Taylor NM, Mauk MD. (2000). Timing mechanisms in the cerebellum: testing predictions of a large-scale computer simulation. J Neurosci. **20**:5516–5525.

Medina JF, Mauk MD. (1999). Simulations of cerebellar motor learning: computational analysis of plasticity at the mossy fiber to deep nucleus synapse. J Neurosci. **19**:7140–7151.

Merolla PA, Arthur JV, Alvarez-Icaza R, Cassidy AS, Sawada J, Akopyan F, et al. (2014). A million spiking-neuron integrated circuit with a scalable communication network and interface. Science. 345:668–673.

Miall RC, Christensen LO, Cain O, Stanley J. (2007). Disruption of state estimation in the human lateral cerebellum. PLoS Biol. 5:e316.

Miall RC, Weir DJ, Wolpert DM, Stein JF. (1993). Is the cerebellum a Smith predictor? J Mot Behav. 25:203–216.

Miles FA, Lisberger SG. (1981). Plasticity in the vestibulo-ocular reflex: a new hypothesis. Annu Rev Neurosci. 4:273–299.

Minsky M, Papert S. (1969). Perceptrons: An Introduction to Computational Geometry. Cambridge, MA: MIT Press.

Minsky M, Papert S. (1988). Perceptrons: An Introduction to Computational Geometry (expanded edition). Cambridge, MA: MIT Press.

Nambu T, Sakurai T, Mizukami K, Hosoya Y, Yanagisawa M, Goto K. (1999). Distribution of orexin neurons in the adult rat brain. Brain Res. 827:243–260.

Nisimaru N, Mittal C, Shirai Y, Sooksawate T, Anandaraj P, Hashikawa T, et al. (2013). Orexin-neuromodulated cerebellar circuit controls redistribution of arterial blood flows for defense behavior in rabbits. Proc Natl Acad Sci U S A. 110:14124–14131.

Okamoto T, Endo S, Shirao T, Nagao S. (2011). Role of cerebellar cortical protein synthesis in transfer of memory trace of cerebellum-dependent motor learning. J Neurosci. 31:8958–8966.

Piaget J. (1951). Principal factors determining intellectual evolution from childhood to adult life. In: Organization and pathology of thought, pp. 154–175. New York: Columbia University Press.

Pellerin JP, Lamarre Y. (1997). Local field potential oscillations in primate cerebellar cortex during voluntary movement. J Neurophysiol. 78:3502–3507.

Pellionisz A, Szentagothai J. (1973). Dynamic single unit simulation of a realistic cerebellar network model. Brain Res. 49:83–99.

Piaget J (1951). Principal factors idetermining intellectual evolution from childhood to adult life.

Pugh JR, Raman IM. (2006). Potentiation of mossy fiber EPSCs in the cerebellar nuclei by NMDA receptor activation followed by postinhibitory rebound current. Neuron. 51:113–123.

Raichle ME, Fiez JA, Videen TO, MacLeod A-MK, Pardo JV, et al. (1994). Practice-related changes in human brain functional anatomy during nonmotor learning. Cereb Cortex. 4:8–26.

Ramnani N. (2006). The primate cortico-cerebellar system: anatomy and function. Nat Rev Neurosci. 7:511–522.

Rancillac A, Crépel F. (2004). Synapses between parallel fibres and stellate cells express long-term changes in synaptic efficacy in rat cerebellum. J Physiol. 554:707–720.

Rosenblatt F. (1958). The perceptron: a probabilistic model for information storage and organization in the brain. Psychol Rev. 65:386.

Rosenblatt F. (1962). Principles of Neurodynamics: Perceptrons and the Theory of Brain Mechanisms. Washington, DC: Spartan.

Sakurai M. (1987). Synaptic modification of parallel fibre-Purkinje cell transmission in in vitro guinea-pig cerebellar slices. J Physiol. 394:463–480.

Schmahmann JD, Sherman JC. (1998). The cerebellar cognitive affective syndrome. Brain. 121 (Pt 4):561–579.

Schonewille M, Gao Z, Boele HJ, Veloz MF, Amerika WE, Simek AA, et al. (2011). Reevaluating the role of LTD in cerebellar motor learning. Neuron. 70:43–50.

Schweighofer N, Doya K, Kuroda S. (2004). Cerebellar aminergic neuromodulation: towards a functional understanding. Brain Res Rev. **44**:103–116.

Shepherd G, Grillner S. (2010). Handbook of Brain Microcircuits. Oxford: Oxford University Press.

Shibuki K, Okada D. (1992). Cerebellar long-term potentiation under suppressed postsynaptic Ca^{2+} activity. Neuroreport. **3**:231–234.

Shutoh F, Ohki M, Kitazawa H, Itohara S, Nagao S. (2006). Memory trace of motor learning shifts transsynaptically from cerebellar cortex to nuclei for consolidation. Neuroscience. **139**:767–777.

Solinas S, Nieus T, D'Angelo E. (2010). A realistic large-scale model of the cerebellar granular layer predicts circuit spatio-temporal filtering properties. Front Cell Neurosci. **4**:12.

Steinberg JP, Huganir RL, Linden DJ. (2004). N-ethylmaleimide-sensitive factor is required for the synaptic incorporation and removal of AMPA receptors during cerebellar long-term depression. Proc Natl Acad Sci U S A. **101**:18212–18216.

Steuber V, Mittmann W, Hoebeek FE, Silver RA, De Zeeuw CI, Häusser M, De Schutter E. (2007). Cerebellar LTD and pattern recognition by Purkinje cells. Neuron. **54**:121–136.

Stoodley CJ, Schmahmann JD. (2010). Evidence for topographic organization in the cerebellum of motor control versus cognitive and affective processing. Cortex. **46**:831–844.

Šveljo O, Ćulić M, Koprivšek K, Lučić M. (2014). The functional neuroimaging evidence of cerebellar involvement in the simple cognitive task. Brain Imaging Behav. **8**:480–486.

Thompson RF, Steinmetz JE. (2009). The role of the cerebellum in classical conditioning of discrete behavioral responses. Neuroscience. **162**:732–755.

Toyama K, Tsukahara N, Kosaka K, Matsunami K. (1970). Synaptic excitation of red nucleus neurones by fibres from interpositus nucleus. Exp Brain Res. **11**:187–198.

Tsukahara N, Kosaka K. (1968). The mode of cerebral excitation of red nucleus neurons. Exp Brain Res. **5**:102–117.

Tyrrell T, Willshaw D. (1992). Cerebellar cortex: its simulation and the relevance of Marr's theory. Philos Trans R Soc Lond B Biol Sci. **336**:239–257.

Walter JT, Khodakhah K. (2006). The linear computational algorithm of cerebellar Purkinje cells. J Neurosci. **26**:12861–12872.

Walter JT, Khodakhah K. (2009). The advantages of linear information processing for cerebellar computation. Proc Natl Acad Sci U S A. **106**:4471–4476.

Wang D, Song C, Barabasi AL. (2013). Quantifying long-term scientific impact. Science. **342**:127–132.

Wang SS, Denk W, Hausser M. (2000). Coincidence detection in single dendritic spines mediated by calcium release. Nat Neurosci. **3**:1266–1273.

Wang W, Nakadate K, Masugi-Tokita M, Shutoh F, Aziz W, Tarusawa E, et al. (2014). Distinct cerebellar engrams in short-term and long-term motor learning. Proc Natl Acad Sci U S A **111**:E188–193.

Welsh JP, Yamaguchi H, Zeng XH, Kojo M, Nakada Y, Takagi A, et al. (2005). Normal motor learning during pharmacological prevention of Purkinje cell long-term depression. Proc Natl Acad Sci U S A. **102**:17166–17171.

Wiesendanger R, Wiesendanger M, Ruegg DG. (1979). An anatomical investigation of the corticopontaine projection in the primate (*Macaca fascicularis* and *Saimiri sciureus*)—II. The projection from frontal and parental association areas. Neuroscience. **4**:747–765.

Winkelman B, Frens M. (2006). Motor coding in floccular climbing fibers. J Neurophysiol. **95**:2342–2351.

Wolpert DM, Miall RC. (1996). Forward models for physiological motor control. Neural Netw. **9**:1265–1279.

Yamaguchi K, Itohara S, Ito M. Reassessment of long-term depression in cerebellar Purkinje cells in mice carrying mutated GluA2 - C terminus. Proc Natl Acad Sci U S A. In press.

Yamazaki T, Igarashi J. (2013). Realtime cerebellum: a large-scale spiking network model of the cerebellum that runs in realtime using a graphics processing unit. Neural Netw. **47**:103–111.

Yamazaki T, Nagao S. (2012). A computational mechanism for unified gain and timing control in the cerebellum. PloS ONE. **7**:e33319.

Yamazaki T, Nagao S, Lennon W, Tanaka S. (2015). Modeling memory consolidation during posttraining periods in cerebellovestibular learning. Proc Natl Acad Sci U S A. **112**:3541–3546.

Yamazaki T, Tanaka S. (2005). Neural modeling of an internal clock. Neural Comput. **17**:1032–1058.

Yamazaki T, Tanaka S. (2007a). The cerebellum as a liquid state machine. Neural Netw. **20**:290–297.

Yamazaki T, Tanaka S. (2007b). A spiking network model for passage-of-time representation in the cerebellum. Eur J Neurosci. **26**:2279–2292.

Yeo CH, Hesslow G. (1998). Cerebellum and conditioned reflexes. Trends Cogn Sci. **2**:322–330.

Yuzaki M. (2013). Cerebellar LTD vs. motor learning-lessons learned from studying GluD2. Neural Netw. **47**:36–41.

Zhang W, Linden DJ. (2006). Long-term depression at the mossy fiber–deep cerebellar nucleus synapse. J Neurosci. **26**:6935–6944.

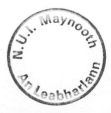

Chapter 3

Challenging Marr's theory of the cerebellum

Egidio D'Angelo

Introduction to motor learning theory

There have been successive attempts to understand the relationships between the structure, function, and dynamics in neuronal circuits (Arbib et al., 1998) in the hope of explaining behavior. At different times these attempts have been based on the available experimental data and conceptual tools and have been synthesized into various theories and models. One of the most famous is Marr's theory of the cerebellum, the so-called motor learning theory (MLT; Marr, 1969), which was developed in the late 1960s and has since then dominated the view of how the cerebellum might function. To be fair we must say that the MLT was extended by Albus two years later (Albus, 1971) and then further developed by Ito in the subsequent decades (Ito, 1972; Ito, 1984; Ito, 1993, 2006, 2008). Thus, it is appropriate to consider it as the Marr–Albus–Ito theory. The MLT was based purely on statistical connectivity rules, so that, unavoidably, it did not take into account the myriad biological parameters that are now considered critical to guarantee cerebellar network functioning. Therefore, over the years Marr's theory has been repeatedly challenged by new experimental findings and concepts. In this chapter, I analyze the major aspects of the MLT, how it has been challenged experimentally, and how it has contributed to our understanding of the structure–function relationship of the cerebellar circuit and the adaptive behaviors that are dependent on the cerebellum.

The foundations of Marr's theory of cerebellum

The MLT was based on two series of anatomical observations: the number of neurons of a given species and the divergence/convergence ratios between these neurons. In addition, the excitatory or inhibitory nature of neuronal connections was known, largely based on the work of Eccles and collaborators (summarized in Eccles et al. (1967)). This made it possible to set up a statistical model of connectivity and to draw a general picture of the presumed role of neurons in the circuit. A critical element in the theory was that the weight of specific parallel fiber–Purkinje cell connections could be tuned depending on error signals coming from the inferior olive through the climbing fibers.

In the MLT, the granular layer performed an operation of expansion recoding of contextual information and the molecular layer an operation of learning of this information depending on climbing fiber activity. As a whole, the cerebellar cortex was viewed as a perceptron-like structure, with Purkinje cells operating like integrators and regulating the output through the deep cerebellar nuclei. The sign of learning was predicted to be long-term potentiation (LTP), although in the Albus version this was converted into long-term depression (LTD).

The MLT was attractive because the cerebellum, embedded in the sensorimotor control system, could exploit the massive mossy fiber input to extract the contextual information it needs to produce accurate movements from high-level motor commands.

> It is reasonably certain that patterns of activity on mossy fibers represent to the cerebellum the position, velocity, tension, and so on of the muscles, tendons, and joints. This is feedback information that is required to control precise or sequential movements, or both. This information must modulate signals to the muscles to achieve precise movement under varying load conditions. (Albus, 1971, p.59)

Moreover, if the teaching signal conveyed through climbing fibers was a motor error, then the cerebellum could implement motor adaptation depending on the precision of movement execution. Recast in modern terms, the MLT predicts that the cerebellum could implement the long-sought forward controller operation needed to regulate movement in a predictive manner. The MLT has been later generalized from motor execution to motor planning and cognitive control (Ito, 1993, 2008), implying that the cerebellum could play a role in higher brain functions.

The MLT principles have been included into models of signal processing (e.g., Tyrrell and Willshaw, (1992)). In the Adaptive Filter Model (AFM) (Fujita, 1982), the consequences of MLT have been developed in mathematical form (Dean and Porrill, 2010, 2011; Dean et al., 2010). The MLT principles have also been implemented in robotic models (Kawato and Gomi, 1992; Schweighofer et al., 1998a, 1998b; Wolpert et al., 1998; Imamizu et al., 2000; Kawato et al., 2003; Imamizu and Kawato, 2009, 2012; Kawato et al., 2011). These illustrate the variety of ways in which the MLT scheme might be used in adaptive control. The evolution of these concepts is explained in the following sections of this chapter.

Critical experimental evidence from cellular neurophysiology

Recent experimental studies in cellular neurophysiology have provided results which have confronted the MLT, since they could either provide proofs in favor or undermine the foundations of the theory itself. The most critical advances have been done in three fields—neuronal dynamics, local network connectivity, and synaptic plasticity. These provide new clues on microcircuit functions and raise specific issues for the Marr theory that can be summarized as follows:

◆ The cerebellar granular layer does not simply perform pattern discrimination (see Chapter 2), expansion recoding (see Chapter 4) and gain regulation of mossy fiber inputs.

- There are different coding schemes: spike-timing versus spike-rate coding.
- There are microcircuit structures that go beyond simple statistical rules.
- The olivo-cerebellar loop performs complex timing operations.
- The Purkinje cell and other cerebellar neurons are not simple linear integrators.
- Learning in the circuit is not solely related to parallel fiber LTD under climbing fiber control.
- Oscillation and resonance, together with nonlinear neuronal and synaptic time-dependent properties, could design dynamic spatiotemporal geometries in the circuit.

The extended function of the granular layer

Marr noticed that, since granule cells are much more numerous than mossy fibers, incoming signals should diverge over many more lines than in the input, allowing decorrelation of common components. The main role envisaged by Marr for the Golgi cells was that of controlling the transmission gain along these lines. There is now evidence that the cerebellar granular layer does not simply perform a combinatorial decorrelation of the inputs but rather it performs complex nonlinear spatiotemporal transformations under the guidance of local synaptic plasticity.

The mossy fibers were shown to activate independent synapses on granule cell dendrites (D'Angelo et al., 1995) and this was also subsequently shown for Golgi cell inhibitory synapses (Mapelli et al., 2009) providing evidence in favor of the decorrelation hypothesis. Moreover, the convergence/divergence ratio at the mossy fiber–granule cell relay was shown to enable efficient lossless sparse encoding (Billings et al., 2014). These concepts are consistent with MLT predictions. Nonetheless, at least 50% of the information carried through the mossy fiber–granule cell relay is carried by first-spike timing and the rest by as few as another 1–3 spikes (Arleo et al., 2010). Other experiments have shown that several forms of plasticity can change transmission at the mossy fiber–granule cell relay (D'Angelo et al., 1999; Armano et al., 2000; Nieus et al., 2006). Therefore, signal transfer through the granular layer is probably only partly explained by the anatomical circuit arrangement and can be modified by intrinsic neuronal responsiveness and synaptic plasticity (see "Numerous forms of synaptic plasticity in addition to parallel fiber LTD").

A tonic component of synaptic inhibition in the cerebellar glomerulus was shown to regulate mossy fiber–granule cell gain (Mitchell and Silver, 2003). This result attracted considerable interest as it supported Marr's prediction. However, the impact of dynamic inhibitory transmission was neglected, although this is several times more potent than tonic inhibition and plays a critical role in controlling the information transmitted through the mossy fiber–granule cell relay during impulsive signaling. The dynamic role of inhibition in controlling granule cell spike patterning was demonstrated about 10 years later (Nieus et al., 2014). These observations therefore indicate that Marr's predictions on gain control have a biological underpinning but also indicate that this latter is much more complex than predicted by the MLT. Actually, gain control turned out to be highly nonlinear and input pattern-dependent (Mapelli et al., 2010a).

Another relevant observation was that most granule cells in vivo are inactive at rest (Chadderton et al., 2004). This result was used to support the concept of sparseness: that is, that only a minor proportion of granule cells have to be active at a time in order to allow efficient input pattern decorrelation. However, since no activity patterns were actually conveyed through the circuit, the concept of sparseness in those experiments appears hard to evaluate. In a more effective assessment obtained in response to punctuate stimulation, granule cells were activated in dense clusters with an estimated spike generation probability of about 10% (Diwakar et al., 2011). This result was deemed to support the sparseness hypothesis in relation to inputs activating local signal processing. In no case, however, has the sparseness hypothesis ever been tested during effective behaviors in alert animals.

Finally, the signals transferred through the granular layer were shown to follow complex spatiotemporal rearrangements leading to combinatorial operations and frequency-dependent gain control (Mapelli and D'Angelo, 2007; Mapelli et al., 2010a, 2010b). These results showed that the concept of expansion recoding could be interpreted in terms of local signal processing depending on molecular properties of ionic channels and synaptic receptors and the local geometry of circuit connections.

Spike patterns in time and space

Marr's theory of the cerebellum is characterized by the absence of explicit representation of time and geometrical organization. The statistical nature of model connectivity generates a topological map and the coding scheme that seems to best approximate Marr's idea is that of rate-coding, i.e. of a continuously modulated spike discharge flowing through the various network elements.

Early in the 1980s, the nature of mossy fiber discharges was demonstrated during eye movements: some fibers carry on–off spike burst while others carry protracted frequency-modulated spike discharges (Kase et al., 1980; van Kan et al., 1993). These patterns have more recently been supported by whole-cell recordings in vivo showing that granule cells respond to mossy fiber activity by generating spike bursts following punctuate sensory stimulation (Chadderton et al., 2004; Rancz et al., 2007) and by generating protracted discharges during head rotation in a vestibulo-ocular reflex (VOR) protocol (Arenz et al., 2008). Therefore, the two modalities coexist and the cerebellum is able to process both spike patterns simultaneously.

The implications of spike-burst coding are broad and go beyond Marr's intuition, introducing unpredicted consequences for signal processing. By virtue of Golgi cell lateral inhibition, the granular layer response to mossy fiber bursts becomes spatially organized in a center–surround pattern with a radius of about 50 μm, in which excitation prevails in the center and inhibition in the surround (Mapelli and D'Angelo, 2007). By virtue of Golgi cell feedforward inhibition, the granular layer generates a time-window effect limiting the duration and intensity of the output (Nieus et al., 2006; D'Angelo and De Zeeuw, 2009). The molecular properties at granular layer synapses add further complexity. In response to specific burst patterns, NMDA and GABA receptors control the induction of long-term synaptic plasticity at the mossy fiber–granule cell synapse. Since induction is regulated by synaptic inhibition (which controls membrane depolarization and therefore the level of NMDA channel unblocking and calcium influx), LTP dominates in the center and LTD in the surround of the response fields, consolidating specific geometries of activity. In these structures, the NMDA and GABA receptors generate a high-pass filter allowing bursts over 50 Hz to be optimally transmitted (Mapelli et al., 2010a, 2010b; Gandolfi et al., 2014).

As a whole, the granular layer appears to transform incoming signals by making use of specific cellular mechanisms translating incoming spike patterns into local responses (Farrant and Nusser, 2005; D'Angelo, 2008; D'Angelo et al., 2013; Mapelli et al., 2014). The emerging view is that the granular layer network behaves as a complex set of filters operating in the space and time domains, and that this filter can be adapted through long-term synaptic plasticity (Garrido et al., 2013a; Nieus et al., 2014), Thus, the original idea of input decorrelation should be extended to the spatiotemporal dynamics of circuit activity, an aspect that deserves specific future investigations. A way to test this would require independent measurement of multiple neurons in active clusters at high temporal resolution, for example applying multiphoton recording techniques in vivo (Gandolfi et al., 2014).

Microcircuit structure beyond statistical connectivity rules

Since Marr's theory is based on statistics rather than the geometry of connectivity, it is challenged by discoveries revealing critical spatial structures in the circuit. There is indeed a fundamental property that needs to be revisited. The parallel fibers, after dividing into two opposite branches originating from the ascending axon of granule cells, travel transversly for millimeters, contacting numerous Purkinje cells. This fact has inspired the idea that signals generated by granule cells activate beams of Purkinje cells (Eccles et al., 1967; Eccles, 1973; Braitenberg et al., 1997). In Marr's theory, this is translated into the idea that Purkinje cells operate as perceptrons, homogeneously receiving the sparse signal representation generated by granule cells. Actually, beam activation can be easily demonstrated by direct parallel fiber stimulation (e.g. Vranesic et al., 1994; Baginskas et al., 2009; Reinert et al., 2011). However, when cerebellar activation is elicited by natural stimuli, the activation of parallel fiber beams is less evident and spots of activity are more likely to be observed (Cohen and Yarom, 1998, 1999). This is possibly in relation to the center–surround organization of granular layer responses to high-frequency mossy fiber bursts (Gandolfi et al., 2014) and the low-pass filtering exerted by the molecular layer interneuron network. This allows only low frequencies to be transmitted along the parallel fibers; Mapelli et al., (2010a)), although further experiments are needed to confirm this hypothesis.

As seen earlier, activation of granule cells by punctate sensory stimulation occurs in dense clusters, reflecting activity of mossy fiber bundles in the afferent trigemino-cerebellar sensory pathway and in the associated thalamo-cortico-ponto-cerebellar channel (Diwakar et al., 2011). As indicated by experiments in vitro, this effect would correspond to the formation of center–surround structures in the granular layer (Mapelli and D'Angelo, 2007; Mapelli et al., 2010a, 2010b; Gandolfi et al., 2014) with the effect that signals are focused and contrasted before being retransmitted to the molecular layer. Recently, another discovery has lent support to this geometrical organization: the Golgi cells receive over 50% of their connections from neighboring granule cells (Cesana et al., 2013; D'Angelo et al., 2013), suggesting that their inhibition is closely related to local activity clusters. There are indications that a similar effect could also occur in Purkinje cells (Llinas and Sugimori, 1980a, 1980b).

Actually, punctate sensory stimulation in vivo causes a prominent "vertical" pattern of cerebellar cortex activation, in which Purkinje cells overlying the active granular layer clusters are organized in spots rather than beams. The formation of these spots could be reinforced in the molecular layer by various mechanisms including higher synaptic density, lower activation times, higher spike frequency transmission, and lower synaptic inhibition in the spot than in the associated parallel fiber beam (Bower and Woolston, 1983; Cohen and Yarom, 1998; Hartmann and Bower, 1998; Lu et al., 2005; Rokni et al., 2007; Santamaria et al., 2007; Bower, 2010). Moreover, although the synapses formed by granule cell ascending axon and parallel fibers on Purkinje cells were shown to be functionally equivalent (Isope and Barbour, 2002; Walter et al., 2009), differences in terms of long-term synaptic plasticity have been reported (Sims and Hartell, 2005, 2006).

Another relevant case concerns the olivo-cerebellar loop, in which inhibitory connections have been reported between the deep cerebellar nuclei and the inferior olive, an issue that is considered in the next section. Thus, there is a conspicuous body of experiments supporting a specific geometrical organization that could involve formation of multiple vertical columns of active cells communicating though the parallel fibers, a concept resembling the organization of the cerebral cortex. Computation may then be reflected in the geometry of neuronal activation rather than statistics of neuronal connectivity.

Timing in the olivo-cerebellar loop

A critical issue in Marr's theory is the role attributed to climbing fibers. Marr's intuition was that climbing fibers had to be functional to instruct the cerebellar cortex on the need to generate long-term synaptic plasticity at the parallel fiber–Purkinje cell synapses and, as a consequence, for motor learning. However, some investigations have challenged the teaching role of climbing fibers and some remarkable aspects of microcircuit spatiotemporal organization have emerged that could be important in explaining the function of the olivo-cerebellar loop.

The olivo-cerebellar loop was reported to perform complex timing operations by dynamically wiring groups of Purkinje cells (Llinas, 1988; Welsh et al., 1995). This observation led to the hypothesis that the olivo-cerebellar loop operates as a generator of temporal patterns encoded by complex spikes (Yarom and Cohen, 2002; Jacobson et al., 2008, 2009) and was proposed as an alternative to the teaching role of climbing fibers. The basis of this hypothesis is that inferior olivary neurons form a network of electrically coupled cells and this coupling is modulated by inhibitory inputs from the deep cerebellar nuclei.

It has been proposed that, when Purkinje cells inhibit the deep cerebellar nuclei neurons, these latter modify the oscillatory state of inferior olive neuronal clusters, which in turn can recruit different groups of Purkinje cells. Thus, a "request" for specific patterns delivered via the mossy fiber system could be translated into patterns of inferior olive activity, which could in turn reorganize activity in specific sections of the cerebellar cortex by sending climbing fiber signals to Purkinje cells organized in sagittal bands (Yarom and Cohen, 2002). Although attractive, this hypothesis lacks experimental validation at present and its relationship to cerebellar learning remains unknown.

The most conservative conclusion is that, while the intuition of parallel fiber plasticity remains, it should be coupled to the dynamic assembly of spatiotemporal geometries in the inferior olive and to the concept that the the inferior olive, deep cerebellar nuclei, and Purkinje cell neurons form a dynamics subcircuit. These concepts are further expanded in the next section.

Complex dynamics in Purkinje cells and other cerebellar neurons

On the basis of the histological observation that Purkinje cells receive the signals generated by about 200 000 granule cells, Marr hypothesized that these neurons operate as perceptrons through a linear integration process of parallel fiber inputs. Actually, a more recent investigation has proved that Purkinje cells can optimally store information through changes in their parallel fiber synapses, supporting their perceptron capabilities (Brunel et al., 2004). The simplest implementation of the cerebellar perceptron would be that Purkinje cells operate as linear integrators (Dean and Porrill, 2011). However, computational modeling suggests that Purkinje cells, by generating local regenerative currents at the level of dendritic spines, could express properties going beyond those of a linear integrator (De Schutter and Bower, 1994a, 1994b; Masoli et al., 2015).

Purkinje cells have a large dendritic tree receiving synaptic inputs and a somato-axonal section (including the initial segment and first Ranvier nodes) responsible for action potential generation (Llinas and Sugimori, 1980a, 1980b; Churchland, 1998). While synaptic potentials, generated by both parallel and climbing fibers, can easily reach the soma, spikes cannot travel efficiently into the dendritic tree. Moreover, these neurons have a complex set of ionic channels distributed unequally over the compartments, generating a rich repertoire of electroresponsive properties including, bursting, rebounds, and pauses. The Purkinje cells generate simple and complex spikes in response to parallel fiber and climbing fiber inputs. These synaptically driven events modulate a basal activity state generating bursts and pauses.

Moreover, recent observations have raised the possibility that Purkinje cells operate as bistable elements (Loewenstein et al., 2005), although the occurrence of this observation in vitro as well as in vivo is still under debate (Schonewille et al., 2006; Yartsev et al., 2009) as it could be related to the level of anesthesia and the action of certain drugs (Zhou et al., 2015). The membrane potential could switch between two stable levels, partially (but not strictly) under the control of simple and complex spikes. Current injections as well as synaptic inputs (either excitatory from parallel and climbing fibers or inhibitory from molecular layer interneurons) can bidirectionally shift the Purkinje cell states (Rokni et al., 2009).

Hence, the current view is that spontaneous firing of Purkinje cells sets the baseline activity of deep cerebellar nuclear neurons and that this activity is modulated by accelerating and decelerating firing frequency (burst–pause behavior) under control of synaptic inputs. Therefore, the existence of complex Purkinje cell firing dynamics replaces the concepts of continuous spike frequency modulation and simple linear integrator envisaged by Marr. The concept of spike timing, i.e. that the precise relative positioning of a spike is important to generate the neural code (Rieke et al., 1997), is also applicable to other neurons like granule cells (Nieus et al., 2006; Diwakar et al., 2009; D'Angelo and Solinas, 2011), Golgi cells (Solinas et al., 2007a; Solinas et al., 2007b), unipolar brush cells (Subramaniyam et al., 2014), inferior olive cells (De Gruijl et al., 2012), and deep cerebellar nuclei cells (Steuber et al., 2011), which all take part in reshaping the spike discharge in the cerebellar circuit.

Numerous forms of synaptic plasticity in addition to parallel fiber LTD

One major prediction of the MLT was that cerebellar learning should occur through some form of plasticity between parallel fibers and Purkinje cells under climbing fiber control. The climbing fibers originating from the inferior olive were assumed to play a teaching role, instructing the cerebellar cortex to modify its connectivity in order to cope with new motor demands. Parallel fiber–Purkinje cell LTP was predicted by Marr and reversed into LTD by Albus: LTD was in fact discovered more than a decade later by Ito (Ito et al., 1982). The resonance of this discovery can be compared to that of LTP in the hippocampus (Bliss and Lomo, 1973), which followed Hebb's postulate on brain plasticity (Hebb, 1949). In 1984, the Nobel prizewinner J.C. Eccles said:

> For me the most significant property of the cerebellar circuitry would be its plastic ability, whereby it can participate in motor learning, that is the acquisition of skills. This immense neuronal machine with the double innervation of Purkinje cells begins to make sense if it plays a key role in motor learning … it could be optimistically predicted that the manner of operation of the cerebellum in movement and posture would soon be known in principle (from the foreword to Ito, 1984).

For more than a decade after this, the dominant idea was that LTD was not just the most important but also probably the only relevant form of plasticity in the cerebellum. However, LTP was subsequently induced by parallel fiber stimulation without the need for climbing fiber activity (Sakurai, 1987) and a solitary role for LTD was also challenged computationally since supervised learning schemes require both LTD and LTP (Doya (1999)).

Following these fundamental discoveries, the physiological relevance of LTP and LTD at the parallel fiber–climbing fiber synapse has been evaluated experimentally, leading to contrasting conclusions. Some authors simply dismissed the relevance of parallel fiber–climbing fiber LTD for behavioral learning (De Schutter, 1995; Raymond et al., 1996; Coesmans et al., 2004; De Zeeuw and Yeo, 2005) while others concluded that learning had to occur in deeper structures, like the deep cerebellar nuclei and vestibular nuclei (Raymond et al., 1996). At the same time, several novel forms of plasticity have been demonstrated (for review see Hansel et al., 2001; De Zeeuw et al., 2011; Gao et al., 2012; D'Angelo, 2014; Galliano and De Zeeuw, 2014). Various forms of LTP and LTD have been demonstrated at the mossy fiber–granule cell synapses, at synapses between both mossy fiber and Purkinje cells to deep cerebellar nuclei, and at molecular layer interneuron synapses. Moreover, plasticity of intrinsic excitability has been shown in granule cells, Purkinje cells, and deep cerebellar nuclei cells. It should also be noted that several forms of plasticity exist at parallel fiber synapses, some of which are bidirectional and depend solely on parallel fiber (but not climbing fiber) activity.

Thus, the cerebellar network is plastic in a much more extended sense than originally envisaged. The functional meaning of this extended plasticity in computational terms remains largely to be assessed, although critical experimental and modeling investigations have been carried out (see "The final challenges"). The plasticity issue requires further comments. Just because a synapse is shown to express forms of plasticity does not necessarily mean that it is involved in "learning" in the classical sense. It is likely that at some level, all synapses in the brain are plastic; the question is for what functional purpose. For example, the classical parallel fiber–Purkinje cell LTD is Hebbian and supervised in nature, while the aforementioned mossy fiber–granule cell LTP and LTD are Hebbian but unsupervised with a fundamentally different impact on learning and behavior. In fact, as far as we understand, plasticity in the granular layer could tune the response timing of specific granule cells and therefore the activation patterns of Purkinje cells rather than implementing "motor learning" directly. In general, multiple forms of plasticity may be needed to operate in concert in order to generate biological learning properties (D'Angelo, 2014).

Oscillation and resonance could design a functional geometry

As noted, the MLT copes with a homogeneous cerebellar structure with prewired anatomical circuits. However, recent experimental evidence suggests that oscillatory and resonant properties in cerebellar neurons could help setting up coherent patterns of activity.

The inferior olivary neurons are electrically coupled (Sotelo and Llinas, 1972), and can generate rhythmic activities propagating to the cerebellar cortex through climbing fiber connections to Purkinje cells and to the deep cerebellar nuclei (reviewed in De Zeeuw et al., 2008; D'Angelo et al., 2009). A similar architecture made up of oscillatory neurons coupled through gap junctions has been recognized in Golgi cells in the granular layer (Dieudonne, 1998; Forti et al., 2006; Dugue et al., 2009; Vervaeke et al., 2010) and in stellate cells in the molecular layer (Mann-Metzer and Yarom, 2000). These oscillations therefore pervade the whole cerebrocerebellar system. The cerebellum has also been involved in large-scale low-frequency oscillation (Gross et al., 2005; Schnitzler et al., 2006) spreading through cerebrocerebellar loops involving various cerebral cortical areas (prefrontal cortex, premotor cortex, primary sensorimotor cortex and posterior parietal cortex) (Schnitzler et al., 2009).

Therefore, some circuit elements of the cerebrocerebellar loops can intrinsically generate and sustain the rhythm, while others are probably entrained by circuit activity. These two mechanisms, entraining and being entrained, are probably not disjoined because large-scale brain oscillations are collective processes, in which coalitions of neurons transiently reinforce their reciprocal interaction (Buzsaki, 2006). Voluntary movement causes oscillatory activity in the prefrontal areas, which propagates to the premotor, motor, and posterior parietal areas and is then relayed to the cerebellum through the pontine nuclei. The cerebellum may therefore initially be entrained and then participate to reinforce theta-band oscillations in the cerebrocerebellar loop. Both the granular and molecular layers can be entrained into theta-frequency cycles driven by the cerebral cortex (Courtemanche et al., 2009; Ros et al., 2009); the granular layer is resonant at the theta frequency and this may help the entrainment of the cerebellum into such rhythms (Gandolfi et al., 2013).

The double oscillatory system in the granular layer and in the inferior olive could provide the necessary coherence for multiple inputs occurring in different regions of the cerebellum. This involves an extension of the concepts of congruence of climbing and mossy fiber signals (Brown and Bower, 2002; Kistler and De Zeeuw, 2003). The result is also to generate functional assemblies of neurons with variable spatiotemporal geometry (D'Angelo et al., 2009; D'Angelo, 2011).

The final challenges

As we have seen, the main challenge for Marr's MLT is provided by circuit spatiotemporal dynamics. Will Marr's now venerable model survive or not after dynamic behaviors of the cerebellar circuit are taken into consideration?

The cerebellar circuit has now been modeled in detail using biophysically precise models of neurons and synapses and reproducing several aspects of spatiotemporal circuit processing (Maex and De Schutter, 1998; Medina and Mauk, 1999, 2000; Medina et al., 2000; Solinas et al., 2010; D'Angelo and Solinas, 2011; Jaeger, 2011; De Gruijl et al., 2012). A recent attempt has seemed to provide a favorable answer by incorporating realistic neuronal and synaptic dynamics, previously developed in a highly detailed granular layer model (Solinas et al., 2010), into the AFM (Rossert et al., 2014). The realistic granular layer, once incorporated into the AFM, still performed linear signal transduction under sustained frequency-modulated mossy fiber inputs, supporting Marr's hypothesis. Moreover, synaptic strength at mossy fiber–granule cell synapses exerted a remarkable regulation of transmission gain and phase. Therefore, Marr's hypothesis for the granular layer still holds in the presence of complex nonlinear neuronal and synaptic properties. The best guess to explain the evolutionary relevance of these last properties is that they are required to process complex spatiotemporal sequences when the input is organized in spike bursts.

Another series of observations directly supports the central tenet that supervised learning has to occur at the parallel fiber–Purkinje cell synapse under climbing fiber control. It has been recently possible to incorporate a spiking cerebellar network, endowed with reversible forms of long-term synaptic plasticity at three synaptic sites (parallel fiber–Purkinje cell, Purkinje cell–deep cerebellar nuclei, mossy fiber–deep cerebellar nuclei) into the control system of a robot (Casellato et al., 2012, 2013; Garrido et al., 2013b; Casellato et al., 2014; Luque et al., 2014). Importantly, the presence of the supervised parallel fiber–Purkinje cell plasticity under climbing fiber control remained critical in order to exploit granular layer expansion recoding and to bind learning to sensorimotor errors. The Purkinje cell–deep cerebellar nuclei and mossy fiber–deep cerebellar nuclei plasticities made it possible to generate learning on multiple timescales, to prevent saturation and to determine rescaling and generalization. Therefore, the critical intuition on parallel fiber LTD/LTP remains viable though additional forms of plasticity seem to be required to build up the remaining biological aspects of learning.

Conclusion

Although almost half a century has passed since its formulation, Marr's MLT is still fascinating for its conceptual elegance and remains a fundamental basis for research on the functions of the cerebellum and of the whole brain. Considering that cerebellar computations are based on geometry and timing, the validity of the MLT may have to be confined to homogeneous cerebellar substructures during limited time-periods dominated by modulated firing frequency. In order to understand how the cerebellar network operates, in view of recent discoveries, Marr's MLT is not sufficient in itself. A new comprehensive theory will require extensive experimental research and computational modeling integrated with closed-loop robotic simulations. At present, this is far from achieved.

References

Albus JS. (1971). The theory of cerebellar function. Math Biosci. 10:25–61.

Arbib MA, Erdi P, Szentagothai J. (1998). Neural Organization: Structure, Function, and Dynamics. Cambridge, MA: MIT Press.

Arenz A, Silver RA, Schaefer AT, Margrie TW. (2008). The contribution of single synapses to sensory representation in vivo. Science. 321:977–980.

Arleo A, Nieus T, Bezzi M, D'Errico A, D'Angelo E, Coenen OJ. (2010). How synaptic release probability shapes neuronal transmission: information-theoretic analysis in a cerebellar granule cell. Neural Comput. 22:2031–2058.

Armano S, Rossi P, Taglietti V, D'Angelo E. (2000). Long-term potentiation of intrinsic excitability at the mossy fiber-granule cell synapse of rat cerebellum. J Neurosci. 20:5208–5216.

Baginskas A, Palani D, Chiu K, Raastad M. (2009). The H-current secures action potential transmission at high frequencies in rat cerebellar parallel fibers. Eur J Neurosci. 29:87–96.

Billings G, Piasini E, Lorincz A, Nusser Z, Silver RA. (2014). Network structure within the cerebellar input layer enables lossless sparse encoding. Neuron. 83:960–974.

Bliss TV, Lomo T. (1973). Long-lasting potentiation of synaptic transmission in the dentate area of the anaesthetized rabbit following stimulation of the perforant path. J Physiol. 232:331–356.

Bower JM. (2010). Model-founded explorations of the roles of molecular layer inhibition in regulating Purkinje cell responses in cerebellar cortex: more trouble for the beam hypothesis. Front Cell Neurosci. 4:27.

Bower JM, Woolston DC. (1983). Congruence of spatial organization of tactile projections to granule cell and Purkinje cell layers of cerebellar hemispheres of the albino rat: vertical organization of cerebellar cortex. J Neurophysiol. **49**:745–766.

Braitenberg V, Heck D, Sultan F. (1997). The detection and generation of sequences as a key to cerebellar function: experiments and theory. Behav Brain Sci. **20**:229–245; discussion 245–277.

Brown IE, Bower JM. (2002). The influence of somatosensory cortex on climbing fiber responses in the lateral hemispheres of the rat cerebellum after peripheral tactile stimulation. J Neurosci. **22**:6819–6829.

Brunel N, Hakim V, Isope P, Nadal JP, Barbour B. (2004). Optimal information storage and the distribution of synaptic weights: perceptron versus Purkinje cell. Neuron. **43**:745–757.

Buzsaki G. (2006). Rhythms of the Brain. New York: Oxford University Press.

Casellato C, Garrido JA, Franchin C, Ferrigno G, D'Angelo E, Pedrocchi A. (2013). Brain-inspired sensorimotor robotic platform: learning in cerebellum-driven movement tasks through a cerebellar realistic model. In: Challenges in Neuroengineering—SSCN–NCTA, Villamuora, Algarve, Portugal, pp. 568–573.

Casellato C, Pedrocchi A, Garrido JA, Luque NR, Ferrigno G, D'Angelo E, Ros E. (2012). An integrated motor control loop of a human-like robotic arm: Feedforward, feedback and cerebellum-based learning. In: Biomedical Robotics and Biomechatronics (BioRob), 2012 4th IEEE RAS & EMBS International Conference, pp. 562–567.

Casellato C, Antonietti A, Garrido JA, Carrillo RR, Luque NR, Ros E, Pedrocchi A, D'Angelo E. (2014). Adaptive robotic control driven by a versatile spiking cerebellar network. PLoS ONE. **9**:e112265.

Cesana E, Pietrajtis K, Bidoret C, Isope P, D'Angelo E, Dieudonne S, Forti L. (2013). Granule cell ascending axon excitatory synapses onto Golgi cells implement a potent feedback circuit in the cerebellar granular layer. J Neurosci. **33**:12430–12446.

Chadderton P, Margrie TW, Hausser M. (2004). Integration of quanta in cerebellar granule cells during sensory processing. Nature. **428**:856–860.

Churchland P. (1998). Toward a Neurobiology of the Mind. London: MIT Press.

Coesmans M, Weber JT, De Zeeuw CI, Hansel C. (2004). Bidirectional parallel fiber plasticity in the cerebellum under climbing fiber control. Neuron. **44**:691–700.

Cohen D, Yarom Y. (1998). Patches of synchronized activity in the cerebellar cortex evoked by mossy-fiber stimulation: questioning the role of parallel fibers. Proc Natl Acad Sci U S A. **95**:15032–15036.

Cohen D, Yarom Y. (1999). Optical measurements of synchronized activity in isolated mammalian cerebellum. Neuroscience. **94**:859–866.

Courtemanche R, Chabaud P, Lamarre Y. (2009). Synchronization in primate cerebellar granule cell layer local field potentials: basic anisotropy and dynamic changes during active expectancy. Front Cell Neurosci. **3**:6.

D'Angelo E. (2008). The critical role of Golgi cells in regulating spatio-temporal integration and plasticity at the cerebellum input stage. Front Neurosci. **2**:35–46.

D'Angelo E. (2011). Neural circuits of the cerebellum: hypothesis for function. J Integr Neurosci. **10**:317–352.

D'Angelo E. (2014). The organization of plasticity in the cerebellar cortex: from synapses to control. Prog Brain Res. **210**:31–58.

D'Angelo E, De Zeeuw CI. (2009). Timing and plasticity in the cerebellum: focus on the granular layer. Trends Neurosci. **32**:30–40.

D'Angelo E, De Filippi G, Rossi P, Taglietti V. (1995). Synaptic excitation of individual rat cerebellar granule cells in situ: evidence for the role of NMDA receptors. J Physiol. **484** (Pt 2):397–413.

D'Angelo E, Rossi P, Armano S, Taglietti V. (1999). Evidence for NMDA and mGlu receptor-dependent long-term potentiation of mossy fiber-granule cell transmission in rat cerebellum. J Neurophysiol. **81**:277–287.

D'Angelo E, Solinas S, Mapelli J, Gandolfi D, Mapelli L, Prestori F. (2013). The cerebellar Golgi cell and spatiotemporal organization of granular layer activity. Front Neural Circuits. **7**:93.

D'Angelo E, Koekkoek SK, Lombardo P, Solinas S, Ros E, Garrido J, et al. (2009). Timing in the cerebellum: oscillations and resonance in the granular layer. Neuroscience. **162**:805–815.

De Gruijl JR, Bazzigaluppi P, de Jeu MT, De Zeeuw CI. (2012). Climbing fiber burst size and olivary sub-threshold oscillations in a network setting. PLoS Comput Biol. **8**:e1002814.

De Schutter E. (1995). Cerebellar long-term depression might normalize excitation of Purkinje cells: a hypothesis. Trends Neurosci. **18**:291–295.

De Schutter E, Bower JM. (1994a). An active membrane model of the cerebellar Purkinje cell II. Simulation of synaptic responses. J Neurophysiol. **71**:401–419.

De Schutter E, Bower JM. (1994b). An active membrane model of the cerebellar Purkinje cell. I. Simulation of current clamps in slice. J Neurophysiol. **71**:375–400.

De Zeeuw CI, Yeo CH. (2005). Time and tide in cerebellar memory formation. Curr Opin Neurobiol. **15**:667–674.

De Zeeuw CI, Hoebeek FE, Schonewille M. (2008). Causes and consequences of oscillations in the cerebellar cortex. Neuron. **58**:655–658.

De Zeeuw CI, Hoebeek FE, Bosman LW, Schonewille M, Witter L, Koekkoek SK. (2011). Spatiotemporal firing patterns in the cerebellum. Nat Rev Neurosci. **12**:327–344.

Dean P, Porrill J. (2010). The cerebellum as an adaptive filter: a general model? Funct Neurol. **25**:173–180.

Dean P, Porrill J (2011) Evaluating the adaptive-filter model of the cerebellum. J Physiol. **589**:3459–3470.

Dean P, Porrill J, Ekerot CF, Jorntell H. (2010). The cerebellar microcircuit as an adaptive filter: experimental and computational evidence. Nat Rev Neurosci. **11**:30–43.

Dieudonne S. (1998). Submillisecond kinetics and low efficacy of parallel fibre-Golgi cell synaptic currents in the rat cerebellum. J Physiol. **510** (Pt 3):845–866.

Diwakar S, Magistretti J, Goldfarb M, Naldi G, D'Angelo E. (2009). Axonal Na$^+$ channels ensure fast spike activation and back-propagation in cerebellar granule cells. J Neurophysiol. **101**:519–532.

Diwakar S, Lombardo P, Solinas S, Naldi G, D'Angelo E. (2011). Local field potential modeling predicts dense activation in cerebellar granule cells clusters under LTP and LTD control. PLoS ONE. **6**:e21928.

Doya K. (1999). What are the computations of the cerebellum, the basal ganglia and the cerebral cortex? Neural Netw. **12**:961–974.

Dugue GP, Brunel N, Hakim V, Schwartz E, Chat M, Levesque M, et al. (2009). Electrical coupling mediates tunable low-frequency oscillations and resonance in the cerebellar Golgi cell network. Neuron. **61**:126–139.

D'Angelo E, Solinas S. (2011). Realistic modeling of large-scale networks: spatio-temporal dynamics and long-term synaptic plasticity in the cerebellum. In: Advances in Computational Intelligence (Cabestany J, Rojas I, Joya G, eds), pp. 547–553. Berlin: Springer.

Eccles JC. (1973). The cerebellum as a computer: patterns in space and time. J Physiol. **229**:1–32.

Eccles JC, Ito M, Szentagothai J. (1967). The Cerebellum as a Neural Machine. Berlin: Springer-Verlag.

Farrant M, Nusser Z. (2005). Variations on an inhibitory theme: phasic and tonic activation of GABA(A) receptors. Nat Rev Neurosci. **6**:215–229.

Forti L, Cesana E, Mapelli J, D'Angelo E. (2006). Ionic mechanisms of autorhythmic firing in rat cerebellar Golgi cells. J Physiol. **574**:711–729.

Fujita M. (1982). Adaptive filter model of the cerebellum. Biol Cybernet. **45**:195–206.

Galliano E, De Zeeuw CI. (2014). Questioning the cerebellar doctrine. Prog Brain Res. **210**:59–77.

Gandolfi D, Lombardo P, Mapelli J, Solinas S, D'Angelo E. (2013). Theta-frequency resonance at the cerebellum input stage improves spike timing on the millisecond time-scale. Front Neural Circuits. **7**:64.

Gandolfi D, Pozzi P, Tognolina M, Chirico G, Mapelli J, D'Angelo E. (2014). The spatiotemporal organization of cerebellar network activity resolved by two-photon imaging of multiple single neurons. Front Cell Neurosci. **8**:92.

Gao Z, van Beugen BJ, De Zeeuw CI. (2012). Distributed synergistic plasticity and cerebellar learning. Nat Rev Neurosci. **13**:619–635.

Garrido JA, Ros E, D'Angelo E. (2013a). Spike timing regulation on the millisecond scale by distributed synaptic plasticity at the cerebellum input stage: a simulation study. Front Comput Neurosci. **7**:64.

Garrido JA, Luque NR, D'Angelo E, Ros E. (2013b). Distributed cerebellar plasticity implements adaptable gain control in a manipulation task: a closed-loop robotic simulation. Front Neural Circuits. **7**:159.

Gross J, Pollok B, Dirks M, Timmermann L, Butz M, Schnitzler A. (2005). Task-dependent oscillations during unimanual and bimanual movements in the human primary motor cortex and SMA studied with magnetoencephalography. Neuroimage. **26**:91–98.

Hansel C, Linden DJ, D'Angelo E. (2001). Beyond parallel fiber LTD: the diversity of synaptic and nonsynaptic plasticity in the cerebellum. Nat Neurosci. **4**:467–475.

Hartmann MJ, Bower JM. (1998). Oscillatory activity in the cerebellar hemispheres of unrestrained rats. J Neurophysiol. **80**:1598–1604.

Hebb DO. (1949). The Organization of Behavior: A Neuropsychological Theory. New York: Wiley.

Imamizu H, Kawato M. (2009). Brain mechanisms for predictive control by switching internal models: implications for higher-order cognitive functions. Psychol Res. **73**:527–544.

Imamizu H, Kawato M (2012) Cerebellar internal models: implications for the dexterous use of tools. Cerebellum. **11**:325–35.

Imamizu H, Miyauchi S, Tamada T, Sasaki Y, Takino R, Putz B, et al. (2000). Human cerebellar activity reflecting an acquired internal model of a new tool. Nature. **403**:192–195.

Isope P, Barbour B. (2002). Properties of unitary granule cell→Purkinje cell synapses in adult rat cerebellar slices. J Neurosci. **22**:9668–9678.

Ito M. (1972). Neural design of the cerebellar motor control system. Brain Res. **40**:81–84.

Ito M. (1984). The Cerebellum and Neural Control. New York: Raven Press.

Ito M. (1993). Movement and thought: identical control mechanisms by the cerebellum. Trends Neurosci. **16**:448–450; discussion 453–444.

Ito M. (2006). Cerebellar circuitry as a neuronal machine. Prog Neurobiol. **78**:272–303.

Ito M. (2008). Control of mental activities by internal models in the cerebellum. Nat Rev Neurosci. **9**:304–313.

Ito M, Sakurai M, Tongroach P. (1982). Climbing fibre induced depression of both mossy fibre responsiveness and glutamate sensitivity of cerebellar Purkinje cells. J Physiol. **324**:113–134.

Jacobson GA, Rokni D, Yarom Y. (2008). A model of the olivo-cerebellar system as a temporal pattern generator. Trends Neurosci. **31**:617–625.

Jacobson GA, Lev I, Yarom Y, Cohen D. (2009). Invariant phase structure of olivo-cerebellar oscillations and its putative role in temporal pattern generation. Proc Natl Acad Sci U S A. **106**:3579–3584.

Jaeger D. (2011). Mini-review: synaptic integration in the cerebellar nuclei—perspectives from dynamic clamp and computer simulation studies. Cerebellum. **10**:659–66.

Kase M, Miller DC, Noda H. (1980). Discharges of Purkinje cells and mossy fibres in the cerebellar vermis of the monkey during saccadic eye movements and fixation. J Physiol. 300:539–555.

Kawato M, Gomi H. (1992). A computational model of four regions of the cerebellum based on feedback-error learning. Biol Cybernet. 68:95–103.

Kawato M, Kuroda S, Schweighofer N. (2011). Cerebellar supervised learning revisited: biophysical modeling and degrees-of-freedom control. Curr Opin Neurobiol. 21:791–800.

Kawato M, Kuroda T, Imamizu H, Nakano E, Miyauchi S, Yoshioka T. (2003). Internal forward models in the cerebellum: fMRI study on grip force and load force coupling. Prog Brain Res. 142:171–188.

Kistler WM, De Zeeuw CI. (2003). Time windows and reverberating loops: a reverse-engineering approach to cerebellar function. Cerebellum. 2:44–54.

Llinas R, Sugimori M. (1980a). Electrophysiological properties of in vitro Purkinje cell dendrites in mammalian cerebellar slices. J Physiol. 305:197–213.

Llinas R, Sugimori M. (1980b). Electrophysiological properties of in vitro Purkinje cell somata in mammalian cerebellar slices. J Physiol. 305:171–195.

Llinas RR. (1988). The intrinsic electrophysiological properties of mammalian neurons: insights into central nervous system function. Science. 242:1654–1664.

Loewenstein Y, Mahon S, Chadderton P, Kitamura K, Sompolinsky H, Yarom Y, Hausser M. (2005). Bistability of cerebellar Purkinje cells modulated by sensory stimulation. Nat Neurosci. 8:202–211.

Lu H, Hartmann MJ, Bower JM. (2005). Correlations between purkinje cell single-unit activity and simultaneously recorded field potentials in the immediately underlying granule cell layer. J Neurophysiol. 94:1849–1860.

Luque NR, Garrido JA, Carrillo RR, D'Angelo E, Ros E. (2014). Fast convergence of learning requires plasticity between inferior olive and deep cerebellar nuclei in a manipulation task: a closed-loop robotic simulation. Front Comput Neurosci. 8:97.

Maex R, De Schutter E. (1998). Synchronization of golgi and granule cell firing in a detailed network model of the cerebellar granule cell layer. J Neurophysiol. 80:2521–2537.

Mann-Metzer P, Yarom Y. (2000). Electrotonic coupling synchronizes interneuron activity in the cerebellar cortex. Prog Brain Res. 124:115–122.

Mapelli J, D'Angelo E. (2007). The spatial organization of long-term synaptic plasticity at the input stage of cerebellum. J Neurosci. 27:1285–1296.

Mapelli J, Gandolfi D, D'Angelo E. (2010a). High-pass filtering and dynamic gain regulation enhance vertical bursts transmission along the mossy fiber pathway of cerebellum. Front Cell Neurosci. 4:14.

Mapelli J, Gandolfi D, D'Angelo E. (2010b). Combinatorial responses controlled by synaptic inhibition in the cerebellum granular layer. J Neurophysiol. 103:250–261.

Mapelli L, Solinas S, D'Angelo E. (2014). Integration and regulation of glomerular inhibition in the cerebellar granular layer circuit. Front Cell Neurosci. 8:55.

Mapelli L, Rossi P, Nieus T, E. DA. (2009). Tonic activation of GABAB receptors reduces release probability at inhibitory connections in the cerebellar glomerulus. J Neurophysiol. 101:3089–3099.

Marr D. (1969). A theory of cerebellar cortex. J Physiol. 202:437–470.

Masoli S, Solinas S, D'Angelo E. (2015). Action potential processing in a detailed Purkinje cell model reveals a critical role for axonal compartmentalization. Front Cell Neurosci. 9:47.

Medina JF, Mauk MD. (1999). Simulations of cerebellar motor learning: computational analysis of plasticity at the mossy fiber to deep nucleus synapse. J Neurosci. 19:7140–7151.

Medina JF, Mauk MD. (2000). Computer simulation of cerebellar information processing. Nat Neurosci. 3(Suppl):1205–1211.

Medina JF, Garcia KS, Nores WL, Taylor NM, Mauk MD. (2000). Timing mechanisms in the cerebellum: testing predictions of a large-scale computer simulation. J Neurosci. 20:5516–5525.

Mitchell SJ, Silver RA. (2003). Shunting inhibition modulates neuronal gain during synaptic excitation. Neuron. 38:433–445.

Nieus T, Sola E, Mapelli J, Saftenku E, Rossi P, D'Angelo E. (2006). LTP regulates burst initiation and frequency at mossy fiber-granule cell synapses of rat cerebellum: experimental observations and theoretical predictions. J Neurophysiol. 95:686–699.

Nieus TR, Mapelli L, D'Angelo E. (2014). Regulation of output spike patterns by phasic inhibition in cerebellar granule cells. Front Cell Neurosci. 8:246.

Rancz EA, Ishikawa T, Duguid I, Chadderton P, Mahon S, Hausser M. (2007). High-fidelity transmission of sensory information by single cerebellar mossy fibre boutons. Nature. 450:1245–1248.

Raymond JL, Lisberger SG, Mauk MD. (1996). The cerebellum: a neuronal learning machine? Science. 272:1126–1131.

Reinert KC, Gao W, Chen G, Wang X, Peng YP, Ebner TJ. (2011). Cellular and metabolic origins of flavoprotein autofluorescence in the cerebellar cortex in vivo. Cerebellum. 10:585–599.

Rieke F, Warland D, de Ruyter van Steveninck R, Bialek W. (1997). Spikes: Exploring the Neural Code. Cambridge, MA: MIT Press.

Rokni D, Llinas R, Yarom Y. (2007). Stars and stripes in the cerebellar cortex: a voltage sensitive dye study. Front Syst Neurosci. 1:1.

Rokni D, Tal Z, Byk H, Yarom Y. (2009). Regularity, variability and bi-stability in the activity of cerebellar purkinje cells. Front Cell Neurosci. 3:12.

Ros H, Sachdev RN, Yu Y, Sestan N, McCormick DA. (2009). Neocortical networks entrain neuronal circuits in cerebellar cortex. J Neurosci. 29:10309–10320.

Rossert C, Solinas S, D'Angelo E, Dean P, Porrill J. (2014). Model cerebellar granule cells can faithfully transmit modulated firing rate signals. Front Cell Neurosci. 8:304.

Sakurai M. (1987). Synaptic modification of parallel fibre-Purkinje cell transmission in in vitro guinea-pig cerebellar slices. J Physiol. 394:463–480.

Santamaria F, Tripp PG, Bower JM. (2007). Feedforward inhibition controls the spread of granule cell-induced Purkinje cell activity in the cerebellar cortex. J Neurophysiol. 97:248–263.

Schnitzler A, Timmermann L, Gross J. (2006). Physiological and pathological oscillatory networks in the human motor system. J Physiol Paris. 99:3–7.

Schnitzler A, Munks C, Butz M, Timmermann L, Gross J. (2009). Synchronized brain network associated with essential tremor as revealed by magnetoencephalography. Mov Disord. 24:1629–1635.

Schonewille M, Khosrovani S, Winkelman BH, Hoebeek FE, De Jeu MT, Larsen IM, et al. (2006). Purkinje cells in awake behaving animals operate at the upstate membrane potential. Nat Neurosci. 9:459–461; author reply 461.

Schweighofer N, Arbib MA, Kawato M. (1998a). Role of the cerebellum in reaching movements in humans. I. Distributed inverse dynamics control. Eur J Neurosci. 10:86–94.

Schweighofer N, Spoelstra J, Arbib MA, Kawato M. (1998b). Role of the cerebellum in reaching movements in humans. II. A neural model of the intermediate cerebellum. Eur J Neurosci. 10:95–105.

Sims RE, Hartell NA. (2005). Differences in transmission properties and susceptibility to long-term depression reveal functional specialization of ascending axon and parallel fiber synapses to Purkinje cells. J Neurosci. 25:3246–3257.

Sims RE, Hartell NA. (2006). Differential susceptibility to synaptic plasticity reveals a functional specialization of ascending axon and parallel fiber synapses to cerebellar Purkinje cells. J Neurosci. 26:5153–5159.

Solinas S, Nieus T, D'Angelo E. (2010). A realistic large-scale model of the cerebellum granular layer predicts circuit spatio-temporal filtering properties. Front Cell Neurosci. 4:12.

Solinas S, Forti L, Cesana E, Mapelli J, De Schutter E, D'Angelo E. (2007a). Computational reconstruction of pacemaking and intrinsic electroresponsiveness in cerebellar Golgi cells. Front Cell Neurosci. 1:2.

Solinas S, Forti L, Cesana E, Mapelli J, Schutter ED, Angelo ED. (2007b). Fast-reset of pacemaking and theta-frequency resonance patterns in cerebellar Golgi cells: Simulations of their impact in vivo. Front Cell Neurosci. 1:4.

Sotelo C, Llinas R. (1972). Specialized membrane junctions between neurons in the vertebrate cerebellar cortex. J Cell Biol. 53:271–289.

Steuber V, Schultheiss NW, Silver RA, De Schutter E, Jaeger D. (2011). Determinants of synaptic integration and heterogeneity in rebound firing explored with data-driven models of deep cerebellar nucleus cells. J Comput Neurosci. 30:633–658.

Subramaniyam S, Solinas S, Perin P, Locatelli F, Masetto S, D'Angelo E. (2014). Computational modeling predicts the ionic mechanism of late-onset responses in unipolar brush cells. Front Cell Neurosci. 8:237.

Tyrrell T, Willshaw D. (1992). Cerebellar cortex: its simulation and the relevance of Marr's theory. Philos Trans R Soc Lond B Biol Sci. 336:239–257.

van Kan PL, Gibson AR, Houk JC. (1993). Movement-related inputs to intermediate cerebellum of the monkey. J Neurophysiol. 69:74–94.

Vervaeke K, Lorincz A, Gleeson P, Farinella M, Nusser Z, Silver RA. (2010). Rapid desynchronization of an electrically coupled interneuron network with sparse excitatory synaptic input. Neuron. 67:435–451.

Vranesic I, Iijima T, Ichikawa M, Matsumoto G, Knopfel T. (1994). Signal transmission in the parallel fiber-Purkinje cell system visualized by high-resolution imaging. Proc Natl Acad Sci U S A. 91:13014–13017.

Walter JT, Dizon MJ, Khodakhah K. (2009). The functional equivalence of ascending and parallel fiber inputs in cerebellar computation. J Neurosci. 29:8462–8473.

Welsh JP, Lang EJ, Suglhara I, Llinas R. (1995). Dynamic organization of motor control within the olivocerebellar system. Nature. 374:453–457.

Wolpert DM, Miall RC, Kawato M. (1998). Internal models in the cerebellum. Trends Cogn Sci. 2:338–347.

Yarom Y, Cohen D. (2002). The olivocerebellar system as a generator of temporal patterns. Ann N Y Acad Sci. 978:122–134.

Yartsev MM, Givon-Mayo R, Maller M, Donchin O. (2009). Pausing purkinje cells in the cerebellum of the awake cat. Front Syst Neurosci. 3:2.

Zhou H, Voges K, Lin Z, Ju C, Schonewille M. (2015). Differential Purkinje cell simple spike activity and pausing behavior related to cerebellar modules. J Neurophysiol. 113:2524–2536.

Chapter 4

The importance of Marr's three levels of analysis for understanding cerebellar function

Paul Dean and John Porrill

Introduction to the Marrian framework

This chapter attempts to use a conceptual framework particularly associated with David Marr (Marr and Poggio, 1977; Marr, 1982) to evaluate current research on the cerebellum. The central feature of the Marrian framework is the claim that complex information processing systems have be analyzed at different levels. Usually three levels of analysis, sometimes referred to as levels of description or of understanding, are chosen (e.g., Frisby and Stone, 2012):

1 Computational level: What task is the system carrying out?

2 Algorithmic level: What method does the system use?

3 Implementational level: How is the algorithm carried out by the available hardware?

Reasons for using this framework can perhaps best be illustrated by applying it first of all to a very simplified version of a problem in cerebellar research, in this case the problem of how the cerebellum makes sure that reaching is accurate.

Reaching and the cerebellum

It has long been known from clinical investigation that inaccurate reaching is one of the symptoms of cerebellar damage (e.g., Holmes, 1939), but what the cerebellum actually does to ensure accuracy is not well understood (e.g., Bhanpuri et al., 2014). One of the problems to be solved is illustrated in simplified form in Figure 4.1A.

This shows the geometry of a two-joint "arm" operating in the horizontal plane. It is apparent that the position in space of its "hand" is determined by the angles of the two joints, which means that getting that hand to a particular point in space entails knowing what the correct joint angles are for that location. How can this be achieved? Even for the schematic arm shown in Figure 4.1A this is not an obvious question, and it is in fact representative of a very important class of problems in motor control (e.g., Jordan and Rumelhart, 1992; Shadmehr and Wise, 2005).

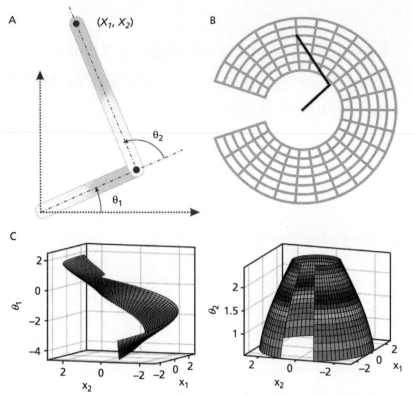

Figure 4.1 Geometry of planar "arm" with two degrees of freedom. (A) The position of the "hand" x_1, x_2 is specified by the joint angles θ_1, θ_2 and the lengths l_1 and l_2 of the upper and lower arm. (B) Work space where accurate reaching is required. (C) Joint angles as functions of hand position in the work space. Shades of grey illustrate different values of the joint angles θ_1 and θ_2.

Panels A and B adapted from Figure 2 of Porrill and Dean (2007b): John Porrill and Paul Dean, "Recurrent Cerebellar Loops Simplify Adaptive Control of Redundant and Nonlinear Motor Systems," Neural Computation, 19:1 (January, 2007), pp. 170–193. © 2006 by the Massachusetts Institute of Technology.

Computational level

The reaching problem in its simple form is well understood at the computational level (e.g., Snyder, 1985; Jordan and Rumelhart, 1992; Jordan, 1996; Porrill and Dean, 2007b). The equations relating joint angles θ_1, θ_2 to hand position x_1, x_2 can be derived geometrically (assuming the arm is stiff, i.e., the lengths l_1, l_2 of its components do not change).

$$x_1 = l_1 \cos \theta_1 + l_2 \cos(\theta_1 + \theta_2)$$
$$x_2 = l_1 \sin \theta_1 + l_2 \sin(\theta_1 + \theta_2) \tag{1}$$

Reaching accurately therefore requires selecting the correct joint angles. It also requires selecting the appropriate motor commands m_1 and m_2 that will produce those joint angles, a calculation that is simplified here by assuming a simple linear relationship between motor commands and joint angles (e.g., $m_i = k\theta_i$). With this simplification the control problem effectively becomes that of solving equations (1) for θ_1, θ_2 given desired x_1, x_2. This is a problem that has to be dealt with by any arm control system, whether biological or robotic, and so can initially be treated independently of how the control system is implemented.

Algebraic manipulation allows equations (1) to be recast in the desired form:

$$\theta_1 = \tan^{-1}\frac{x_1}{x_2} - \tan^{-1}\frac{l_2 \sin\xi\varphi}{l_1 + l_2 \sin\xi\varphi}$$

$$\theta_2 = \xi\varphi \quad \text{where} \quad \varphi = \cos^{-1}\frac{x_1^2 + x_2^2 - l_1^2 - l_2^2}{2 l_1 l_2}$$

(2)

The choice $\xi = \pm 1$ determines the arm configuration, so there are two solutions for each position in space, an example of redundancy which although important for control is not considered further here. These equations may seem surprisingly complex given the apparent simplicity of the arm, and the relations of θ_1, θ_2 to x_1, x_2 in fact are strongly non-linear. This can be seen in Figure 4.1C, which plots the required values of θ_1, θ_2 for desired x_1, x_2 over the work space shown in Figure 4.1B. Nonetheless, for robots these equations can easily be coded in a computer-based control system.

However, a precoded solution ceases to ensure accuracy if the arm (and hence equations 2) change in any way, for example as a result of wear or damage. This may be a serious issue for autonomous robots, and certainly is a central one for biological systems, where the body changes almost continually. Arm control in animals requires constant calibration as the equations change, and so any candidate algorithm for ensuring accurate reaching has to adapt to changing circumstances

Algorithm level

A simple scheme that could achieve such adaptive control is illustrated in Figure 4.2A. The signal x_d, arriving perhaps from motor cortex, represents the desired location of the hand. It is transformed by an adaptive element **C** (i.e., the cerebellum) into a signal representing the motor command **m** (assumed here to be simply proportional to the joint angles θ). This is sent to the arm **P**, which transforms it into hand location **x** according to equations (1) and (2). The signal $\mathbf{m}_d$ represents the correct motor command, and if the actual motor command **m** is incorrect, the error signal $\delta\mathbf{m} = \mathbf{m} - \mathbf{m}_d$ is sent to **C**. The task of the adaptive element **C** is to use this error signal to learn the correct motor command, so that after enough examples it learns the equations (2) that link desired end-effector locations and correct commands. An algorithm that can achieve this learning is available (the adaptive filter model), and is described in the section on Cerebellar microcircuit, Algorithm level below.

Here we point out that, at a very general level, the Marrian framework makes explicit how the simple architecture for Figure 4.2A fails to meet two different kinds of constraint. The first is implementational: extensive evidence indicates that cerebellar lesions result in inaccurate movements, not paralysis. However, if **C** were removed from Figure 4.2A, no

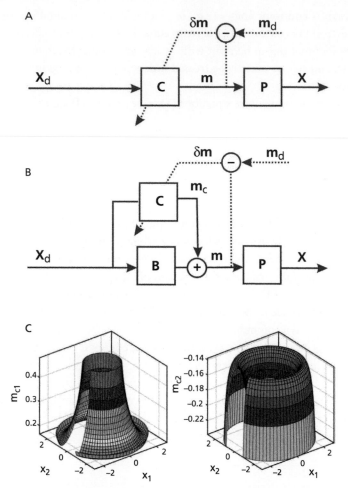

Figure 4.2 Algorithms for learning correct motor commands for two-joint arm, shown schematically. (A) The adaptive element **C** receives a signal x_d representing the desired location of the hand (i.e., the desired x_1, x_2). It converts these into a motor command **m** (i.e., m_1, m_2) which acts on the plant **P** to produce the actual hand location **x** (x_1, x_2) as indicated by equations (1) and (2). Learning in **C** is driven by the error signal δ**m** (δm_1, δm_2), which is the difference between the actual motor command **m** and the desired command $\mathbf{m_d}$ (desired m_1, m_2). (B) The adaptive element **C** now acts in parallel with circuitry in brainstem and spinal cord **B**. This circuitry produces an approximate solution to equations (3) and (4), which is refined by addition of the output of **C**, $\mathbf{m_c}$. The summed command **m** acts on **P** as before, and again learning is driven by the error signal δ**m**. (C) The required corrective commands m_{c1} and m_{c2} as a function of desired hand location x_1, x_2.

motor commands would reach the arm. The algorithm must therefore incorporate parallel pathways for movement control independent of the cerebellum, as indicated in Figure 4.2B, where box **B** represents these parallel pathways through brainstem and spinal cord. It would appear from the effects of cerebellar damage that signal processing in these brainstem pathways results in an approximate solution to equations (2), so that the real task of the cerebellum is not to learn the entire equations but to fine-tune the brainstem solution by providing a correction to the motor commands m_c. The addition of **B** can in principle alter the mapping the **C** has to learn very substantially. Figure 4.2C illustrates this for the situation where **B** produces the correct motor commands for the original arm lengths, but these are then changed by 10%. The required outputs of **C** are now much smaller than for the original problem (Figure 4.1C) as would be expected, but in addition the nature of the nonlinearity, especially for the command to the upper arm, has changed substantially.

The second constraint is computational. Algorithms that learn the correct motor commands are needed because they operate in circumstances where those commands are not known in advance. Yet in Figures 4.2A and 4.2B the correct motor commands are needed to derive the error signal that drives cerebellar learning. Avoiding this circularity requires a procedure for using the available sensory errors $x - x_d$ (i.e., how far the hand is from the target) rather than the unavailable motor errors $m - m_d$.

Such a procedure is available for the simplified arm (Porrill and Dean, 2007b), and is illustrated schematically in Figure 4.3A. The input to the adaptive element **C** is now an

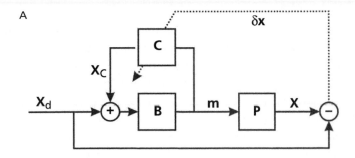

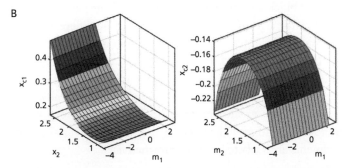

Figure 4.3 Algorithms for solving the arm control problem. (A) Recurrent architecture. Here the motor commands generated by the fixed element **B** are the input to the adaptive element **C**. The output of **C** is then used as a correction to the input to **B**. In this configuration, the sensory error δx can be used to direct learning. (B) Mapping between motor commands and the required correction to input signal for 10% changes in arm length.

efferent copy of the motor commands $\mathbf{m}$, and its output a correction $\mathbf{x}_c$ to the desired hand location $\mathbf{x}_d$. The error signal which drives learning is the difference $\delta\mathbf{x}$ between desired and actual hand location $\mathbf{x}$, that is a sensory signal readily available to the system. The scheme shown in Figure 4.3A has been termed a recurrent architecture, and when $\mathbf{C}$ is modeled as an adaptive filter it is able to use sensory error to learn the calibration necessary for accurate movement (Dean et al., 2002; Porrill et al., 2004; Porrill and Dean, 2007b). Figure 4.3B shows the task that $\mathbf{C}$ is now required to learn, indicating once more the dependence of the task on details of the external circuitry.

Details of both the adaptive filter model and the recurrent architecture are considered further in the section on Cerebellar microcircuit, Algorithm level below. At this stage Figure 4.3 is used to illustrate an important outcome of applying the Marrian framework to control of the simplified arm, namely that any algorithm for autonomous motor control must specify not only how the cerebellar microcircuit works (i.e., how can $\mathbf{C}$ learn equations in general), but also how it interacts with circuitry external to the cerebellum (i.e., what particular equations does $\mathbf{B}$ require $\mathbf{C}$ to learn, and how can $\mathbf{B}$ and $\mathbf{C}$ be connected to ensure appropriate signals are available to drive the learning).

Implementation level

The question of whether an algorithm works, in the sense of solving the computational problem of interest, is crucially distinct from the question of whether it is implemented biologically. For example, it is relatively straightforward to show that the algorithm embodied in the circuit of Figure 4.3 is computationally effective. But determining whether (i) the adaptive filter model of the cerebellum microcircuit, and (ii) the recurrent architecture connecting cerebellum and other neural structures, are consistent with experimental evidence on reaching are much more difficult undertakings.

One reason for this difficulty is that the relevant evidence comes in very different forms. Basic clinical observations were sufficient to show that the simple architecture of Figure 4.2A needed amendment. In contrast, technically demanding measurements of complex intracellular biochemistry may be needed to test the particular forms of synaptic plasticity required by the algorithm. The existence of these different levels of detail suggests a possible way of approaching the implementation question, which is to think of a candidate algorithm being required to pass a series of tests, starting with the simplest. This is the approach attempted here, both for the cerebellum itself, and for the circuits of which it is a part. The intention is that at each level it will become apparent how algorithms can be used to make predictions that can be falsified by experimental evidence. This allows candidate algorithms to be rejected or refined, and may be useful for indicating which experiments are likely to be most informative.

Implications

The application of Marr's levels-of-analysis framework to a simplified motor control problem involving the cerebellum makes clear a distinction often made implicitly in the literature. Understanding cerebellar function requires not only elucidation of the cerebellum's intrinsic information processing role, but also how this fits in with the relevant circuitry extrinsic to the cerebellum. This distinction suggests it may be helpful, at least initially, to evaluate cerebellar research separately under these two headings, and this is the organization adopted in this chapter.

The intrinsic versus extrinsic framework immediately points to a major difference between the wide variety of tasks thought to involve the cerebellum, and the apparent homogeneity of the cerebellar microcircuit. For the specific example of arm control, we have argued, it is necessary to understand the basic arm control circuitry (B in Figure 4.2B), and how it is connected to the cerebellum (Figure 4.3A). However, the cerebellum is involved in a huge array of motor control tasks, involving limbs, head, eyes, posture, and general coordination. It also plays a part in autonomic control (Nisimaru et al., 2013), is important for sensory prediction (e.g., Bastian, 2011; Roth et al., 2013), and is involved in a wide range of apparently nonsensorimotor functions that includes verbal working memory, emotional control, and social cognition (e.g., Stoodley and Schmahmann, 2009; Schmahmann, 2010; Keren-Happuch et al., 2014; Van Overwalle et al., 2014).

In sharp contrast to the multiplicity of what might be termed extrinsic functions, the intrinsic signal processing function of the cerebellum itself is widely thought to remain constant whatever the external circuitry in which it is embedded. This view is based on studies indicating that the anatomical and electrophysiological properties of cerebellar cortex appear almost uniform over its entire extent (e.g., Herrick, 1924; Eccles et al., 1967; Ito, 1984). The difference between intrinsic and extrinsic functionality (Ito, 1970) has been captured by the metaphor of the cerebellar chip (e.g., Ito, 1997; Porrill et al., 2013), as illustrated in Figure 4.4. A particular functional subregion of cerebellar cortex is represented by the chip, which is assumed to have identical properties for all cortex. In contrast, the outputs of each functional subregion are unique, consistent with anatomical evidence that different areas of cortex receives climbing-fiber inputs from a different regions of the inferior olive (Figure 4.5), and project to distinct areas of the deep cerebellar nuclei. Finally, the total set of mossy-fiber inputs is unique to each subregion, though often a subset will be shared with other subregions.

The chip metaphor strongly emphasizes the distinction between the intrinsic function of the cerebellar microcircuit, and the multiple extrinsic functions of the each microzone with its external circuitry. We therefore apply the Marrian framework to these two kinds of cerebellar "function" separately. We start with the intrinsic functions of the cerebellar microcircuit.

Cerebellar microcircuit

Circuit diagrams such as those shown in Figures 4.2 and 4.3 clarify the difference between the function of the circuit as a whole, which is directly represented in behavior, and the function of the component C, which is not. This distinction, also relevant to the

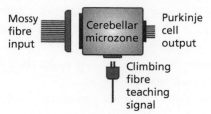

Figure 4.4 The cerebellar "chip" metaphor. The arrangement of neurons and their connections within cerebellar cortex appear similar over the entire cortex, whereas individual regions of cerebellar cortex have unique patterns of connections with external neural structures. This combination has suggested what has been termed the "chip" metaphor of cerebellar organization, shown here in simplified form. The climbing-fiber and output connections are unique to each functional subregion or microzone, whereas mossy-fiber inputs may be shared with other microzones. The climbing-fiber teaching signal specifies the learning goals of a particular microzone, and historically this connectivity has been central to defining zones and microzones (e.g., Voogd, 2011). The Purkinje-cell output must then be connected to a target region in the deep cerebellar or vestibular nuclei which contributes to achieving this goal, and for which the learning procedure hardwired into the chip is stable and convergent. This provides a strong constraint on the output connectivity. The mossy fiber input connections are the least constrained. They can be regarded as a wide "bus" of possibly relevant sensory and motor signals, from which those signals actually relevant to the task will be chosen by the learning procedure.

From Figure 58.9 of Handbook of the Cerebellum and Cerebellar Disorders, Adaptive Filter Models, 2013, pp.1315–1335, Dean P, Jörntell H, Porrill J, © 2013 Springer Science+Business Media Dordrecht. With permission of Springer.

interpretation of lesion studies (e.g., Dean, 1982) and more widely to other aspects of neuroscience (e.g., Willems, 2011) was familiar to Marr:

> In my own case, the cerebellar study … disappointed me, because even if the theory was correct, it did not enlighten one about the motor system—it did not, for example, tell one how to go about programming a mechanical arm. (Marr, 1982, p. 15).

One implication of the distinction is that the function of the cerebellar chip cannot be described in familiar whole-circuit terms (e.g., "sensory," "motor," or "cognitive"), but only in computational terms that may be rather less familiar.

Before exploring this issue further, a qualification needs to be made. The assumption of completely uniform intrinsic processing in all areas of cerebellar cortex is almost certainly too simple. Accumulating electrophysiological and anatomical evidence (for a recent review see Cerminara et al., 2015) points to the strong likelihood of processing differences between areas. At present, however, the computational significance and nature of these differences is not at all clear. We therefore proceed here with the assumption of uniform processing, while bearing in mind the likely need for refinement at a later date.

Computational level

The simplified reaching example makes it clear that the particular task confronting the cerebellum depends on external circuitry (Figures 4.1C, 4.2C, 4.3B). However, in general

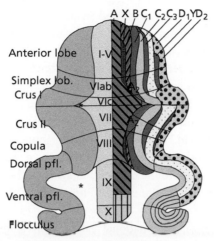

Figure 4.5 Schematic diagram of flattened cerebellar cortex in rat. The left-hand side shows the cerebellar lobules I–X (I–V anterior lobe, VI–X posterior lobe) labelled in the vermis, together with the names given to their hemispheric extensions HI–HX lateral to the vermis (details of nomenclature given in e.g., Glickstein and Voogd, 1995; Glickstein et al., 2011). The lobules run approximately mediolaterally. The right-hand side shows the organization of cerebellar zones A–D2, strips of cortex that (again approximately) run rostrocaudally. A given zone receives climbing-fiber input from a particular region of the inferior olive, and projects solely to a particular region of the deep cerebellar nuclei. (Further details of cerebellar zonal organization are available in e.g., Sugihara and Shinoda, 2004; Voogd and Ruigrok, 2004; Apps and Hawkes, 2009; Marzban and Hawkes, 2011).

terms it can said that the cerebellum is required to learn the mapping between a set of input variables and an output, using information about the consequences of the cerebellum's output to drive the learning. The use of an external signal to control learning makes this an example of supervised learning, and the general idea that the cerebellum is a supervised learning system is familiar as the Marr–Albus–Ito framework (e.g., Doya, 1999).

Although there have been alternative suggestions for the computational role of the cerebellum, including the generation of temporal patterns (Jacobson et al., 2008), as a universal motor control system (Llinás et al., 2004) and the timing of motor and cognitive processes (Ashe and Bushara, 2014), at present these appear not have been formulated precisely enough to provide the basis for a computationally effective algorithm.

Algorithm level

A number of related algorithms have been proposed for how the cerebellum might learn input–output mappings. For reasons of space we select here one particular example, the algorithm embodied in the adaptive filter that was first put forward as a model of the cerebellum by Fujita (1982). The adaptive filter is particularly suited for dealing with signals that vary in time, and has been shown to be computationally very powerful and versatile in engineering applications (e.g., Widrow and Stearns, 1985). It is also typically used to model the role of the cerebellum in a variety of behavioral tasks (Dean et al., 2010).

Figure 4.6A shows a simplified diagram of an adaptive filter, in which a time-varying input $y(t)$ is recoded into a larger number of internal signals $p_1(t) \ldots p_n(t)$. These signals are weighted ($w_1 \ldots w_n$) and summed to give the filter's output $z(t)$. The weights are altered by the error signal $e(t)$ until $z(t)$ becomes the desired output $z_d(t)$. Since a major reason for proposing this model was its apparent resemblance to the cortical microcircuit, a sketch of this is shown in Figure 4.6B. The filter's inputs $y(t)$ correspond to mossy-fiber signals, which are recoded by the granule cells to give signals in the parallel fibers $p(t)$. The weights w correspond to the efficacies of synapses between parallel fibers and Purkinje cells, and the summing is done by the Purkinje cells. Error signals are conveyed by climbing fibers.

We focus here on one central computational feature of this algorithm, namely the learning rule that is used to adjust the weights. Other related models of the cerebellum, such as the CMAC (Albus, 1971) use variants of this rule. The learning rule is a central feature of the algorithm because the algorithm is only effective if the rule used to change the weights does in fact bring the filter's output closer to the desired value. A rule with this property can be derived for the case when information about the desired output is directly available (see Appendix), and it takes the form:

$$\delta w_i = -\beta \langle e(t) p_i(t) \rangle \tag{3}$$

where δw_i denotes the change to the weight w_i that is applied to the recoded signal p_i, $e(t)$ denotes the error signal, and the angle brackets denote expected or mean values. The error signal is the difference between the actual and desired filter output, $z(t) - z_d(t)$. One way of interpreting this rule is to note that if a particular signal p_i is positively correlated with the error, the corresponding weight w_i is reduced; conversely, if the correlation is negative, the weight is increased. It is as if correlation means cause, a suitable assumption here since the filter output does in fact influence the error signal appropriately. In that case the rule reduces weights on those recoded signals that increase the error, while increasing those that reduce it (Dean et al., 2002). The learning rule shown in equation (3) has a number of names, for example covariance, delta, Widrow–Hoff, and least mean squares (LMS). Because it can be shown to be optimum in the sense of minimizing the mean square difference between desired and actual output, it is used in many engineering applications of the adaptive filter (e.g., Widrow and Stearns, 1985).

As described in the next section, even in the abstract form of equation (3) the LMS rule makes important general predictions about synaptic function in the cerebellar microcircuit. However, for more detailed predictions about synaptic plasticity it must be recast in a form that connects with the relevant experimental evidence. The immediate problem is that the derivation of the learning rule in equation (3) assumes that the signals in the model of Figure 4.6A can treated as continuous variables (Appendix). But in the cerebellum these signals are carried by spiking neurons. Relating the learning rule to

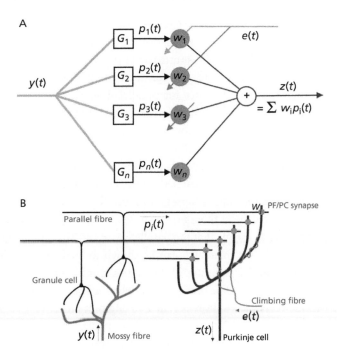

Figure 4.6 (A) Adaptive filter model of cerebellar microcircuit. The filter's input $y(t)$ is recoded by a bank of causal filters G_i so that the parallel fibers carry signals which form an expansion recoding $p_i = G_i[y]$. Filter output is the weighted sum $z(t) = \sum w_i p_i(t)$ of the recoded inputs, implementing a linear-in-weights filter $C = \sum w_i G_i$. The training signal $e(t)$ which adapts synaptic weights w_i using the LMS learning rule derived in the Appendix. (B) Schematic diagram of basic features of the cerebellar cortical microcircuit. Mossy-fiber inputs corresponding to $y(t)$ are distributed over many granule cells G_i, whose axons bifurcate to produce parallel fibers carrying signals $p_i(t)$. These fibers form synapses with weights w_i on Purkinje cells. Each Purkinje cell also receives a climbing-fiber signal $e(t)$, which in Marr–Albus models is assumed to alter the weights w_i. In these models Purkinje cell output $z(t)$ is assumed to be simple spike firing, with the effects of complex spikes produced by climbing-fiber input usually neglected. Not shown in the diagram: (i) Purkinje cell output is inhibitory, and acts via neurons in the deep cerebellar nuclei (and vestibular nuclei); (ii) granule cell axons also form synapses on molecular-layer interneurons (stellate and basket cells) which in turn form inhibitory synapses on Purkinje cells. In this way granule cells influence Purkinje cells via both an excitatory direct and an inhibitory indirect pathway.
A: Adapted from Fig 1B of Porrill et al. (2004); B: Adapted from Fig 1A of Porrill et al. (2004).

experimental evidence therefore requires its translation into a form suitable for signals that are carried by neuronal spike trains, that is in a spike-timing dependent plasticity (STDP) form.

Equation (3) implies that when both parallel-fiber and climbing-fiber signals have higher than normal values in a small time range, the efficacy of the parallel-fiber–Purkinje-cell synapse should decrease (be depressed). Conversely, if the parallel fiber fires without corresponding change in CF firing, the synapse should potentiate. This combination of depression and potentiation can be summarized in the STDP profile illustrated in Figure 4.7B, in which the strong depression for nearly coincident spikes is surrounded by much weaker potentiating side lobes for parallel-fiber spikes that are not coincident with a climbing-fiber spike. It can be demonstrated that this STDP profile implements the decorrelation learning rule for suitable rate-coding schemes (cf. Menzies et al., 2010).

Although Figure 4.7B captures the basic shape of the STDP learning rule, it is misleading in that it assumes the error signal carried by the climbing fibers is instantaneously available for learning at the relevant synapses. However, for some regions of the cerebellum the error signal can be subject to large transmission delays (for example 50–100 ms for visual processing), which means that the parallel-fiber and climbing-fiber signals will not match exactly in time. This mismatch can be shown to lead to unstable learning at high frequencies (Porrill and Dean, 2007a). Since the climbing-fiber signal cannot be advanced, unstable learning has to be prevented by delaying the effect of the parallel-fiber signal. A filter which effects such a delay is called an eligibility trace (Figure 4.7C), and it can be incorporated into the STDP profile by situating the depression dip at an interspike time corresponding to the transmission delay (Figure 4.7D).

Implementation level

One advantage of the adaptive filter, and related algorithms derived from the Marr–Albus–Ito framework, is that they account at a very general level for a distinctive feature of the cerebellar microcircuit. Purkinje cells receive two very different kinds of input. One is from granule cells, whose parallel fiber axons form approximately 150 000 synapses on the Purkinje cell's dendritic tree. There are an enormous number of granule cells, currently estimated to make up about 80% of all neurons in the human brain (Herculano-Houzel, 2009), and at least 100 times more numerous than mossy fibers. In the model these are needed to recode the mossy-fiber input to cerebellar cortex. Purkinje cells fire spontaneously ("simple spikes" at ~40 spikes/s), and this firing rate is altered by granule cell input.

In contrast, each Purkinje cell receives input from only one climbing fiber, the axon of a cell in the inferior olive. The climbing fiber wraps around the dendritic tree, forming about 250 excitatory synapses (Brown et al., 2012), so that each time the climbing fiber fires the Purkinje cell fires also, though in this case with an unusually shaped complex spike as opposed to a simple spike. A central feature of complex-spike firing is its low spontaneous rate, about 1 spike/s. These distinctive features of climbing-fiber input correspond to the requirements of the adaptive filter's error signal. The low frequency (and possibly also the randomness—see Keating and Thach, 1995) mean that the error signal interferes only slightly with the filter's output, and the extensive synaptic input allows the error signal to affect all the parallel-fiber synapses. The ability of Marr–Albus models to account for these general microcircuit features is of course not coincidental, but follows

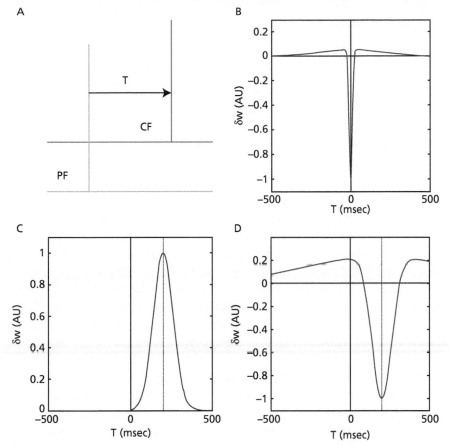

Figure 4.7 Spike-timing dependent plasticity (STDP) implementation of LMS learning rule. (A) Incremental changes in the weights of synapses between parallel fibers and Purkinje cells depend on the relative timing *T* of parallel-fiber and climbing-fiber action potentials. Positive *T* is chosen to represent climbing-fiber spikes arriving after parallel-fiber spikes, so that the parallel-fiber contribution to Purkinje cell input could have causally affected the component of the teaching signal carried by that climbing-fiber spike. (B) The decorrelation learning rule can be induced by the spike timing dependent plasticity profile shown in this plot. Nearly coincident parallel-fiber and climbing-fiber spikes produce long-term depression (LTD), whereas widely separated parallel-fiber and climbing-fiber spikes produce a much smaller amount of long-term potentiation (LTP). The total amount of LTD and LTP must balance in order to produce the symmetric behaviour required by the learning rule. To obtain an exact correlational rule the dip must be infinitesimally wide and infinitely high (a delta function) and the surround LTP lobes must be infinitely wide and infinitesimally high. The more realistic smooth profile shown here will restrict learning performance by causing it to fall off at very high and very low frequencies (further details in Menzies et al., (2010)). (C) The symmetric STDP profile in panel (B) does not respect causality since LTD can be produced by parallel-fiber spikes arriving after climbing-fiber spikes. The expected delay between climbing-fiber spike and the parallel-fiber spike which could be responsible (about 100 ms when the teaching signal is, e.g., retinal slip) can be incorporated into the learning rule by incorporating an eligibility trace induced by the parallel-fiber spike which describes the eligibility for learning of subsequent climbing-fiber spikes. Here this is chosen to be causal and peak at the expected delay. (D) The eligibility trace can be combined with the STDP profile in panel B to produce a causal STDP profile tuned to the expected delay in the teaching signal. The LTD dip produces maximum learning at the expected delay, and the broad dip limits high frequency learning, reducing instabilities caused by any inaccuracy in the estimated delay.

from the fact these models were inspired by the anatomy and physiology of the microcircuit (Eccles et al., 1967).

At a more detailed level, there are a number of important implementational issues the adaptive filter needs to address. Here we focus on just one, the implementation of the LMS learning rule.

In the system-level model shown in Figure 4.6A, the weights that correspond to synapses between parallel fibers and Purkinje cells can switch between negative and positive values. Since actual synapses are either positive or negative, the model predicts a second inhibitory pathway between the granule cells and Purkinje cells. In fact the inhibitory effects of parallel-fiber inputs on Purkinje cells are be mediated by just such a pathway, in which parallel fibers contact inhibitory stellate and basket cells (molecular layer interneurons, MLIs) that in turn project to Purkinje cells (e.g., Albus, 1971). The synaptic weights between parallel fibers and MLIs thus correspond to negative weights in the model, and so according to the LMS rule should be modifiable, with a form of plasticity that is the mirror image of Figure 4.7. Experimental evidence indicates that the synapses between parallel fibers and MLIs are indeed plastic (Jörntell and Ekerot, 2003; Jörntell et al., 2010; Jirenhed et al., 2013), and their general properties appear to be those required by the LMS learning rule (Ekerot and Jörntell, 2003; Porrill and Dean, 2008; Dean et al., 2010).

A second prediction of the LMS rule is that after long periods of training parallel fibers that transmit irrelevant signals will have their synapses on both Purkinje cells and molecular layer interneurons driven to silence (Porrill and Dean, 2008). In qualitative terms, the reason for this is that if their synaptic weights are not zero, irrelevant parallel-fiber signals will produce an erroneous Purkinje cell output, which will therefore in turn produce an error signal in the climbing fibers. The parallel-fiber signal will therefore be correlated with the error signal, and according to the LMS rule its weight will be reduced until the correlation vanishes, i.e., the weight becomes zero. Given the very large number of parallel-fiber signals available to a Purkinje cell, it is likely that a high proportion of their signals are irrelevant, and therefore that a high proportion of parallel-fiber synapses on Purkinje cells and molecular layer interneurons are silent. Experimental evidence is consistent with this prediction, suggesting that as many as 98% of parallel-fiber synapses are silent (e.g., Ekerot and Jörntell, 2001; Isope and Barbour, 2002; Jörntell and Ekerot, 2002, 2003).

Translating the LMS learning rule into the spike-timing dependent form shown in Figure 4.7D permits more detailed comparison with experimental evidence. One prediction is that if a parallel fiber fires shortly before the climbing fiber fires, the efficacy of the synapse between the parallel fiber and the Purkinje cell should be reduced. Such a reduction, known as long-term depression (LTD), was first demonstrated by Ito, Sakurai and Tongroach (1982) and has been very extensively investigated since (for recent review see Ito et al., 2014). A second prediction is that an increase in synaptic efficacy (long-term potentiation, LTP) will be produced by stimulation of parallel fibers alone (Figure 4.7B, D). Postsynaptic LTP has been described by Lev-Ram et al. (2002), and shown to be capable of reversing the effects of LTD (Lev-Ram et al., 2003; Coesmans et al., 2004; Jörntell and Hansel, 2006). A particularly dramatic demonstration of apparent LTP is the finding that parallel-fiber stimulation without conjunctive climbing-fiber stimulation can greatly enlarge the tactile receptive fields of Purkinje cells in the C3 zone of the cerebellum in vivo (Jörntell and Ekerot, 2002, 2011; Ekerot and Jörntell, 2003).

However, experimental investigation of the cellular mechanisms that underlie LTD and LTP has produced a puzzling set of results. Extensive work in vitro has suggested that LTD may result from the internalization of AMPA receptors at the synapses between parallel fibers and Purkinje cells. Consistent with this view, in three different mutant mice where this internalization was blocked, in-vitro LTD was not observed (Schonewille et al., 2011) (though see Honda and Ito, Chapter 2 of this volume, for caveats). However, these mice were not impaired on traditional cerebellar learning tasks such as eyeblink classical conditioning or adaptation of the vestibulo-ocular reflex (VOR) (details of these tasks given in section on External circuitry below). Moreover, the detailed properties of in-vitro LTD appear incompatible with some behavioral observations. For example, in-vitro studies typically find some learning when parallel-fiber and climbing-fiber inputs arrive simultaneously, whereas studies of eyeblink-conditioning find no learning for simultaneously presented conditioned and unconditioned stimuli (Hesslow et al., 2013).

It might be possible to explain part of this discrepancy if in-vivo cerebellar learning sometimes depended on plasticity at synapses between parallel fibers and molecular layer interneurons, or on LTP rather than LTD at the synapses between parallel fibers and Purkinje cells. In particular, the finding that many parallel-fiber synapses are silent points to a fundamental role for LTP, and LTP at synapses on molecular layer interneurons could mimic the effects of LTD on Purkinje cell synapses. Identifying the synapses at which behaviorally relevant plasticity takes place is a crucial precursor to identifying the mechanisms underlying that plasticity.

A second factor contributing to the discrepancy between in-vitro and in-vivo findings is the complexity of synapses between parallel fibers and Purkinje cells, and their ability to display numerous forms of both LTD and LTP in vitro (e.g., Ito, 2012; Honda and Ito, Chapter 2 of this volume). It usually unclear how far a particular form of plasticity has a computational role, how far it is an artifact of the in-vitro preparation, or how far it is serving a biologically important but noncomputational role, such as preserving tonic firing rates within a suitable range (De Schutter, 1995; Hansel et al., 2001; Gao et al., 2012; D'Angelo, 2014, and Chapter 3 of this volume ; Mapelli et al., 2015). In this context Ito et al. (2014) have stressed the importance of developing experimental approaches that would allow characterization of synaptic plasticity in awake, behaving animals. More recently, two types of cerebellar LTD have been postulated in a model of adaptation of the optokinetic reflex (Yamazaki et al., 2015), only one of which has a role in learning while the other is the one abolished in the mutant mice of Schonewille et al. (2011).

In summary, present evidence suggests that bidirectional plasticity of the general form shown in Figure 4.7 could underlie in-vivo electrophysiological results for synapses between parallel fibers and Purkinje cells, and in converse form could underlie results for synapses between parallel fibers and molecular-layer interneurons. In a broad sense, therefore, the predictions of the adaptive filter algorithm appear consistent with experimental evidence. However, at a more detailed level it appears that for particular behavioral tasks the synaptic sites of plasticity may need to be identified, as do the precise mechanisms that mediate behaviorally relevant LTP and LTD in each of the two pathways between granule and Purkinje cells (see also Boyden et al., 2006; Belmeguenai et al., 2010; Schonewille et al., 2010).

Conclusions

The algorithm proposed to account for the functions of the cerebellar microcircuit was initially cast in an abstract system-level form. As its predictions at this level appeared to be confirmed, so the model needed to incorporate more biological features to confront more detailed physiological and anatomical evidence. At present, evaluation of its predictions concerning STDP await identification of the relevant processes in awake, behaving animals.

It has not been possible to address here other implementational aspects of the adaptive filter model. Perhaps the most important of these at present concerns signal processing by the granular layer. There is extensive and as yet unresolved debate about how far this layer implements expansion recoding, and if so what the underlying neural mechanisms might be (see e.g., D'Angelo and De Zeeuw, 2009; D'Angelo et al., 2009, 2013; Yamazaki and Tanaka, 2009; Dean et al., 2010; Gao et al., 2012; Spanne and Jörntell, 2013; Rössert et al., 2014). The potentially very important role of plasticity in the granular layer is addressed by D'Angelo in Chapter 3 of this volume.

External circuitry—cerebellum as component

As indicated in Figure 4.5, cerebellar cortex can be divided into parasagittal zones based on its connectivity with the inferior olive and deep cerebellar (and vestibular) nuclei (e.g., Apps and Hawkes, 2009; Voogd, 2011). These zones can be further subdivided into microzones, defined as a coherent strip of cerebellar cortex in which the Purkinje cells receive input from climbing fibers that are driven by essentially identical peripheral inputs (e.g., Andersson and Oscarsson, 1978; Ekerot et al., 1991; Manni and Petrosini, 2004; Apps and Garwicz, 2005; Apps and Hawkes, 2009). The number of microzones in cat can be very approximately estimated as 5000 (Dean et al., 2010). Presumably there are many more microzones in the human cerebellum, but as far as we know their number has yet to be guessed at.

The anatomical evidence for multiple microzones combined with clinical, behavioral and imaging evidence for cerebellar involvement in an increasingly wide range of motor, sensory, and cognitive tasks (see earlier section on Implications) suggests that there may be a very large number of different functional cerebellar chips. An important question therefore is the extent to which the external circuits of these chips can be classified into a small number of "canonical" patterns, each carrying out a distinctive, basic, signal-processing function (e.g., D'Angelo and Casali, 2013). A number of candidate canonical circuits have been proposed, and we have argued elsewhere (Porrill et al., 2013) that two in particular look promising. These are (i) a circuit for predicting the sensory effects of one's own actions as applied to the reafference problem, and (ii) a circuit for maintaining accurate movement in the face of changes in the body, the plant compensation problem.

The reafference problem

Historically, on the basis of available anatomical, clinical, and lesion evidence, the cerebellum was associated with motor control (e.g., Dow and Moruzzi, 1958; Ito, 1984; Glickstein et al., 2009). More recent investigations have indicated that the cerebellum is also involved in certain forms of sensory processing where the acquisition of sensory information is dependent on the organism's own activities (e.g., Bower, 1997a,1997b; Bower and Parsons, 2003). A central feature of active sensing is the ability to predict the sensory consequences of movement (e.g., Wolpert et al., 1998; Imamizu, 2010; Bastian, 2011; Medina, 2011; Ito, 2012). The predicted sensory consequences of movements can be used to help solve a variety of different sensorimotor problems.

One of these is the reafference problem, which occurs when the sensory signals produced by the organism's own movement interfere with sensory signals coming from the outside world. This problem has long been recognized (for review see e.g., Wolpert et al., 1998; Cullen, 2004), and is sometimes referred to as the reafference problem because it requires distinguishing between "reafferent" (internally generated) and "exafferent" (externally generated) signals. It occurs in a wide variety of contexts, and has been linked to deep questions such as the establishment of personal identity, for example by recognizing inner speech as one's own (e.g., Scott, 2013).

Computational level

The particular mapping the cerebellum needs to learn here is that between information concerning a movement, and the sensory consequences of that movement. A favored source of information about the movement is an efference copy of the motor command, since this occurs earlier in time than e.g., proprioceptive signals. The precise mapping to be learned depends of course on the particular movement in question; for example the visual consequences of an arm movement depend on the relation between motor command and hand location (see Figure 4.1).

Algorithm level

The reafference problem is closely related to a generic application of the adaptive filter algorithm in engineering, namely adaptive noise or interference cancellation (Figure 4.8A).

Here an external signal of interest s is corrupted by additive noise n, and the task of the algorithm is to remove this noise in order to provide an accurate an estimate s_{est} as possible (Widrow and Stearns, 1985). However, the noise cannot be measured directly but has itself to be estimated (n_{est}) from information r that is related to the noise, but in an unknown way, e.g., in the case of electrical noise interfering with electrocardiogram

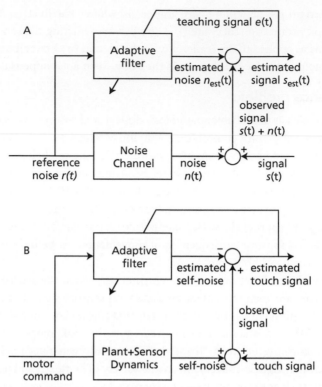

Figure 4.8 Noise cancellation and the reafference problem. (A) If a signal of interest s is contaminated by additive noise n, the observable signal becomes $s + n$. The noise component n may not itself be observable, but may be known to be generated by a noise channel whose input r, called the reference noise, is observable. If an adaptive filter can be trained to mimic the properties of the noise channel, it can be applied to the reference noise to obtain an estimate n_{est} of n. Subtracting this estimated noise from the observed signal $s + n$ then gives an estimate $s_{est} = s + n - n_{est}$ of the signal of interest. (B) The noise cancellation architecture can be applied directly to situations where noise is generated by self-motion, e.g., to removing the component of whisker sensor signals generated by whisker self-motion. Whisker sensory signals are a combination of "touch" signals generated by deflections on contact with objects, and the "self-noise" signals generated by free whisking. These self-noise signals are generated via motor commands to whiskers, and these commands can be regarded as a reference noise signal. The adaptive filter learns a model of the plant dynamics which transforms motor commands into sensory self-noise signals.

signals (Huhta and Webster, 1973). The process that transforms r into n is termed the noise channel, and the task of the adaptive element is to learn to mimic the properties of the channel, that is to learn the mapping of r onto n. If this is achieved, the filter transforms its input r into n exactly as the noise channel does, so that when its output n_{est} (estimated or predicted noise) from the noisy sensory signal $(s + n)$ the result $(s_{est} = s + n - n_{est})$

corresponds exactly to the original signal s. Perfect noise cancellation has been achieved, and the original signal recovered.

The adaptive filter can learn to mimic the noise channel because of the properties of the LMS learning rule (equation 3). The output s_{est} of the noise-canceller is used as the teaching signal. If it contains any contamination by noise, then there will be residual correlations between system output s_{est} and components of the filter input r. The learning rule is designed to remove any such correlation, so that when learning is complete, there will no longer be any contamination of s_{est} by noise (provided suitable component filters G are available).

The architecture shown in Figure 4.8A for generic noise cancellation can be transferred directly to the problem of predicting the sensory effects of movement in biological systems, shown in Figure 4.8B. The signal of interest now comes from a biological sensor, for example one that contains information about deflection of the whiskers (Anderson et al., 2010, 2012). The task is to detect whisker deflections that are produced by contact with objects in the outside world, but the sensory "touch signal" (s) is contaminated by "self-noise" signals (n) that are generated by the animal's own movements of the whiskers. The nature of this contamination cannot be known directly, but there is information about the whisking movements themselves, provided by the motor commands sent to the muscles that move the whiskers. This "efference copy" information is in effect reference information r about the noise source, and so can be used as input to an adaptive filter (in the cerebellum) that learns to mimic the transformation of motor commands into sensory signals from the whiskers. Thus, the cerebellum learns a model of the box labeled "Plant + Sensor Dynamics" in Figure 4.8B, which refers to the mechanical properties of the whisker muscles and whiskers (lumped into the "plant") together with the sensory apparatus which detects whisker deflections. These include the basic properties of elasticity, viscosity, and inertia, and any postprocessing in the sensory apparatus, whose combination can be represented by an appropriate fixed filter—just like the noise channel in Figure 4.8A.

Once learning has been achieved, the adaptive filter mimics this fixed filter, and its output n_{est} becomes an explicit prediction of the effects of the animal's own movements on the sensory signal provided by the whiskers. This prediction is then subtracted from the raw sensory input to provide an estimate s_{est} of the whisker signal generated by objects in the outside world.

Implementation level

Evidence suggesting cerebellar involvement in the reafference problem was initially provided by studies of tickling (Blakemore et al., 1998, 1999, 2000, 2001). Tickling by others is perceived as more effective than tickling by oneself (Weiskrantz et al., 1971), and both imaging and clinical studies indicate cerebellar involvement in this effect.

However, it has proved difficult to move from evidence of cerebellar involvement to evidence about details of the underlying circuitry, for example identifying the cerebellar microzones involved and the comparator where estimated noise is subtracted from the external signal (Figure 4.8B). A circuit has been proposed for the case of rat whisking (Anderson et al., 2012), which specifies zone A2 of cerebellar cortex as the relevant zone, and the superior colliculus as the comparator. However, although the structure of the basic circuit is consistent with experimental evidence, and the role of the superior colliculus in orienting to unexpected whisker deflection is well established (references in Anderson et al., 2012), as yet the nature of the signals conveyed by different parts of the circuit remains unknown. Conversely, in the case of primate head movements, electrophysiological investigation has revealed the existence of neurons in the rostral fastigial nucleus involved in removing the effects of the movements on disturbances of the retinal image (Brooks and Cullen, 2013). However, the underlying circuitry has yet to be fully identified.

There remains an instance of a well-investigated circuit whose relevance to the reafference problem looks plausible but is still uncertain. This is the circuit that mediates delay eyeblink conditioning (Figure 4.9). Here, the relevant area of cerebellar cortex is located primarily in zone C3 (see Figure 4.5), confined to the hemispheric part of lobule VI (Mostofi et al., 2010, for rabbit). In eyeblink conditioning a conditioned stimulus (often a tone) is presented shortly before an unconditioned stimulus (e.g., mild shock to the skin

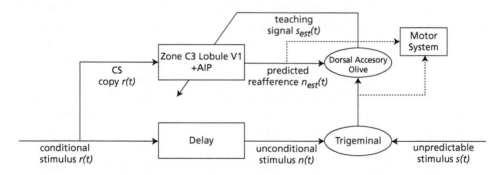

Figure 4.9 Circuitry for classical conditioning of the eyeblink, drawn to resemble the architecture for solving the eraffarence problem. The conditional stimulus $r(t)$ in effect acts to produce a painful unconditional stimulus $n(t)$ to the eye or surrounding tissue after an unknown delay. A copy of $r(t)$ is sent as mossy-fiber input to zone C3 of lobule HVI. The output of this eyeblink region acts via the anterior interpositus nucleus (AIP) as a prediction $n_{est}(t)$ of the unconditional stimulus. This prediction is sent by the nucleo-olivary pathway to part of the dorsal accessory olive, where it is subtracted from the sensory signal provided by part of the trigeminal nucleus. The output of the olive can be regarded as an estimate $s_{est}(t)$ of any unpredicted painful stimulus $s(t)$ to the eye or surrounding tissue, and is used as a teaching signal sent via climbing fibers to the eyeblink region of cerebellar cortex. Learning in the eyeblink region proceeds until $n_{est}(t) = n(t)$ so there is no longer any correlation between $r(t)$ and $s_{est}(t)$. In typical classical conditioning experiments $s(t)$ is set to zero, so learning proceeds until the teaching signal $s_{est}(t)$ is also zero.

Reprinted from Progress in Brain Research, Volume 210, Paul Dean and John Porrill, Decorrelation Learning in the Cerebellum: Computational Analysis and Experimental Questions, pp.157–192, © 2014, with permission from Elsevier.

round the eye) that elicits an eyeblink, the unconditioned response. After a number of such pairings the tone itself elicits a blink (conditioned response) whose peak amplitude occurs approximately at the same time as the unconditioned response is delivered. Very extensive experimental investigation (reviewed in e.g., Hesslow and Yeo, 2002; De Zeeuw and Yeo, 2005; Thompson and Steinmetz, 2009) has revealed that mossy-fiber input to the eyeblink zone conveys information about the conditioned stimulus, climbing-fiber input conveys information about the unconditioned stimulus, and the output of the eyeblink zone is related to the conditioned response.

One difference between the circuits of Figure 4.8B and 4.9 is that the mossy-fiber input to the latter is a sensory stimulus, not an efference copy of a motor command. However, as far as the adaptive element in Figure 4.8B is concerned, the critical computational feature of its inputs is that they predict future sensory signals. It has been argued that reafference problems in general can be solved by the most suitable mixture of efference copy and relevant sensory signals (Cullen, 2004; Abrahamsson et al., 2012). Whether there are efference copy inputs to the eyeblink microzone remains to be established, but they could play an important functional role in preventing the organism's own movements from damaging its eyes (Dean et al., 2013a).

In other respects the eyeblink circuitry has promising features with respect to the reafference algorithm. Although cerebellar output in eyeblink conditioning is usually considered in terms of motor commands, it is well known to have a sensory predictive component. For example, in classical conditioning the unconditioned stimulus is delivered regardless of the organism's response, yet the climbing-fiber signal to cerebellar cortex, which in eyeblink conditioning is driven by inescapable periorbital shock, nonetheless diminishes as acquisition proceeds (e.g., Sears and Steinmetz, 1991; Hesslow and Ivarsson, 1996; Rasmussen et al., 2008; Abrahamsson et al., 2012). The climbing-fiber signal appears to be *predicted* shock, and models of eyeblink conditioning have therefore typically used a comparator in which cerebellar output is compared with the unconditioned stimulus signal, just as in Figure 4.8B (e.g., Grossberg and Schmajuk, 1989; Moore et al., 1989; Medina et al., 2000; Lepora et al., 2010; Abrahamsson et al., 2012). The use of predicted shock explains a number of phenomena in eyeblink conditioning, including the cessation of acquisition even though the unconditioned stimulus continues to be delivered, extinction, blocking and other trial-level phenomena (e.g., Rescorla and Wagner, 1972; Kim et al., 1998; Lepora et al., 2010).

Moreover, a number of studies have suggested that in the specific case of eyeblink conditioning an excellent candidate for the comparator is the inferior olive itself (e.g., Andersson et al., 1988; Sears and Steinmetz, 1991; Kim et al., 1998; Medina et al., 2002; Nicholson and Freeman, 2003; Bengtsson and Hesslow, 2006; Bengtsson et al., 2007; Jirenhed et al., 2007; Rasmussen et al., 2008; Lepora et al., 2010). A subset of neurons in the relevant part of the deep cerebellar nuclei (the anterior interpositus nucleus) send inhibitory projections to the relevant region of the inferior olive (dorsal accessory olive), and these nucleo-olivary neurons would provide a natural substrate for the cerebellar signal $n_{est}(t)$ in Figure 4.8A. The issue is not settled: it is unclear whether other comparators are located elsewhere (e.g., the red nucleus), or whether an olivary comparator function has to be combined with tonic regulation of Purkinje cell simple-spike firing rates (references in Lepora et al., 2010). Nonetheless, experimental studies of eyeblink conditioning have made considerable progress in identifying a vital component of the circuit shown in Figure 4.8B.

Conclusions

Evidence for the implementation of the algorithm of Figure 4.8B by the cerebellum and associated circuitry is still circumstantial. Although the eyeblink-conditioning circuit (Figure 4.9) appears similar in some respects to the theoretical circuit, the sensory prediction task it carries out may not be to do with reafference. A further problem is that the circuit is also involved directly in motor control, since produces eyeblinks. If the unconditioned stimulus is an avoidable corneal airpuff rather than an unavoidable periorbital shock, then the situation becomes more complicated still, since for avoidable stimuli the "comparator" is in effect located in the outside world (Lepora et al., 2010; Dean and Porrill, 2014). These complications are not currently well understood.

In contrast, very detailed evidence is available for the part played by precerebellar structures in electric fish in reafference. These structures resemble the cerebellar microcircuit in certain respects, and extensive experimental investigation has demonstrated that some do indeed adaptively remove reafferent interference from sensory signals. Moreover, they appear to use a form of the LMS learning rule to do so (e.g., Bell et al., 1997, 2008; Requarth and Sawtell, 2011; Montgomery et al., 2012). However, in precerebellar structures the comparator stage occurs inside the structure itself, rather than outside as in Figure 4.8B (e.g., Porrill et al., 2013). The evidence concerning the role of precerebellar structures in the reafference problem can therefore only be suggestive of a similar role for the cerebellum, though it does indicate that the basic cerebellar microcircuit has the required computational capacity, and that solving the reafference problem may have been an evolutionarily ancient cerebellar function.

The plant compensation problem

In the simplified arm control example (Figure 4.1), the cerebellum learned to modify the motor commands sent to the arm ("plant") to restore movement accuracy after a change in arm length. Since the body changes in many ways as a result of growth and wear, the plant compensation problem is a generic one, and in the general case involves signals that vary in time.

Computational level

The precise mapping to be learned by the cerebellum for plant compensation depends on the nature of the plant changes, and also on how the cerebellum is connected to noncerebellar circuitry (e.g., Figures 4.2, 4.3). We focus here on the type of mapping produced by the recurrent architecture (Figure 4.3).

Algorithm level

The recurrent architecture shown in Figure 4.3A embodies an algorithm that successfully solves the plant compensation problem. Its key features are that the input to the adaptive element is a copy of the motor commands sent to the plant, and that the error signal is a sensory measure of movement inaccuracy. It therefore requires only signals that are available to an autonomous agent, and it can be shown that learning using sensory error in this algorithm is stable, for example by Lyapounov analysis (Porrill and Dean, 2007b). The algorithm therefore meets the criterion of computational adequacy.

Implementation level

The problem of plant compensation has perhaps been most extensively addressed for the oculomotor system. In the case of the VOR, an unintended head movement produces an equal and opposite eye movement, thus ensuring the visual image does not move across the retina and so degrade vision. The required eye-movement command depends upon the mechanics of the oculomotor plant (eye muscles and orbital tissue), as recognized by Skavenski and Robinson (1973). If the mechanics change, then the eye movements become inaccurate, and the image does move across the retina ("retinal slip"). However, in the course of time the VOR adapts, and accuracy is restored. The dependence of VOR adaptation on the cerebellum, and its suitability as a task for investigating cerebellar function, were first recognized by Ito (1970), and the role of the cerebellum in oculomotor calibration acknowledged by Robinson's description of it as the "repair shop" of the oculomotor system (Robinson, 1975).

Figure 4.10 shows a highly simplified diagram of the circuitry involved in VOR adaptation. A possible mapping onto the recurrent architecture of Figure 4.3A is as follows. The brainstem **B** corresponds to secondary vestibular and oculomotor neurons (together with neurons in the nucleus prepositus hypoglossi, not shown). **P** is the oculomotor plant, as described above. The input to **B** is a head velocity command, relayed via sensory processing in the semicircular canals. **C** is the flocculus (Figure 4.5) which receives as mossy-fiber input an efference copy of the motor commands sent to the eye muscles. Its climbing-fiber input signals retinal slip.

A number of lines of evidence are consistent with this mapping. The involvement of the flocculus in VOR adaptation is well established, by both classical inactivation and lesion studies in a variety of species, and more recent studies in mutant mice (e.g., De Zeeuw and Yeo, 2005). Mossy-fiber inputs to the flocculus carry an extensive array of eye-movement related signals (e.g., Miles et al., 1980), and its climbing-fiber inputs convey information related to retinal slip (e.g., Simpson et al., 1996). Floccular Purkinje cells project to ocular motoneurons, with the most direct projections having either two or three synapses. Their simple-spike firing rates are related to eye movements (more than 30 in-vivo studies in primates alone), with a number of studies providing detailed quantitative analyses of firing rates in relation to eye position, velocity, and acceleration (e.g., Gomi et al., 1998). Finally, the recurrent architecture has been shown to be capable of plant compensation in simulated VOR adaptation (Dean et al., 2002; Porrill et al., 2004).

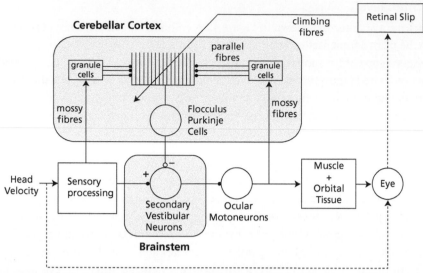

Figure 4.10 Simplified diagram of the circuitry that mediates the VOR. Head velocity signals are processed by the semicircular canals and primary vestibular neurons, relayed to secondary vestibular neurons in the brainstem, and then passed to ocular motoneurons (the classic three-neuron arc). Motor command signals from the motoneurons control the oculomotor plant, i.e., eye muscles plus orbital tissue, in order to produce eye movements that counteract the effects of the head velocity on the retinal image. Inaccurate eye movements produce retinal slip, which is detected by the visual system. A side-loop to the main three-neuron arc passes through the floccular region of the cerebellum. This region of cerebellar cortex receives as mossy-fiber input vestibular information and a copy of the motor command sent to the eye muscles. Its output is transmitted to a subset of secondary vestibular neurons (floccular target neurons) in the brainstem. The flocculus also receives a retinal slip signal as climbing-fiber input. The simplified diagram shows the efference copy of the motor commands as originating from the oculomotor neurons themselves. In reality this signal appears to originate from a number of areas, in particular the secondary vestibular nuclei, and the cell groups of the paramedian tracts (Dean and Porrill, 2008).
From Porrill and Dean (2007a), Fig 1.

However, despite these encouraging similarities, it has proved difficult to make more detailed predictions concerning, for example, changes in Purkinje cell firing during VOR adaptation. One important complicating factor has been the discovery of a site of synaptic plasticity in the brainstem (Miles and Lisberger, 1981). It appears that floccular output itself can act as a teaching signal to guide this plasticity (Lisberger, 1998; Boyden et al., 2004; Lisberger, 2009; Menzies et al., 2010; Nguyen-Vu et al., 2013). The computational role of brainstem plasticity may be a relatively straightforward transfer of high-frequency VOR gain to the brainstem (Porrill and Dean, 2007a), but the relative contributions of floccular and brainstem plasticity depend on precise experimental conditions, making the interpretation of experimental results potentially very difficult. For example, in some circumstances brainstem plasticity can be responsible for VOR adaptation on its own, with no apparent learning in cerebellar cortex (Boyden et al., 2004; Porrill and Dean, 2007a; Ke et al., 2009; McElvain et al., 2010; Menzies et al., 2010). Unraveling the experimental conditions in which different forms of plasticity are activated is proving a formidable challenge (e.g., Shin et al., 2014).

A second complicating factor is that the flocculus has functions besides plant compensation, for example improving the performance of the optokinetic reflex which is driven by retinal slip, and in primates generating smooth pursuit movements of the eye (references in e.g., Lisberger, 2009). Since these movements can themselves be adapted, interpreting changes in Purkinje cell firing requires very close attention to experimental detail. Unless special care is taken to use training conditions that rule out contributions of brainstem plasticity and the optokinetic reflex, such as adapting the VOR with high-frequency (~5 Hz) stimuli (Raymond and Lisberger, 1998; Boyden et al., 2004), interpreting experimental findings can requires increasingly complex models (e.g., Haith and Vijayakumar, 2009; Clopath et al., 2014).

Conclusions

Current evidence from studies of VOR adaptation appears compatible with the algorithm for plant compensation embodied in the recurrent architecture of Figure 4.3A, but only as part of a wider and more complex picture. The VOR has turned out not to be as simple as originally hoped, and it seems that only by understanding its complexities can even simple algorithms be evaluated. The importance of such evaluation is underscored by the apparent prevalence of recurrent loops in cerebellar connectivity. For example, a number of cerebellar regions project via the deep cerebellar nuclei and thalamus to specific areas of the cerebral cortex, which in turn project via the pons to the parent region of cerebellar cortex (reviewed by e.g., Ramnani, 2006; Bostan et al., 2013). At present the functions of these loops are unknown, but the computational analysis presented here provides a possible answer: cerebellar loops allow stable adaptive learning using only observable sensory errors. This allows the cerebellar microcircuit to be treated as a "cerebellar chip" which can be plugged into a motor system to improve performance.

An alternative solution to the "motor error" problem (Figure 4.3A) has been proposed by Kawato and coworkers (e.g., Gomi and Kawato, 1992) in which sensory errors are converted approximately to motor errors, that are then used for both adaptive learning and online feedback control. How the feedback–error–learning scheme compares with the one considered here is discussed in Porrill et al. (2013) and Haith and Vijayakumar (2009). Related issues have also been addressed in recent work exploring cerebellar-inspired control in robotics (Garrido et al., 2013; Casellato et al., 2014, 2015; Luque et al., 2014).

External circuitry: conclusions

The two examples considered here are probably the most extensively studied of all circuits involving the cerebellum. Yet the sites of synaptic plasticity within the cerebellum that underlie eyeblink conditioning and VOR adaptation have yet to be unequivocally localized. For both tasks the initial apparent simplicity proved deceptive, masking just how much experimental work was needed to establish even the basic features of the circuit.

However, at least for these circuits the effects of Purkinje cell output on climbing-fiber input appear to be relatively well understood, and seem consistent with the requirement of the LMS learning rule that the changes in synaptic plasticity it specifies do in fact reduce predictable climbing-fiber modulation. Moreover, in the case of the VOR, genetically reversing this relationship produces very severe disturbances in performance and learning (Badura et al., 2013). But it is not clear that even this basic relationship has been established for any other functional subregions of cerebellar cortex. Perhaps the third most intensively studied area is the oculomotor vermis (zone A, lobules VIb, c and VII, Figure 4.5), known to be involved in maintaining the accuracy of saccadic eye movements (Hopp and Fuchs, 2004; Iwamoto and Kaku, 2010). Here some experiments indicate that the climbing-fiber input to the oculomotor vermis conveys the information about saccadic inaccuracy required by the LMS learning rule (e.g., Soetedjo and Fuchs, 2006), but others suggest to the contrary that the climbing-fiber signal increases as adaptation proceeds (Catz et al., 2005). This controversy has yet to be fully resolved (Iwamoto and Kaku, 2010).

For the less well studied functional subregions of cerebellar cortex—numbering possibly in the thousands—the information needed to close the loop between Purkinje cell output and climbing-fiber input seems to be too meager even to generate a controversy.

Implications of the Marrian framework

Applying the Marrian framework to current research on the cerebellum suggests the following conclusions.

1 The computational task facing the cerebellar cortical microcircuit differs from those facing different areas of cortex with their unique external connections. This distinction is already familiar as the cerebellar chip metaphor (Figure 4.4).

2 The role of the microcircuit appears at this stage to be that of learning input–output mappings. A powerful algorithm is available for such learning, dependent upon the LMS learning rule. For time-varying inputs this algorithm is represented by the adaptive filter model.

3 There may be many different algorithms embodied in the distinct external connections of what is probably a very large number of functional cerebellar subregions. However, it is possible that a relatively small number of "canonical" circuits are employed a wide variety of different contexts. One candidate circuit carries out an algorithm for solving the reafference problem, which is linked to the general problem of sensory prediction; a second carries out an algorithm for solving the plant compensation problem, linked to general problems of motor control.

4 At the implementational level, a major question for the cerebellar microcircuit is whether the synaptic plasticity found there does conform to the LMS learning rule.

This question cannot be answered definitively at present, partly because the relevant sites of plasticity have not yet been localized, and partly because synaptic plasticity in vivo appears not to be simply related to forms of synaptic plasticity characterized in vitro.

5 For the proposed external circuits, evidence from apparently simple cerebellar tasks (eyeblink conditioning and VOR adaptation) indicates that their neural substrates are more complex than the algorithms would seem to require. This additional complexity makes it difficult to design experiments that can isolate different functional aspects of these circuits.

Simple algorithm, complex implementation

The problem of complexity at the implementational level is rather more severe now than it was when the Marrian framework was formulated. For example, a recent study of synaptic boutons led to the generation of "a three-dimensional model of an average synapse, displaying the 300,000 proteins in atomic detail" (Wilhelm et al., 2014, Figure 3). Whereas very large-scale detailed models may well be required to understand particular forms of neuronal dysfunction, the hope is that only some of this detail will be needed to understand normal function. Thus, many implementational features may not be concerned directly with computation, but rather with, for example, ensuring the neuron stays alive. The potential value of the Marrian approach is that it can serve as a guide through otherwise impenetrable thickets of implementational complexity.

In the case of the cerebellum where powerful algorithms are available, it is possible to start from system-level models with known computational power, and step by step add the features required for implementation by neurons and synapses. This method allows the predictions of the model to start with the simple (e.g., Figures 4.2A and 4.2B), then progress to the more detailed as the relevant evidence becomes available. A contrasting approach is to try and extract computational insights from very detailed models. The difficulties here resemble those that Marr drew attention to in the context of visual electrophysiology (Marr, 1982). However, in the case of modeling it may prove easier to combine the two approaches by exploring intermediate-level models that combine both computational power and biological detail. The case for multiscale modeling has been made at length (e.g., Sejnowski et al., 1988; Noble, 2002; Hunter and Nielsen, 2005).

Using the Marrian framework

Explicit use of the Marrian framework with its three levels of analysis is not especially common in neuroscience. A similar situation has been described for vision by Frisby and Stone (2010), who suggest two possible reasons. One is that many vision scientists may have a different view of what constitutes a theory of perception. For example, in Frisby and Stone's words "finding a link between a given visual phenomenon and a neurophysiological process amounts to *Job Done*" (p. 548). A second is that using Marr's approach requires a combination of skills that is difficult to acquire, for example competence in mathematics and understanding of techniques in electrophysiology. This latter problem seems only likely to grow, as both mathematical analysis (of e.g., machine learning) and experimental techniques grow in sophistication. As Frisby and Stone suggest, it may be that "for many the computational approach can best be pursued in a multi-disciplinary manner" (p. 548) for both vision in particular, and computational neuroscience in general.

Appendix

Derivation of the supervised learning rule

If the desired output of the filter (Figure 4.6A) is $z_d(t)$ and its actual output $z(t)$, we can define the neuron output error as the difference between actual and desired neuron output:

$$e(t) = z(t) - z_d(t) = \sum w_i p_i(t) - z_d(t) \tag{A1}$$

The mean square output error over time interval T,

$$\langle e^2 \rangle = \frac{1}{T} \int_{t_0}^{t_0+T} e(t)^2 \, dt \tag{A2}$$

provides a well-behaved measure of performance over that time (we use angle brackets to express expected or mean values). Hence we can define a cost function

$$E(w) = \frac{1}{2} \langle e^2 \rangle \tag{A3}$$

which quantifies the performance of the neuron for any given value of the weight vector $w = (w_1, w_2, \ldots, w_n)$. The optimal weight estimate (in the sense of least squares, for these data) minimizes this cost function. While many direct techniques are available to solve such minimization problems, we are looking specifically for a biologically plausible algorithm that can be implemented as a synaptic learning rule.

For a learning rate parameter β which is chosen positive and small enough, weight changes given by the gradient descent learning rule

$$\delta w_i = -\beta \frac{\partial E}{\partial w_i} \tag{A4}$$

are guaranteed to reduce the cost function (unless the gradient is zero, in which case we are already at the global minimum for the quadratic cost function we have chosen). The gradient of the cost function is

$$\frac{\partial E}{\partial w_i} = \frac{1}{2} \left\langle \frac{\partial e^2}{\partial w_i} \right\rangle = \left\langle e \frac{\partial e}{\partial w_i} \right\rangle = \langle e p_i \rangle \tag{A5}$$

hence the gradient descent learning rule can be written as

$$\delta w_i = -\beta \langle e p_i \rangle \tag{A6}$$

Since this change in weight is proportional to the correlation of $p_i(t)$ and $e(t)$, learning stops when parallel-fiber activity has zero correlation with climbing-fiber activity, hence this process is also called decorrelation learning (Dean et al., 2002).

Acknowledgments

The writing of this was supported by EPSRC grant no. EP/IO32533/1 to John Porrill.

References

Abrahamsson T, Cathala L, Matsui K, Shigemoto R, DiGregorio DA. (2012). Thin dendrites of cerebellar interneurons confer sublinear synaptic integration and a gradient of short-term plasticity. Neuron. 73:1159–1172.

Albus JS. (1971). A theory of cerebellar function. Math Biosci. 10:25–61.

Anderson SR, Pearson MJ, Pipe A, Prescott T, Dean P, Porrill J. (2010). Adaptive cancelation of self-generated sensory signals in a whisking robot. IEEE Trans Robot. 26:1065–1076.

Anderson SR, Porrill J, Pearson MJ, Pipe A, Prescott T, Dean P. (2012). An internal model architecture for novelty detection: Implications for cerebellar and collicular roles in sensory processing. PLoS ONE 7:e44560.

Andersson G, Garwicz M, Hesslow G. (1988). Evidence for a GABA-mediated cerebellar inhibition of the inferior olive in the cat. Exp Brain Res. 72:450–456.

Andersson G, Oscarsson O. (1978). Climbing fiber microzones in cerebellar vermis and their projection to different groups of cells in lateral vestibular nucleus. Exp Brain Res. 32:565–579.

Apps R, Garwicz M. (2005). Anatomical and physiological foundations of cerebellar information processing. Nat Rev Neurosci. 6:297–311.

Apps R, Hawkes R. (2009). Cerebellar cortical organization: a one-map hypothesis. Nat Rev Neurosci. 10:670–681.

Ashe J, Bushara K. (2014). The olivo-cerebellar system as a neural clock. In: Neurobiology of Interval Timing (Merchant H, de Lafuente V, eds), pp. 155–165. New York: Springer.

Badura A, Schonewille M, Voges K, Galliano E, Renier N, Gao ZY, et al. (2013). Climbing fiber input shapes reciprocity of Purkinje cell firing. Neuron. 78:700–713.

Bastian AJ. (2011). Moving, sensing and learning with cerebellar damage. Curr Opin Neurobiol. 21:596–601.

Bell C, Bodznick D, Montgomery J, Bastian J. (1997). The generation and subtraction of sensory expectations within cerebellum-like structures. Brain Behav Evol. 50:17–31.

Bell CC, Han V, Sawtell NB. (2008). Cerebellum-like structures and their implications for cerebellar function. Ann Rev Neurosci. 31:1–24.

Belmeguenai A, Hosy E, Bengtsson F, Pedroarena CM, Piochon C, Teuling E, et al. (2010). Intrinsic plasticity complements long-term potentiation in parallel fiber input gain control in cerebellar Purkinje cells. J Neurosci. 30:13630–13643.

Bengtsson F, Hesslow G. (2006). Cerebellar control of the inferior olive. Cerebellum. 5:7–14.

Bengtsson F, Jirenhed DA, Svensson P, Hesslow G. (2007). Extinction of conditioned blink responses by cerebello-olivary pathway stimulation. Neuroreport. 18:1479–1482.

Bhanpuri NH, Okamura AM, Bastian AJ. (2014). Predicting and correcting ataxia using a model of cerebellar function. Brain. **137**:1931–1944.

Blakemore SJ, Frith CD, Wolpert DM. (2001). The cerebellum is involved in predicting the sensory consequences of action. Neuroreport. **12**:1879–1884.

Blakemore SJ, Wolpert D, Frith C. (1998). Central cancellation of self-produced tickle sensation. Nat Neurosci. **1**:635–640.

Blakemore SJ, Wolpert D, Frith C. (1999). The cerebellum contributes to somatosensory cortical activity during self-produced tactile stimulation. Neuroimage. **10**:448–459.

Blakemore SJ, Wolpert D, Frith C. (2000). Why can't you tickle yourself? Neuroreport. **11**:R11–R16.

Bostan AC, Dum RP, Strick PL. (2013). Cerebellar networks with the cerebral cortex and basal ganglia. Trends Cogn Sci. **17**:241–254.

Bower JM. (1997a). Control of sensory data acquisition. Int Rev Neurobiol. **41**:489–513.

Bower JM. (1997b). Is the cerebellum sensory for motor's sake or motor for sensory's sake: the view from the whiskers of a rat? Prog Brain Res. **114**:463–496.

Bower JM, Parsons LM. (2003). Rethinking the "lesser brain." Sci Am. **289**(Aug):40–47.

Boyden ES, Katoh A, Pyle JL, Chatila TA, Tsien RW, Raymond JL. (2006). Selective engagement of plasticity mechanisms for motor memory storage. Neuron. **51**:823–834.

Boyden ES, Katoh A, Raymond JL. (2004). Cerebellum-dependent learning: the role of multiple plasticity mechanisms. Ann Rev Neurosci. **27**:581–609.

Brooks JX, Cullen KE. (2013). The primate cerebellum selectively encodes unexpected self-motion. Curr Biol. **23**:947–955.

Brown KM, Sugihara I, Shinoda Y, Ascoli GA. (2012). Digital morphometry of rat cerebellar climbing fibers reveals distinct branch and bouton types. J Neurosci. **32**:14670–14684.

Casellato C, Antonietti A, Garrido JA, Carrillo RR, Luque NR, Ros E, et al. (2014). Adaptive robotic control driven by a versatile spiking cerebellar network. PLoS ONE. **9**:e112265.

Casellato C, Antonietti A, Garrido JA, Ferrigno G, D'Angelo E, Pedrocchi A. (2015). Distributed cerebellar plasticity implements generalized multiple-scale memory components in real-robot sensorimotor tasks. Front Comput Neurosci. **9**:24.

Catz N, Dicke PW, Thier P. (2005). Cerebellar complex spike firing is suitable to induce as well as to stabilize motor learning. Curr Biol. **15**:2179–2189.

Cerminara NL, Lang EJ, Sillitoe RV, Apps R. (2015). Redefining the cerebellar cortex as an assembly of non-uniform Purkinje cell microcircuits. Nat Rev Neurosci. **16**:79–93.

Clopath C, Badura A, De Zeeuw CI, Brunel N. (2014). A cerebellar learning model of vestibulo-ocular reflex adaptation in wild-type and mutant mice. J Neurosci. **34**:7203–7215.

Coesmans M, Weber JT, De Zeeuw CI, Hansel C. (2004). Bidirectional parallel fiber plasticity in the cerebellum under climbing fiber control. Neuron. **44**:691–700.

Cullen KE. (2004). Sensory signals during active versus passive movement. Curr Opin Neurobiol. **14**:698–706.

D'Angelo E. (2014). The organization of plasticity in the cerebellar cortex: from synapses to control. Prog Brain Res. **210**:31–58.

D'Angelo E, Casali S. (2013). Seeking a unified framework for cerebellar function and dysfunction: from circuit operations to cognition. Front Neural Circuits. **6**:116.

D'Angelo E, De Zeeuw CI. (2009). Timing and plasticity in the cerebellum: focus on the granular layer. Trends Neurosci. **32**:30–40.

D'Angelo E, Koekkoek SK, Lombardo P, Solinas S, Ros E, Garrido J, et al. (2009). Timing in the cerebellum: oscillations and resonance in the granular layer. Neuroscience. **162**:805–815.

D'Angelo E, Solinas S, Mapelli J, Gandolfi D, Mapelli L, Prestori F. (2013). The cerebellar Golgi cell and spatiotemporal organization of granular layer activity. Front Neural Circuits. **7**:93.

De Schutter E. (1995). Cerebellar long term depression may normalize excitation of Purkinje cells: A hypothesis. Trends Neurosci. **18**:291–295.

De Zeeuw CI, Yeo CH. (2005). Time and tide in cerebellar memory formation. Curr Opin Neurobiol. **15**:667–674.

Dean P. (1982). Analysis of visual behavior in monkeys with inferotemporal lesions. In: Analysis of Visual Behavior (**Ingle D J** et al., eds), pp. 587–628. Cambridge, MA: MIT Press.

Dean P, Anderson S, Porrill J, Jorntell H. (2013a). An adaptive filter model of cerebellar zone C3 as a basis for safe limb control? J Physiol. **591**:5459–5474.

Dean P, Jörntell H, Porrill J. (2013b). Adaptive filter models. In: Handbook of the Cerebellum and Cerebellar Disorders (**Manto M.** et al., eds), pp. 1315–1335. Heidelberg: Springer.

Dean P, Porrill J. (2008). Oculomotor anatomy and the motor-error problem: the role of the paramedian tract nuclei. Prog Brain Res. **171**:177–186.

Dean P, Porrill J. (2014). Decorrelation learning in the cerebellum: computational analysis and experimental questions. Prog Brain Res. **210**:157–192.

Dean P, Porrill J, Ekerot CF, Jörntell H. (2010). The cerebellar microcircuit as an adaptive filter: experimental and computational evidence. Nat Rev Neurosci. **11**:30–43.

Dean P, Porrill J, Stone JV. (2002). Decorrelation control by the cerebellum achieves oculomotor plant compensation in simulated vestibulo-ocular reflex. Proc R Soc Lond B Biol Sci. **269**:1895–1904.

Dow RS, Moruzzi G. (1958). The Physiology and Pathology of the Cerebellum. Minneapolis, MN: University of Minnesota Press.

Doya K. (1999). What are the computations of the cerebellum, the basal ganglia and the cerebral cortex? Neural Netw. **12**:961–974.

Eccles JC, Ito M, Szentágothai J. (1967). The Cerebellum as a Neuronal Machine. Berlin: Springer-Verlag.

Ekerot CF, Garwicz M, Schouenborg J. (1991). Topography and nociceptive receptive fields of climbing fibres projecting to the cerebellar anterior lobe in the cat. J Physiol. **441**:257–274.

Ekerot CF, Jorntell H. (2001). Parallel fibre receptive fields of Purkinje cells and interneurons are climbing fibre-specific. Eur J Neurosci. **13**:1303–1310.

Ekerot CF, Jörntell H. (2003). Parallel fiber receptive fields: a key to understanding cerebellar operation and learning. Cerebellum. **2**:101–109.

Frisby JP, Stone JV. (2010). Seeing: The Computational Approach to Biological Vision. Cambridge, MA: MIT Press.

Frisby JP, Stone JV. (2012). Marr: An appreciation. Perception. **41**:1040–1052.

Fujita M. (1982). Adaptive filter model of the cerebellum. Biol Cybern. **45**:195–206.

Gao ZY, van Beugen BJ, De Zeeuw CI. (2012). Distributed synergistic plasticity and cerebellar learning. Nat Rev Neurosci. **13**:619–635.

Garrido JA, Luque NR, D'Angelo E, Ros E. (2013). Distributed cerebellar plasticity implements adaptable gain control in a manipulation task: a closed-loop robotic simulation. Front Neural Circuits. **7**:159.

Glickstein M, Strata P, Voogd J. (2009). Cerebellum: history. Neuroscience. **162**:549–559.

Glickstein M, Sultan F, Voogd J. (2011). Functional localization in the cerebellum. Cortex. **47**:59–80.

Glickstein M, Voogd J. (1995). Lodewijk Bolk and the comparative anatomy of the cerebellum. Trends Neurosci. **18**:206–211.

Gomi H, Kawato M. (1992). Adaptive feedback control models of the vestibulocerebellum and spinocerebellum. Biol Cybern. **68**:105–114.

Gomi H, Shidara M, Takemura A, Inoue Y, Kawano K, Kawato M. (1998). Temporal firing patterns of Purkinje cells in the cerebellar ventral paraflocculus during ocular following responses in monkeys I. Simple spikes. J Neurophysiol. **80**:818–831.

Grossberg S, Schmajuk NA. (1989). Neural dynamics of adaptive timing and temporal discrimination during associative learning. Neural Netw. **2**:79–102.

Haith A, Vijayakumar S. (2009). Implications of different classes of sensorimotor disturbance for cerebellar-based motor learning models. Biol Cybern. **100**:81–95.

Hansel C, Linden DJ, D'Angelo E. (2001). Beyond parallel fiber LTD: the diversity of synaptic and non-synaptic plasticity in the cerebellum. Nat Neurosci. **4**:467–475.

Herculano-Houzel S. (2009). The human brain in numbers: a linearly scaled-up primate brain. Front Human Neurosci. **3**:31.

Herrick CJ. (1924). Origin and evolution of the cerebellum. Arch Neurol Psychiatry. **11**:621–652.

Hesslow G, Ivarsson M. (1996). Inhibition of the inferior olive during conditioned responses in the decerebrate ferret. Exp Brain Res. **110**:36–46.

Hesslow G, Jirenhed DA, Rasmussen A, Johansson F. (2013). Classical conditioning of motor responses: What is the learning mechanism? Neural Netw. **47**:81–87.

Hesslow G, Yeo CH. (2002). The functional anatomy of skeletal conditioning. In: A Neuroscientist's Guide to Classical Conditioning (Moore JW, ed.), pp. 86–146. New York: Springer.

Holmes G. (1939). The cerebellum of man. The Hughlings Jackson Memorial Lecture. Brain. **62**:1–30.

Hopp JJ, Fuchs AF. (2004). The characteristics and neuronal substrate of saccadic eye movement plasticity. Prog Neurobiol. **72**:27–53.

Huhta JC, Webster JG. (1973). 60-Hz interference in electrocardiography. IEEE Trans Biomed Eng. **BM20**:91–101.

Hunter P, Nielsen P. (2005). A strategy for integrative computational physiology. Physiology. **20**:316–325.

Imamizu H. (2010). Prediction of sensorimotor feedback from the efference copy of motor commands: A review of behavioral and functional neuroimaging studies. Japanese Psychol Res. **52**:107–120.

Isope P, Barbour B. (2002). Properties of unitary granule cell→Purkinje cell synapses in adult rat cerebellar slices. J Neurosci. **22**:9668–9678.

Ito M. (1970). Neurophysiological aspects of the cerebellar motor control system. Int J Neurol. **7**:162–176.

Ito M. (1984). The Cerebellum and Neural Control. New York: Raven Press.

Ito M. (1997). Cerebellar microcomplexes. Int Rev Neurobiol. **41**:475–487.

Ito M. (2012). The Cerebellum: Brain for an Implicit Self. Upper Saddle River, NJ: FT Press.

Ito M, Sakurai M, Tongroach P. (1982). Climbing fibre induced depression of both mossy fibre responsiveness and glutamate sensitivity of cerebellar Purkinje cells. J Physiol. **324**:113–134.

Ito M, Yamaguchi K, Nagao S, Yamazaki T. (2014). Long-term depression as a model of cerebellar plasticity. Prog Brain Res. **210**:1–30.

Iwamoto Y, Kaku Y. (2010). Saccade adaptation as a model of learning in voluntary movements. Exp Brain Res. **204**:145–162.

Jacobson GA, Rokni D, Yarom Y. (2008). A model of the olivo-cerebellar system as a temporal pattern generator. Trends Neurosci. **31**:617–625.

Jirenhed DA, Bengtsson F, Hesslow G. (2007). Acquisition, extinction, and reacquisition of a cerebellar cortical memory trace. J Neurosci. **27**:2493–2502.

Jirenhed DA, Bengtsson F, Jörntell H. (2013). Parallel fiber and climbing fiber responses in rat cerebellar cortical neurons in vivo. Front Syst Neurosci. **7**:16.

Jordan MI. (1996). Computational aspects of motor control and motor learning. In: Handbook of Perception and Action, Volume 2: Motor Skills (**Heuer H, Keele, S,** eds), pp. 71–120. London: Academic Press.

Jordan MI, Rumelhart DE. (1992). Forward models—Supervised learning with a distal teacher. Cogn Sci. **16**:307–354.

Jörntell H, Bengtsson F, Schonewille M, De Zeeuw CI. (2010). Cerebellar molecular layer interneurons—computational properties and roles in learning. Trends Neurosci. **33**:524–532.

Jörntell H, Ekerot CF. (2002). Reciprocal bidirectional plasticity of parallel fiber receptive fields in cerebellar Purkinje cells and their afferent interneurons. Neuron. **34**:797–806.

Jörntell H, Ekerot CF. (2003). Receptive field plasticity profoundly alters the cutaneous parallel fiber synaptic input to cerebellar interneurons in vivo. J Neurosci. **23**:9620–9631.

Jörntell H, Ekerot CF. (2011). Receptive field remodeling induced by skin stimulation in cerebellar neurons in vivo. Front Neural Circuits. **5**:3.

Jörntell H, Hansel C. (2006). Synaptic memories upside down: bidirectional plasticity at cerebellar parallel fiber-Purkinje cell synapses. Neuron. **52**:227–238.

Ke MC, Guo CC, Raymond JL. (2009). Elimination of climbing fiber instructive signals during motor learning. Nat Neurosci. **12**:1171–1179.

Keating JG, Thach WT. (1995). Nonclock behavior of inferior olive neurons: Interspike interval of Purkinje cell complex spike discharge in the awake behaving monkey is random. J Neurophysiol. **73**:1329–1340.

Keren-Happuch E, Chen SHA, Ho MHR, Desmond JE. (2014). A meta-analysis of cerebellar contributions to higher cognition from PET and fMRI studies. Hum Brain Mapp. **35**:593–615.

Kim JJ, Krupa DJ, Thompson RF. (1998). Inhibitory cerebello-olivary projections and blocking effect in classical conditioning. Science. **279**:570–572.

Lepora N, Porrill J, Yeo CH, Dean P. (2010). Sensory prediction or motor control? Application of Marr-Albus models of cerebellar function to classical conditioning. Front Comput Neurosci. **4**:1–16.

Lev-Ram V, Mehta SB, Kleinfeld D, Tsien RY. (2003). Reversing cerebellar long-term depression. Proc Natl Acad Sci U S A. **100**:15989–15993.

Lev-Ram V, Wong ST, Storm DR, Tsien RY. (2002). A new form of cerebellar long-term potentiation is postsynaptic and depends on nitric oxide but not cAMP. Proc Natl Acad Sci U S A. **99**:8389–8393.

Lisberger SG. (1998). Physiologic basis for motor learning in the vestibulo-ocular reflex. Otolaryngology. **119**:43–48.

Lisberger SG. (2009). Internal models of eye movement in the floccular complex of the monkey cerebellum. Neuroscience. **162**:763–776.

Llinás RR, Leznik E, Makarenko VI. (2004). The olivo-cerebellar circuit as a universal motor control system. IEEE J Ocean Eng. **29**:631–639.

Luque NR, Garrido JA, Carrillo RR, D'Angelo E, Ros E. (2014). Fast convergence of learning requires plasticity between inferior olive and deep cerebellar nuclei in a manipulation task: a closed-loop robotic simulation. Front Comput Neurosci. **8**:97.

Manni E, Petrosini L. (2004). A century of cerebellar somatotopy: a debated representation. Nat Neurosci Rev. **5**:241–249.

Mapelli L, Pagani M, Garrido JA, D'Angelo E. (2015). Integrated plasticity at inhibitory and excitatory synapses in the cerebellar circuit. Front Cell Neurosci. **9**:169.

Marr D. (1982). Vision: A Computational Investigation into the Human Representation and Processing of Visual Information. San Francisco: W. H. Freeman.

Marr DC, Poggio T. (1977). From understanding computation to understanding neural circuitry. Neurosci Res Program Bull. **15**:470–491.

Marzban H, Hawkes R. (2011). On the architecture of the posterior zone of the cerebellum. Cerebellum. **10**:422–434.

McElvain LE, Bagnall MW, Sakatos A, du Lac S. (2010). Bidirectional plasticity gated by hyperpolarization controls the gain of postsynaptic firing responses at central vestibular nerve synapses. Neuron. **68**:763–775.

Medina JF. (2011). The multiple roles of Purkinje cells in sensori-motor calibration: to predict, teach and command. Curr Opin Neurobiol. **21**:616–622.

Medina JF, Nores WL, Mauk MD. (2002). Inhibition of climbing fibres is a signal for the extinction of conditioned eyelid responses. Nature. **416**:330–333.

Medina JF, Nores WL, Ohyama T, Mauk MD. (2000). Mechanisms of cerebellar learning suggested by eyelid conditioning. Curr Opin Neurobiol. **10**:717–724.

Menzies JRW, Porrill J, Dutia M, Dean P. (2010). Synaptic plasticity in medial vestibular nucleus neurons: Comparison with computational requirements of VOR adaptation. PLoS ONE **5**:e13182.

Miles FA, Fuller JH, Braitman DJ, Dow BM. (1980). Long-term adaptive changes in primate vestibuloocular reflex. III. Electrophysiological observations in flocculus of normal monkeys. J Neurophysiol. **43**:1437–1476.

Miles FA, Lisberger SG. (1981). Plasticity in the vestibulo-ocular reflex—a new hypothesis. Ann Rev Neurosci. **4**:273–299.

Montgomery JC, Bodznick D, Yopak KE. (2012). The cerebellum and cerebellum-like structures of cartilaginous fishes. Brain Behav Evol. **80**:152–165.

Moore JW, Desmond JE, Berthier NE. (1989). Adaptively timed conditioned responses and the cerebellum: a neural network approach. Biol Cybern. **62**:17–28.

Mostofi A, Holtzman T, Grout AS, Yeo CH, Edgley SA. (2010). Electrophysiological localization of eyeblink-related microzones in rabbit cerebellar cortex. J Neurosci. **30**:8920–8934.

Nguyen-Vu TDB, Kimpo RR, Rinaldi JM, Kohli A, Zeng HK, Deisseroth K, Raymond JL. (2013). Cerebellar Purkinje cell activity drives motor learning. Nat Neurosci. **16**:1734–1736.

Nicholson DA, Freeman JH. (2003). Addition of inhibition in the olivocerebellar system and the ontogeny of a motor memory. Nat Neurosci. **6**:532–537.

Nisimaru N, Mittal C, Shirai Y, Sooksawate T, Anandaraj P, Hashikawa T, et al. (2013). Orexin-neuromodulated cerebellar circuit controls redistribution of arterial blood flows for defense behavior in rabbits. Proc Natl Acad Sci U S A. **110**:14124–14131.

Noble D. (2002). Modeling the heart—from genes and cells to the whole organ. Science. **295**:1678–1682.

Porrill J, Dean P. (2007a). Cerebellar motor learning: when is cortical plasticity not enough? PLoS Comput Biol. **3**:1935–1950.

Porrill J, Dean P. (2007b). Recurrent cerebellar loops simplify adaptive control of redundant and nonlinear motor systems. Neural Comput. **19**:170–193.

Porrill J, Dean P. (2008). Silent synapses, LTP and the indirect parallel-fibre pathway: computational consequences of optimal noise processing. PLoS Comput Biol **4**:e1000085.

Porrill J, Dean P, Anderson SR. (2013). Adaptive filters and internal models: Multilevel description of cerebellar function. Neural Netw. **47**:134–149.

Porrill J, Dean P, Stone JV. (2004). Recurrent cerebellar architecture solves the motor error problem. Proc R Soc Lond B Biol Sci. **271**:789–796.

Ramnani N. (2006). The primate cortico-cerebellar system: anatomy and function. Nat Rev Neurosci. **7**:511–522.

Rasmussen A, Jirenhed DA, Hesslow G. (2008). Simple and complex spike firing patterns in Purkinje cells during classical conditioning. Cerebellum. **7**:563–566.

Raymond JL, Lisberger SG. (1998). Neural learning rules for the vestibulo-ocular reflex. J Neurosci. 18:9112–9129.

Requarth T, Sawtell NB. (2011). Neural mechanisms for filtering self-generated sensory signals in cerebellum-like circuits. Curr Opin Neurobiol. 21:602–608.

Rescorla RA, Wagner AR. (1972). A theory of Pavlovian conditioning: Variations in the effectiveness of reinforcement and non-reinforcement. In: Classical Conditioning II: Current Research and Theory (Black AH, Prokasy WF, eds), pp. 64–99. New York: Appleton-Century-Crofts.

Robinson DA. (1975). How the oculomotor system repairs itself. Invest Ophthalmol. 14:413–415.

Rössert C, Solinas S, D'Angelo E, Dean P, Porrill J. (2014). Model cerebellar granule cells can faithfully transmit modulated firing rate signals. Front Cell Neurosci. 8:304.

Roth MJ, Synofzik M, Lindner A. (2013). The cerebellum optimizes perceptual predictions about external sensory events. Curr Biol. 23:930–935.

Schmahmann JD. (2010). The role of the cerebellum in cognition and emotion: personal reflections since 1982 on the dysmetria of thought hypothesis, and its historical evolution from theory to therapy. Neuropsychol Rev. 20:236–260.

Schonewille M, Belmeguenai A, Koekkoek SK, Houtman SH, Boele HJ, van Beugen BJ, et al. (2010). Purkinje cell-specific knockout of the protein phosphatase PP2B impairs potentiation and cerebellar motor learning. Neuron. 67:618–628.

Schonewille M, Gao Z, Boele HJ, Vinueza Veloz MF, Amerika WE, Simek AA, et al. (2011). Reevaluating the role of LTD in cerebellar motor learning. Neuron. 70:43–50.

Scott M. (2013). Corollary discharge provides the sensory content of inner speech. Psychol Sci. 24:1824–1830.

Sears LL, Steinmetz JE. (1991). Dorsal accessory olive activity diminishes during acquisition of the rabbit classically conditioned eyelid response. Brain Res. 545:112–122.

Sejnowski TJ, Koch C, Churchland PS. (1988). Computational neuroscience. Science. 241:1299–1306.

Shadmehr R, Wise SP. (2005). The Computational Neurobiology of Reaching and Pointing: A Foundation for Motor Learning. Cambridge, MA: MIT Press.

Shin SL, Zhao GQ, Raymond JL. (2014). Signals and learning rules guiding oculomotor plasticity. J Neurosci. 34:10635–10644.

Simpson JI, Wylie DR, De Zeeuw CI. (1996). On climbing fiber signals and their consequence(s). Behav Brain Sci. 19:384–398.

Skavenski AA, Robinson DA. (1973). Role of abducens neurons in vestibuloocular reflex. J Neurophysiol. 36:724–738.

Snyder WE. (1985). Industrial Robots: Computer Interfacing and Control. Englewood-Cliffs, NJ: Prentice-Hall.

Soetedjo R, Fuchs AF. (2006). Complex spike activity of Purkinje cells in the oculomotor vermis during behavioral adaptation of monkey saccades. J Neurosci. 26:7741–7755.

Spanne A, Jorntell H. (2013). Processing of multi-dimensional sensorimotor information in the spinal and cerebellar neuronal circuitry: a new hypothesis. PLoS Comput Biol 9:e1002979.

Stoodley CJ, Schmahmann JD. (2009). Functional topography in the human cerebellum: a meta-analysis of neuroimaging studies. Neuroimage. 44:489–501.

Sugihara I, Shinoda Y. (2004). Molecular, topographic, and functional organization of the cerebellar cortex: A study with combined aldolase C and olivocerebellar labeling. J Neurosci. 24:8771–8785.

Thompson RF, Steinmetz JE. (2009). The role of the cerebellum in classical conditioning of discrete behavioral responses. Neuroscience. 162:732–755.

Van Overwalle F, Baetens K, Marien P, Vandekerckhove M. (2014). Social cognition and the cerebellum: A meta-analysis of over 350 fMRI studies. NeuroImage. 86:554–572.

Voogd J. (2011). Cerebellar zones: A personal history. Cerebellum. **10**:334–350.

Voogd J, Ruigrok TJH. (2004). The organization of the corticonuclear and olivocerebellar climbing fiber projections to the rat cerebellar vermis: The congruence of projection zones and the zebrin pattern. J Neurocytol. **33**:5–21.

Weiskrantz L, Elliott J, Darlington C. (1971). Preliminary observations of tickling oneself. Nature. **230**:598–599.

Widrow B, Stearns SD. (1985). Adaptive Signal Processing. Englewood Cliffs, NJ: Prentice-Hall.

Wilhelm BG, Mandad S, Truckenbrodt S, Krohnert K, Schafer C, Rammner B, et al. (2014). Composition of isolated synaptic boutons reveals the amounts of vesicle trafficking proteins. Science. **344**:1023–1028.

Willems RM. (2011). Re-appreciating the why of cognition: 35 years after Marr and Poggio. Front Psychol. **2**:244.

Wolpert DM, Miall RC, Kawato M. (1998). Internal models in the cerebellum. Trends Cogn Sci. **2**:338–347.

Yamazaki T, Nagao S, Lennon W, Tanaka S. (2015). Modeling memory consolidation during posttraining periods in cerebellovestibular learning. Proc Natl Acad Sci U S A. **112**:3541–3546.

Yamazaki T, Tanaka S. (2009). Computational models of timing mechanisms in the cerebellar granular layer. Cerebellum. **8**:423–432.

Section 2

Simple memory: A theory for archicortex

Chapter 5

The dentate gyrus: defining a new memory of David Marr

Alessandro Treves

Memory versus space

The 2014 Nobel Prize in Medicine or Physiology, awarded while this volume was in preparation, has been also the conclusion of a long, sweeping gesture to salute David Marr. In a bizarre variant of the *surya namaskara*, the sun salutation, it began in 1971 with the near-simultaneous publication of his theory of simple memory on the one hand, and of the discovery of place cells by John O'Keefe and John Dostrovsky on the other (Marr, 1971; O'Keefe and Dostrovsky, 1971). A discovery leading in an almost orthogonal direction, pointing toward the spatial computations that might lead to place cell coding, rather than toward understanding memory formation. The discovery of associative synaptic plasticity in the hippocampus, first reported also around the same time, may be regarded within the salutation as the forward bend standing with feet firmly on the ground - but that is another story (Bliss and Lomo, 1973).

After the insightful but largely overlooked paper by Tony Gardner-Medwin in 1976, the two hands appeared to come together again with the review by Bruce McNaughton and Richard Morris (1987) in *Trends in Neuroscience* on Hebb–Marr networks and their potential use as models of hippocampal circuits. The leading pioneer of large-scale place cell single-unit recording and the inventor of the water maze for assessing spatial memory were bringing Marr's ideas to the attention of the rodent neuroscience community. Another dramatic discovery that year, to be appreciated only gradually: that of *remapping* by Bob Muller and John Kubie (1987), indicating that the essence of the place cell code was likely not in the exact spatial computations that produce it from an array of sensory inputs but rather in the flexibility with which new representations can be formed when the spatial environment is changed. Could we, then, take place cells as a model for analysing the mechanisms behind this flexibility, and if so serve as an expedient, practical approach toward memory formation?

It was to be only a brief crossover. In the years following 1987 the two hands again swept in orthogonal directions. In Jerusalem, through the interdisciplinary year on Physics and the Brain at the Institute of Advanced Studies, a whole and entirely different community of statistical physicists was embracing models of associative memory and striving to make them neurally plausible, while retaining their amenability to rigorous quantitative analysis (Amit, 1989). They were following the trajectory imagined by David Marr, even though most of them knew little of Marr or of what the hippocampus was, and did not know that place cells had been discovered there without asking for Marr's permission. Attractor neural networks were conceived by the physicists to store discrete patterns of activity, often implemented with binary variables, nothing to do with space or with the representation of continuous variables in general. Simple associative memories had become a theoretical domain in their own right, disengaged from the hippocampus.

On the other hand, the experimental analysis of place cells focused on explaining the dependence of their spatial selectivity on particular sensory components, such as distal versus proximal visual cues or olfactory cues, culminating in the "geometrical determinants" of the boundary vector cell model of O'Keefe and Neil Burgess (1996), which—except in the generic sense discussed by Becker (2015)—has nothing to do with memory. Place cells seemed quintessential to the hippocampus, even though earlier models had suggested that place cell coding per se may not be informative about the logic of hippocampal design (Sharp, 1991; Treves et al., 1992). Furthermore, Edmund Rolls had *not*, over several years of attempts, observed place cells in the monkey hippocampus which, like that of all mammals, has the same design as the rodent one. Instead, he observed spatial view cells (Rolls et al., 1997) but in such low numbers, relative to the prevalence of place cells in rat, as to hardly offer sufficient material to construct a divergent theory of hippocampal function, Rolls has consistently developed a theory in the Marr tradition, extending it to apply to visuospatial memory in primates (Rolls 1989, 1996; Rolls and Kesner, 2006).

Associative memories on the one hand, therefore, and place cells expressing spatial computations on the other. Two perspectives finally reconciled, in a most surprising twist, by the discovery of grid cells (Fyhn et al., 2004, Hafting et al., 2005). By using the O'Keefe approach of recording single cells in rodents and assessing their spatial selectivity, the Mosers (Fyhn et al., 2007; Moser and Moser, 2008) have shown that there are clearly more sophisticated spatial computations; but they occur upstream of the hippocampus in the flow of information, in entorhinal cortex. Unshackled from having to toil over space, the hippocampus remains entitled to use spatial computations produced by other structures, and is now free to focus on memory.

Marr's view of the dentate gyrus

With Marr's memory perspective, and half a century of human neuropsychology, vindicated by the grid cells, the road should have been open to understand hippocampal design in engineering detail. After all, the design is the same across mammals. Marr's approach, with its elaborate set of statements about the properties of different cell types, while not conclusive, could have provided a roadmap. Yet, two problems arise: the lack of a real dentate gyrus in David Marr, and the lack of a real dentate gyrus in vertebrates other than mammals.

Marr characterizes the dentate granule cells in his 1971 paper as "extensions to the dendritic trees of the CA pyramidal cells" (p. 69) and appears to be at a loss assigning them a specific function. Having assumed that nonstructured patterns of activity in the cornu ammonis subfields represent sensory information in the cortex, he states that "simple representations are set up in F[ascia] D[entata] in the same way as in CA1 to CA3" and motivates this somewhat disappointing dismissal with the observation that "the proposed scheme will result in a saving in the total number of cells transmitting simple representations elsewhere" (because granule cells only transmit them locally to CA3) so that "elsewhere" there will be savings "in the numbers of cells and synapses needed to deal with them."

A bit like trainee journalists who are assigned to research on the same topics as the accomplished professionals, but only so that the latter can cherry-pick some of their findings. They are not to write anything of their own, taking up precious space on the paper. The trainees should not feel useless or exploited, Marr condescends, because "if the amount of afferent information to be dealt with requires more cells than this, something like the proposed theory for the [granule cells] becomes the natural scheme to adopt". The trainees can help by filtering out the excess information, which would otherwise waste the time and energy of the real professionals. But while human trainees can perhaps hope, one day, to become professionals, the destitute, basal-dendrite-deprived granule cells had been genetically consigned to the bottom of a very British hierarchy forever.

Yet, the very interneuronal character of the granule cells, with their axonal projections limited to CA3, is one of two striking novel ideas in the evolution of the mammalian nervous system, along with neocortical lamination (Figures 5.1 and 5.2). The homolog small

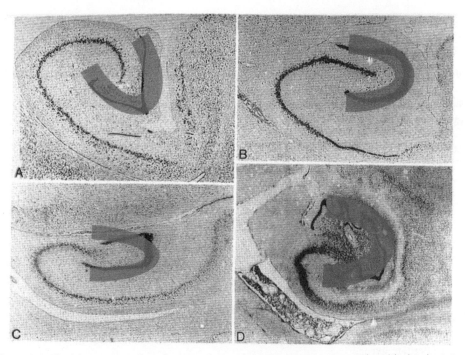

Figure 5.1 The hippocampus has the same internal structure across mammals, with the dentate gyrus, highlighted, as its salient component. Background cross-sections, assembled in the splendid book by Pierre Gloor (1997), from (A) a platypus, (B) a rat, (C) a cat, and (D) a human hippocampus.

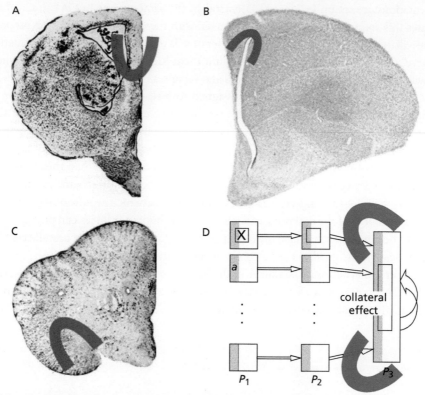

Figure 5.2 A bona fide dentate gyrus is not seen in the hippocampus of other vertebrate classes (A–C), nor in the computational scheme by David Marr (D). Background unilateral cross-sections, with the hypothetical position of the missing dentate gyrus highlighted, through the forebrain of (A) a turtle (from Reiner and Powers, 1983); (B) a pigeon (from Margoliash et al., 2010); (C) a sea bass (from Cerda-Reverter et al., 2001). These cartoons are solely for visual impression; a discussion among avian anatomists is referred to by Treves et al. (2008), and see Gupta et al. (2012) for a thorough study in the chick; see also Herold et al. (2015).

A: Reiner A, Powers AS, The effects of lesions of telencephalic visual structures on visual discriminative performance in turtles. in The Journal of Comparative Neurology © 1983 John Wiley and Sons with permission from John Wiley and Sons.

B: Daniel Margoliash, Wim van Drongelen, and Michael Kohrman, Introducing Songbirds as a Model System for Epilepsy Research, Journal of Clinical Neurophysiology, 27.6 © 2010 with permission from Wolters Kluwer Health.

C: Cerda-Reverter JM, Zanuy S, Munoz-Cueto, JA, Cytoarchitectonic study of the brain of a perciform species, the sea bass. Journal of morphology © 2001 John Wiley and Sons, with permission from John Wiley and Sons.

cells of the reptilian and avian medial pallium are not inserted in the circuitry quite in the same way as their mammalian counterparts (Atoji and Wild, 2004; Treves et al., 2008; Gupta et al., 2012). We are mammals, to a great extent, because we have a modern mammalian dentate gyrus.

And here is the second problem: nonmammals, lacking the dentate gyrus, do not seem to be automatically inferior in spatial memory, subserved by their medial pallium or hippocampal homolog. The most striking evidence is from birds (Sherry and Vaccarino,

1989; Clayton and Krebs, 1995; Gagliardo et al., 2001; Emery and Clayton, 2004; Cnotka et al., 2008), who are similar to mammals in some of the fundamental principles of forebrain organization (Shanahan et al., 2013). There are also, however, indications to the same effect from reptiles and even from fish (Rodríguez et al., 2002). So is the dentate gyrus irrelevant to hippocampal function? And if so, maybe Marr's cavalier attitude was in fact justified?

Learning in associative networks

Marr's 1971 theory was essentially a theory of associative retrieval, which assumed that the representations had been already established to start with. Similarly, the Hopfield (1982) model describes associative retrieval, assuming that p discrete patterns of activity have been encoded in the synaptic weights, and thus turned into dynamical *attractors*, toward which the network converges if stimulated with a partial cue. Amit, Gutfreund, and Sompolinsky (1987) then showed how to use techniques from statistical physics to estimate an upper bound p_c on the number of attractors that can be retrieved, an analysis that can be extended to networks of more neuron-like threshold-linear units (Treves, 1990) but again without detailing how those patterns have been generated in the first place.

This sin of omission is serious because establishing novel representations in a recurrent network is highly nontrivial: the attractors already stored interfere, and the result is new representations which collage fragments of older ones, or at least which encode limited novel information (Treves and Rolls, 1992). Suppressing this interference requires suppressing activity on the recurrent synapses, yet these synapses have to be plastic to undergo the modifications that enable later associative retrieval of the new representation. How can the dilemma be resolved? Marr (1971, p. 35) addresses this only by pointing out that the neural activity for events that are to be stored should be much larger than for events that initiate recall.

The statistical physicists studying the Hopfield model and its variants, on the other hand, did not pay much attention to the dilemma and for two reasons. First, it is common sense to tackle one problem at a time, focusing on retrieval first; second, they had a rudimentary skeleton of a "learning" process in the one-shot encoding of all representations, up front, through the celebrated covariance rule (Sejnowski, 1977) or one of its variants, all of these being models of the mechanism postulated by Donald Hebb (1948). Some attention was also paid to alternative forms of encoding that suppress interference, such as the so-called pseudo-inverse rule (Kanter and Sompolinsky, 1987), but soon it was realized that the covariance rule is as good as any in the relevant regime of sparse activity and similarly sparse synaptic connections or, to use the jargon of the time, *diluted* connectivity (Treves, 1991). The proviso is that it would be necessary for the activity patterns to be fixed or *clamped* without interference from existing memories. Sparsely active encoding schemes present advantages of their own (see Becker, Chapter 7 of this volume), even outside a theory of autoassociative retrieval. The main competing account, the back-propagating networks studied mainly by computer scientists and engineers across the

Atlantic, did not even attempt to portray a neurally plausible learning process. Associative memories in the physics style at least envisaged a plausible ("local") explicit procedure for altering synaptic efficacies, never mind if on the basis of activity patterns clamped by hand (Amit, 1989), as if prescribed by divine fiat.

In the 1990s Mike Hasselmo and collaborators were perhaps the first to point out, from a computational vantage point, that the challenge of establishing new representations while suppressing interference by older ones can be addressed by sprinkling the circuit with acetylcholine. As shown in piriform cortex and then in the hippocampus (Hasselmo and Bower, 1993; Hasselmo and Schnell, 1994, Hasselmo et al., 1995), acetylcholine suppresses transmission along the recurrent collateral connections, those producing the bulk of the interference, while enhancing their plasticity, thus facilitating their future encoding. An amazing trick. Even more amazing, it appears to operate across the board, both across species and across brain structures (Woolf, 1991; Petrillo et al., 1994). In the metaphor already used, acetylcholine encourages the professional journalists to control their opinions and prejudices, so that what they report actually reflects also a modicum of new facts.

That seems like a good strategy in order to acquire new information in a simple, e.g., unimodal, context. But if this is complex multimodal information and it is to be stored for a long time, that is, together with many other items, is it also an effective manner to establish a proper representation? In the mammalian hippocampus, devoted to long-term storage, this generic solution may not suffice.

Since CA3 also receives direct, perforant path connections from entorhinal cortex, the DG inputs to CA3, the mossy fibers, appear to essentially duplicate the information that CA3 can already receive directly from the source. Bruce McNaughton, with his "detonator" synapses, promoted a radically new idea in his 1987 paper with Richard Morris. Although subsequent research has painted a more complex picture (Kerr and Jonas, 2008), let us stick to the simplified detonator idea for the moment, that one mossy fiber can trigger activity in a receiving CA3 cell. If a single dentate granule cell is sufficient to activate a CA3 cell, it is a bit like pairing each professional with a trainee. It is the trainee who dictates the paper to the professional, independently (these particular trainees do not talk to each other). Later, the report composed by the professionals, under dictation by all the trainees, is *redefined* as expressing the novel information with which it is associated.

Prejudices are not just suppressed, they are cleaned away. The report appears as a random collection of disparate statements, but in the end they are just signifiers, and the content to be signified sticks to them through the glue of associative synaptic plasticity. In neuronal terms, the interference problem is resolved because correlations between representations are removed, thanks to the randomizing action of the mossy fibers. If the mossy fiber inputs are those that drive the storage of new representations, the perforant path can then relay the cue that initiates the retrieval of a previously stored representation; the cue is effective because it has been associated in the learning phase with the random pattern in CA3 (Treves and Rolls, 1992). Retrieval can subsequently proceed through attractor dynamics, due largely to recurrent connections in CA3.

Learning new spatial maps

What may seem like an incitement toward dentate anarchy, or outright confabulation, appears in fact to make quantitative sense, at least in a simplified mathematical model based on the storage of discrete memory patterns (Treves and Rolls, 1992). What is critical is the distinction between a storage, or learning, or training phase, and a retrieval phase when the dentate becomes irrelevant. The distinction is missed by connectionist models based on training weights through backpropagation, a rendering of synaptic plasticity so implausible as to be better swept under the carpet.

Many models talk generically about the dentate performing *pattern separation*, without elaborating that pattern separation is only useful during storage. The distinction is easily blurred, however, also in real life, especially in spatially or temporally continuous behaviors. Whereas with strictly discrete events one can think of each of their occurrences as being either storage or retrieval, when for example a rat is continuously exploring an environment, periods when inputs are unequivocal and there is no need to retrieve anything from memory may be admixed with other periods in which inputs temporarily subside, and some degree of *pattern completion* is helpful, and with yet other periods in which new information is stored.

Specifically in rodents, spatial exploration is usually accompanied by prominent theta oscillations in the hippocampus, which may themselves partially separate storage from retrieval, as afferent inputs tend to arrive out of phase with each other and with recurrent activity (see Hasselmo, Chapter 6 of this volume). It would, however, take much stronger theta modulation for a full separation (Stella and Treves, 2011) and the effect is just barely discernible in experimental recordings (Jezek et al., 2011).

Nevertheless, the first attempts to test the idea of a critical dentate role in learning, have come from rodents and in spatial paradigms. Two distinct studies have provided cogent indications, with different techniques, of the necessity for a functioning dentate gyrus to learn either a Morris water maze (Lassalle et al., 2000) or a dry maze (Lee and Kesner, 2004). Once the mazes are learned, DG lesions are ineffective, as they are on retrieving a visual context (Ahn and Lee, 2014). So if the model says that the dentate is needed to establish memories, but the experiments provide tentative evidence that it is needed to establish *spatial* memories, does that mean that it is indeed involved in spatial computations, the role we had dismissed? Does it mean that in order to understand what the dentate does we have to go back to the vectors and bearings and vector sums that we forgot after high school?

If we cannot avoid it, fine, let us think in geometrical terms; but in the abstract, very high-dimensional phase space of the CA3 network. Two-dimensional spatial representations of each position in an environment, to be usable for associative memory, must be compatible with an attractor dynamics scenario. This requires a *multiplicity* of memory states, which approximate one two-dimensional continuous manifold embedded in the phase space, isomorphic to the real spatial environment to be represented. This suggests a memory state up in phase space for each "distinguishable" position down in the environment. Moreover, there has to be a multiplicity of manifolds, to represent distinct environments, with complete remapping from one to the other (Leutgeb et al., 2005). Attractor dynamics then occurs along the dimensions locally *orthogonal* to each manifold, as in the simplified "multi-chart" model (Samsonovich and McNaughton, 1997; Battaglia and Treves, 1998).

Tangentially one expects marginal stability, allowing for small signals related to the movement of the animal, reflecting changing sensory cues as well as path integration, to displace a "bump" of activity on the manifold as appropriate (Samsonovich and McNaughton, 1997; Stringer et al., 2002). Excess forward displacement, that can be produced by adaptation (Treves, 2004), implies coding the position of the animal slightly into the future; and this leads to a capacity for prediction that may be part and parcel of that for associative retrieval (Byrne et al., 2007, and Becker, Chapter 7 of this volume). This dual nature of the dynamics has been captured qualitatively with a highly simplified model, comprised of binary units, in a strikingly beautiful series of mathematical studies (Monasson and Rosay, 2013, 2014, 2015).

To turn these requirements into a somewhat more realistic model, amenable to the extraction of quantitative measures, one needs the experimental discoveries that largely clarified, in the rodent, the nature of the spatial representations in the regions that feed into CA3. First, roughly half of the entorhinal perforant path (PP) inputs, those coming from layer II of the medial portion of entorhinal cortex, were found to be often in the form of "pure" grid cells (Hafting et al., 2005; Sargolini et al., 2006). Second, the other half, those coming from layer II of the lateral entorhinal cortex, were found not to convey precise location specific information, but if anything to code for the spatial context as defined by objects, object novelty, and object–place associations (Deshmukh and Knierim, 2011; Neunuebel et al., 2013; Knierim et al., 2014). Third, and most important, the DG granule cell activity was earlier described as very sparse, with a tendency to fragment into discontiguous subfields (Jung and McNaughton, 1993) and then seen to be concentrated in cells with multiple fields, a bit like grid cells, but irregularly arranged in the environment (Leutgeb et al., 2007).

Subsequently, a new study has observed both cells with single and with multiple fields, but its authors argued that those in the granular layer, likely comprised of most mature granule cells, fire sparsely and with single fields; whereas the units with multiple fields are a physiologically distinct population, possibly including adult-born granule cells (Neunuebel and Knierim, 2012). This intriguing observation has tentatively linked the spatial properties of adult-born granule cells to the other features (Temprana et al., 2015) of their ever-richer phenomenology (Becker, 2005; and see Aimone et al., 2010 for a review), which has been prodding the emergence of a new understanding that makes sense of the fact that the dentate gyrus is one of only two regions to retain adult neurogenesis in both the rodent and human brain (Spalding et al., 2013).

These discoveries inform a quantitative, though simplified, spatial model, which would have otherwise been based on ill-defined assumptions. The role of multiple DG place fields in establishing novel CA3 representations has been treated by Cerasti and Treves

(2010, 2013) and found to be relatively unimportant. What really matters is the sparseness of the activity in the dentate, and the sparseness of the connectivity from the dentate to CA3. Both mathematical analysis and computer simulations of the model show that, while the memory system would still function otherwise, strong connections as sparse as those observed (only about 50 inputs from granule cells to a CA3 pyramidal cell in the rat, compared to several thousand from other sources) make it function optimally, in terms of the bits of information new memories contain (Cerasti and Treves, 2010). The effect of both types of sparsity, in the activity and in the connectivity, is to produce randomness. DG acts in the model as a sort of spatial random number generator, a bit like the trainees generating random statements. Associating these random CA3 codes to the spatial and object ones in entorhinal cortex, through PP synapses, raises them to the status of symbols with high information content. Quantitative analysis of the model shows that much of this information, is, however, encoded in a difficult, "dark" format, suggesting that other regions of the hippocampus, in particular CA1, may have to contribute to decode it. Random codes are not easy to read.

The last suggestions, surprisingly, connects us back to the human hippocampus, where technical improvements in imaging technology allow researchers to examine activity in distinct subregions, and potentially to link observations to those in monkeys and rats (Small et al., 2004). Functional magnetic resonance imaging (fMRI) reflects the mass activity of hundreds of thousands of neurons together, and it is not even possible to disentangle all subregions, e.g., DG from CA3. Nonetheless, with a clever use of the repetition suppression paradigm, Bakker et al. (2008) have shown that the DG/CA3 complex is sensitive to fine differences between two visual stimuli, while CA1 combines them as effectively different versions of the same visual item. Interpreted in this scenario, DG and CA3 produce a new random representation for each visual image, undeterred by the memory of similar ones, while CA1 decodes the mess in terms of previously acquired concepts.

Whether these insights really apply at the microscopic level of individual neurons, however, remains unclear, and it is a difficult question to resolve with studies in humans. Moreover, the critical question is whether they apply to the spatial domain, because in the abstract, ill-defined, perhaps very high-dimensional space of objects used by Bakker et al., random codes are difficult to disentangle from orderly ones, if the latter follow an order of which we are not aware. Note that the storage capacity expected of the human CA3 network, for discrete patterns of activity, is very high, with p_c in the order of tens of thousands or perhaps even hundreds of thousands of discrete patterns, as David Marr had envisaged and a different kind of analysis also indicates (Treves and Rolls, 1991).

A recent rat study, however, has in fact probed the randomness of spatial codes in CA3. Alme et al. (2014) have recorded activity from CA3 cells in rats exposed to as many as 11 environments, 1 familiar and 10 novel, all with near-identical geometric features, similar objects present, and while performing the same nondescript foraging task. It is important to note that despite the very large p_c just mentioned for the human CA3

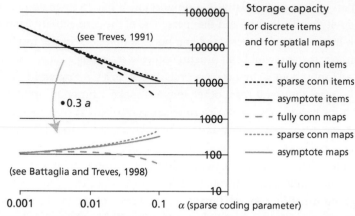

Figure 5.3 In a network of threshold-linear units, the storage capacity for discrete memory items and for spatial maps, or *charts*, can be calculated by solving the same equations. They are written as $A_1^2 - \alpha A_3 = 0$ in the case of a fully connected network and as $A_2^2 - \alpha A_3 = 0$ for a sparsely connected one (see Treves, 1991 and Battaglia and Treves, 1998). The capacity for charts can be obtained from that for discrete items simply by multiplying by $0.3a$, where a is the sparse coding parameter. The numerical values for p_c are plotted assuming the estimated number of connections per pyramidal cell in CA3, $C = 12\ 000$.

network, the maximum capacity in terms of charts in the rodent may be in a much lower range, because each chart is effectively equivalent to many discrete patterns (Battaglia and Treves, 1998; see Figure 5.3). Further, suitable confusing manipulations have been shown, in the "teleportation" experiment, to induce flickering transitions between just 2 charts (Jezek et al., 2011), again suggesting that the capacity for distinct charts may be limited. Strikingly, instead, and despite all their "news unworthiness," the 11 spatial codes observed in each rat were all distinct from each other, effectively random. Statistically, when compared to reshuffled data, these charts remained uncorrelated across all 55 pairs of environments, with only small overlap in the populations of active cells between any 2 charts.

Intriguingly, the small overlap observed might be due to subpopulations of overactive CA3 units that may be those which happen to receive 1 or perhaps 2 mossy fiber inputs from adult-born DG granule cells still in their critical period of enhanced activity (Kaya et al., 2014; see Figure 5.4). Whether or not the small deviation from randomness is due to adult DG neurogenesis, the few cells that are overactive but in different combinations and in different locations are evidence against a conceivable type of CA3 orderly code that would reuse elements, or "spatial motifs", over corresponding positions within the similar environments. Unlike instances in which CA3 apparently succeeds in restoring some order (Neunuebel and Knierim, 2014) here DG has succeeded, it seems, in creating havoc. It is a beneficial havoc, that endows the CA3 autoassociative network with its large storage capacity, and which perhaps can be cleaned up in CA1 (Treves, 2004).

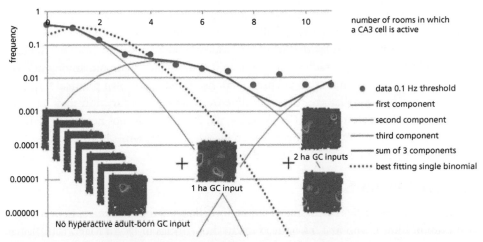

Figure 5.4 The distribution of the relative frequency with which CA3 cells are active in 0, 1, … , 11 distinct environments (note the log scale on the frequency axis; data points from Alme et al., 2014) is very different from the binomial expected if all cells had the same probability of activation (dashed curve). It is better approximated as the sum of 3 binomial components (thick solid curve), each corresponding to a subpopulation of CA3 units with a distinct probability of activation (Kaya et al., 2014). It is conceivable that the largest subpopulation includes the CA3 cells that only receive mossy fiber inputs from mature, sparsely active granule cells (GCs, here represented by single-field firing rate maps, as discussed by Neunuebel and Knierim, 2012); the second subpopulation by those CA3 cells (here 13.5% of the total) that receive just one input from an hyperactive, adult-born DG cell with multiple fields; the third, by those that receive two such inputs (here, 1.2%), and so on.

(note the log scale on the frequency axis; data points from Alme et I, 2014).

Fall like a sparrow, fly like a dove

Something was wrong, all right, with Marr's theory for archicortex. Willshaw and Buckingham (1990) have clarified how, for all his emphasis on the collateral effect, the collateral effect does not really play a useful role in the operation of Marr's model. Quantitatively speaking, the way Marr defined the model, one can safely remove its recurrent collateral synapses. Still, that emphasis, which inspired Bruce McNaughton and Edmund Rolls and then many others to "see" a collateral effect in CA3, was a stroke of Marr's genius.

The network model that articulated the theory at the algorithmic level, or perhaps at the implementational level (the two had luckily not yet divorced at the time, in Marr's mind) was crude and implausible with all its binary variables and even binary synapses (cf. Bartol et al., 2015). Marr analyzed it with calculations that seem primitive and powerless compared with the statistical physics techniques applied to the Hopfield model (Amit, 1989), or with the brute-force computer power applied to a wide variety of more complicated models. Still, Marr analyzed his crude binary model and obtained insights, something which cannot unfortunately be said of much of the subsequent work.

Marr did not find the time to assign something to do to the dentate gyrus, and here his model really falls like a sparrow. Still, I see them as if forever bound to each other. Both the dentate gyrus and David Marr emerged almost out of nowhere. Both the dentate gyrus and David Marr led a radical paradigm shift, among mammals and among neuroscientists. Both establish new, stable representations, despite their own physical fragility. Recent studies indicate that age-related decline in dentate gyrus function may be contrasted with a chocolate-rich diet (Brickman et al., 2014). We do not need chocolate to continue to be inspired by Marr's theory for archicortex. In this sense, his theory flies like a dove (Bingman and Jones, 1994). Toward the sun.

Acknowledgments

I am grateful for extensive discussions with many colleagues over the years, in particular with Edmund Rolls, who first introduced me to the writings of David Marr, with Bruce McNaughton and Carol Barnes and those in their lab in the early 1990s, and with those in the SPACEBRAIN and GRIDMAP collaborations. The criticism by Sophie Rosay of the very compressed first draft of this chapter was particularly helpful, as were those by Sue Becker and Mike Hasselmo.

References

Ahn JR, Lee I. (2014). Intact CA3 in the hippocampus is only sufficient for contextual behavior based on well-learned and unaltered visual background. Hippocampus. 24:1081–1093.

Aimone JB, Deng W, Gage FH. (2010). Adult neurogenesis: integrating theories and separating functions. Trends Cogn Sci. 14:325–337.

Alme CB, Miao C, Jezek K, Treves A, Moser EI, Moser, MB. (2014). Place cells in the hippocampus: Eleven maps for eleven rooms. Proc Natl Acad Sci U S A. 111:18428–18435.

Amit DJ. (1989). Modeling Brain Function: The World of Attractor Neural Networks. Cambridge: Cambridge University Press.

Amit DJ, Gutfreund H, Sompolinsky H. (1987). Statistical mechanics of neural networks near saturation. Ann Phys. 173:30–67.

Atoji Y, Wild JM. (2004). Fiber connections of the hippocampal formation and septum and subdivisions of the hippocampal formation in the pigeon as revealed by tract tracing and kainic acid lesions. J Comp Neurol. 475:426–461.

Bakker A, Kirwan CB, Miller M, Stark, CEL. (2008). Pattern separation in the human hippocampal CA3 and dentate gyrus. Science. 319:1640–2.

Bartol TM, Bromer C, Kinney JP, Chirillo MA, Bourne JN, Harris, KM, Sejnowski TJ. (2015). Hippocampal spine head sizes are highly precise. bioRxiv:016329.

Battaglia FP, Treves A. (1998). Attractor neural networks storing multiple space representations: a model for hippocampal place fields. Phys Rev E. 58:7738–7753.

Becker S. (2005). A computational principle for hippocampal learning and neurogenesis. Hippocampus. 15:722–738.

Bingman VP, Jones TJ. (1994). Sun-compass based spatial learning impaired in homing pigeons with hippocampal lesions. J Neurosci. 14:6687–6694.

Bliss TV, Lomo T. (1973). Long-lasting potentiation of synaptic transmission in the dentate area of the anaesthetized rabbit following stimulation of the perforant path. J Physiol. 232:331–356.

Brickman AM, Khan, UA, Provenzano FA, Yeung LK, Suzuki W, Schroeter, H, et al. (2014). Enhancing dentate gyrus function with dietary flavanols improves cognition in older adults. Nat Neurosci. **17**:1798–1803.

Byrne P, Becker S, Burgess N. (2007). Remembering the past and imagining the future: a neural model of spatial memory and imagery. Psychol Rev. **114**:340–375.

Cerasti E, Treves A. (2010). How informative are spatial CA3 representations established by the dentate gyrus?. PLoS Comput Biol. **6**:e1000759.

Cerasti E, Treves A. (2013). The spatial representations acquired in CA3 by self-organizing recurrent connections. Front Cell Neurosci. **7**:112.

Cerda-Reverter, JM, Zanuy S, Munoz-Cueto, JA. (2001). Cytoarchitectonic study of the brain of a perciform species, the sea bass (*Dicentrarchus labrax*). I. The telencephalon. J Morphol. **247**:217–228.

Clayton NS, Krebs JR. (1995). Memory in food-storing birds: from behaviour to brain. Curr Opin Neurobiol. **5**:149–154.

Cnotka J, Mohle M, Rehkamper G. (2008). Navigational experience affects hippocampus size in homing pigeons. Brain Behav Evol. **72**:233–238.

Deshmukh SS, Knierim JJ. (2011). Representation of non-spatial and spatial information in the lateral entorhinal cortex. Front Behav Neurosci. **5**:69.

Fyhn M, Molden S, Witter MP, Moser EI, Moser MB. (2004). Spatial representation in the entorhinal cortex. Science. **305**:1258–1264.

Fyhn M, Hafting T, Treves A, Moser MB, Moser EI. (2007). Hippocampal remapping and grid realignment in entorhinal cortex. Nature. **446**:190–194.

Gagliardo A, Ioalè P, Odetti F, Bingman VP, Siegel JJ, Vallortigara G. (2001). Hippocampus and homing in pigeons: left and right hemispheric differences in navigational map learning. Eur J Neurosci. **13**:1617–1624.

Gardner-Medwin AR. (1976). The recall of events through the learning of associations between their parts. Proc R Soc London B Biol Sci. **194**:375–402.

Gloor P. (1997). The Temporal Lobe and Limbic System. New York: Oxford University Press.

Gupta S, Maurya R, Saxena M, Sen J. (2012). Defining structural homology between the mammalian and avian hippocampus through conserved gene expression patterns observed in the chick embryo. Dev Biol. **366**:125–141.

Hafting T, Fyhn M, Molden S, Moser M-B, Moser EI. (2005). Microstructure of a spatial map in the entorhinal cortex. Nature. **436**:801–806.

Hasselmo ME, Bower JM. (1993). Acetylcholine and memory. Trends Neurosci. **16**:218–22.

Hasselmo ME, Schnell E. (1994). Laminar selectivity of the cholinergic suppression of synaptic transmission in rat hippocampal region CA1: Computational modeling and brain slice physiology. J Neurosci. **14**:3898–3914.

Hasselmo ME, Schnell E, Barkai E. (1995). Dynamics of learning and recall at excitatory recurrent synapses and cholinergic modulation in rat hippocampal region CA3. J Neurosci. **15**:5249–5262.

Hebb DO. (1948/2005). The Organization of Behavior: A Neuropsychological Theory. Hove, UK: Psychology Press.

Herold C, Coppola VJ, Bingman VP. (2015). The maturation of research into the avian hippocampal formation: recent discoveries from one of Nature's foremost navigators. Hippocampus. **25**:1193–211.

Hopfield JJ. (1982). Neural networks and physical systems with emergent collective computational abilities. Proc Natl Acad Sci U S A. **79**:2554–2558.

Kanter I, Sompolinsky H. (1987). Associative recall of memory without errors. Phys Rev A. **35**: 380–392.

Kaya Z, Cerasti E, Treves A. (2014). Adding new neurons on the tail of a binomial (abstract). SUMMERSOLSTICE 2014, Ljubljana, Slovenia, p. 20.

Kerr AM, Jonas P. (2008). The two sides of hippocampal mossy fiber plasticity. Neuron. **57**:5–7.

Knierim JJ, Neunuebel JP, Deshmukh SS. (2014). Functional correlates of the lateral and medial entorhinal cortex: objects, path integration and local–global reference frames. Philos Trans R Soc Lond B Biol Sci. **369**:20130369.

Jezek K, Henriksen EJ, Treves A, Moser EI, Moser MB. (2011). Theta-paced flickering between place-cell maps in the hippocampus. Nature. **478**:246–249.

Jung MW, McNaughton BL. (1993). Spatial selectivity of unit activity in the hippocampal granular layer. Hippocampus. **3**:165.

Lassalle J-M, Bataille T, Halley H. (2000). Reversible inactivation of the hippocampal mossy fiber synapses in mice impairs spatial learning, but neither consolidation nor memory retrieval, in the Morris navigation task. Neurobiol Learn Mem. **73**:243–257.

Lee I, Kesner RP. (2004). Encoding versus retrieval of spatial memory: Double dissociation between the dentate gyrus and the perforant path inputs into CA3 in the dorsal hippocampus. Hippocampus. **14**:66–76.

Leutgeb S, Leutgeb JK, Barnes CA, Moser EI, McNaughton BL, Moser M-B. (2005). Independent codes for spatial and episodic memory in hippocampal neuronal ensembles. Science. **309**:619–623.

Leutgeb JK, Leutgeb S, Moser M-B, Moser EI. (2007). Pattern separation in the dentate gyrus and CA3 of the hippocampus. Science. **315**:961–966.

Margoliash D, van Drongelen W, Kohrman M. (2010). Introducing songbirds as a model system for epilepsy research. J Clin Neurophysiol. **27**:433–437.

Marr D. (1971). Simple memory: a theory for archicortex. Philos Trans R Soc Lond B Biol Sci. **262**:23–81.

McNaughton BL, Morris RGM. (1987). Hippocampal synaptic enhancement and information storage within a distributed memory system. Trends Neurosci. **10**:408–415.

Monasson R, Rosay S. (2013). Crosstalk and transitions between multiple spatial maps in an attractor neural network model of the hippocampus: Phase diagram. Phys Rev E. **87**:062813.

Monasson R, Rosay S. (2014). Crosstalk and transitions between multiple spatial maps in an attractor neural network model of the hippocampus: Collective motion of the activity. Phys Rev E. **89**:032803.

Monasson R, Rosay S. (2015). Transitions between spatial attractors in place-cell models. Phys Rev Lett. **115**:098101.

Moser EI, Moser MB. (2008). A metric for space. Hippocampus. **18**:1142–1156.

Muller RU, Kubie JL. (1987). The effects of changes in the environment on the spatial firing of hippocampal complex-spike cells. J Neurosci. **7**:1951–1968.

Neunuebel JP, Knierim JJ. (2012). Spatial firing correlates of physiologically distinct cell types of the rat dentate gyrus. J Neurosci. **32**:3848–3858.

Neunuebel JP, Yoganarasimha D, Rao G, Knierim JJ. (2013). Conflicts between local and global spatial frameworks dissociate neural representations of the lateral and medial entorhinal cortex. J Neurosci. **33**:9246–9258.

Neunuebel JP, Knierim, JJ. (2014). CA3 retrieves coherent representations from degraded input: direct evidence for CA3 pattern completion and dentate gyrus pattern separation. Neuron. **81**:416–427.

O'Keefe J, Burgess N. (1996). Geometric determinants of the place fields of hippocampal neurons. Nature. **381**:425–428.

O'Keefe J, Dostrovsky J. (1971). The hippocampus as a spatial map. Preliminary evidence from unit activity in the freely-moving rat. Brain Res. **34**:171–175.

Petrillo M, Ritter CA, Powers AS. (1994). A role for acetylcholine in spatial memory in turtles. Physiol Behav. **56**:135–41.

Reiner A, Powers AS. (1983). The effects of lesions of telencephalic visual structures on visual discriminative performance in turtles (*Chrysemyspicta picta*). J Comp Neurol. **218**:1–24.

Rodríguez F, Carlos López J et al. (2002). Conservation of spatial memory function in the pallial forebrain of reptiles and ray-finned fishes. J Neurosci. **22**:2894–2903.

Rolls ET. (1989). Functions of neuronal networks in the hippocampus and cerebral cortex in memory. In: Models of Brain Function (**Cotterill R**, ed.), pp. 15–33. Cambridge: Cambridge University Press.

Rolls ET. (1996). A theory of hippocampal function in memory. Hippocampus. **6**:601–620.

Rolls ET, Kesner RP. (2006). A computational theory of hippocampal function, and empirical tests of the theory. Progr Neurobiol. **79**:1–48.

Rolls ET, Robertson RG, Georges-Francois P. (1997). Spatial view cells in the primate hippocampus. Eur J Neurosci. **9**:1789–1794.

Samsonovich A, McNaughton BL. (1997). Path integration and cognitive mapping in a continuous attractor neural network model. J Neurosci. **17**:5900–5920.

Sargolini F, Fyhn M, Hafting T, McNaughton BL, Witter MP, Moser MB, Moser EI. (2006). Conjunctive representation of position, direction, and velocity in entorhinal cortex. Science. **312**:758–762.

Sejnowski TJ. (1977). Storing covariance with nonlinearly interacting neurons. J Math Biol. **4**:303–321.

Shanahan M, Bingman VP, Shimizu T, Wild M, Güntürkün O. (2013). Large-scale network organization in the avian forebrain: a connectivity matrix and theoretical analysis. Front Comput Neurosci. **7**:89.

Sharp PE. (1991). Computer simulation of hippocampal place cells. Psychobiology. **19**:103–115.

Sherry DF, Vaccarino AL. (1989). Hippocampus and memory for food caches in black-capped chickadees. Behav Neurosci. **103**:308–318.

Small SA, Chawla MK, Buonocore M, Rapp PR, Barnes CA. (2004). Imaging correlates of brain function in monkeys and rats isolates a hippocampal subregion differentially vulnerable to aging. Proc Natl Acad Sci U S A. **101**:7181–7186.

Spalding KL, Bergmann O, Alkass K, Bernard S, Salehpour M, Huttner HB, et al. (2013). Dynamics of hippocampal neurogenesis in adult humans. Cell. **153**:1219–1227.

Stella F, Treves A. (2011). Associative memory storage and retrieval: involvement of theta oscillations in hippocampal information processing. Neural Plast. **2011**:683961.

Stringer SM, Rolls ET, Trappenberg TP, de Araujo IET. (2002). Self-organizing continuous attractor networks and path integration: two-dimensional models of place cells. Network. **13**:429–446.

Temprana SG, Mongiat LA, Yang SM, Trinchero MF, Alvarez DD, Kropff E, et al. (2015). Delayed coupling to feedback inhibition during a critical period for the integration of adult-born granule cells. Neuron. **85**:116–130.

Treves A. (1990). Threshold-linear formal neurons in auto-associative nets. J Phys A: Math Gen. **23**:2631–2650.

Treves A. (1991). Dilution and sparse coding in threshold-linear nets. J Phys A Math Gen. **24**:327–335.

Treves A. (2004). Computational constraints between retrieving the past and predicting the future, and the CA3-CA1 differentiation. Hippocampus. **14**:539–556.

Treves A, Miglino O, Parisi D. (1992). Rats, nets, maps, and the emergence of place cells. Psychobiology. **20**:1–8.

Treves A, Rolls ET. (1991). What determines the capacity of autoassociative memories in the brain? Network. **2**:371–397.

Treves A, Rolls ET. (1992). Computational constraints suggest the need for two distinct input systems to the hippocampal CA3 network. Hippocampus. **2**:189–199.

Treves A, Tashiro A, Witter MP, Moser EI. (2008). What is the mammalian dentate gyrus good for? Neuroscience. **154**:1155–1172.

Willshaw DJ, Buckingham JT. (1990). An assessment of Marr's theory of the hippocampus as a temporary memory store. Philos Trans R Soc Lond B Biol Sci. **329**:205–215.

Woolf NJ. (1991). Cholinergic systems in mammalian brain and spinal cord. Progr Neurobiol. **37**:475–524.

Chapter 6

Marr's influence on the standard model of hippocampus, and the need for more theoretical advances

Michael E. Hasselmo and James R. Hinman

Introduction to Marr's model of archicortex

This article focuses on the impact of David Marr's 1971 paper entitled "Simple memory: a theory of archicortex." Marr's paper played an essential role in laying the groundwork for an explosion of research on models of the function of the hippocampal formation that have had an ever-expanding influence on experimental research addressing hippocampal function. In this chapter I discuss Marr's paper in the context of the biological dynamics of memory function, with a particular emphasis on understanding how episodic memories are encoded. I will address progress in the following general areas: (1) experimental work on hippocampal function inspired by Marr's framework, (2) further work on the dynamics of associative memory function in cortical structures, (3) subsequent work incorporating network oscillatory dynamics, and (4) the need for a similar theoretical breakthrough that accommodates new knowledge about the dynamics of the hippocampal formation and adjacent structures such as the entorhinal cortex. With regard to the term "archicortex," anatomists use this term to describe the more evolutionarily primitive three-layered cortex at the borders of the neocortex, especially indicating the hippocampus. In this review, rather than using the term archicortex I will primarily use the term "hippocampal formation," which is used most commonly in the field to refer collectively to the subfields of the hippocampus (i.e., cornu ammonis: CA3 and CA1) as well as the dentate gyrus and the entorhinal cortex.

Marr's influence on hippocampal research

Numerous subsequent papers built on many of the ideas from Marr's seminal work. Modeling of the hippocampus has been very successful in guiding experimental work in this area, and a number of experimental studies have tested specific predictions of computational models. In addition to the review presented here, another recent paper also addresses the significant influence of Marr's model on experimental work (Willshaw et al., 2015). Marr's theories of hippocampal function had a slow time constant for their initial influence on experimental work in the field, but ultimately had a remarkable impact. In particular, Marr's 1971 paper is extensively cited with reference to the principle of pattern completion on excitatory recurrent connections. In this paper, Marr describes the phenomenon of completion both in terms of feedfoward connections between layers and with reference to the function of collaterals arising from hippocampal pyramidal cells (his collateral effect). Marr's model does not focus only on the collaterals in region CA3 that have been the focus of most later models of pattern completion. Marr describes the collateral effect as occurring in the output layer (layer $\mathscr{P}_3$) that includes both CA1 and CA3, and also fascia dentata granule cells, which Marr proposes act "as extensions of the dendritic trees of CA pyramidal cells" (Marr, 1971, p. 69).

Marr is also extensively credited with proposing that interference between stored patterns could be reduced by the process of pattern separation. This concept of pattern separation corresponds to Marr's codon hypothesis. Interestingly, as pointed out in a recent review (Willshaw et al., 2015), the codon hypothesis was primarily presented in Marr's earlier papers on the cerebellum (Marr, 1969) and neocortex (Marr, 1970) and is then referred to using the term "codon" in the 1971 paper. Marr states that "codon formation is used to construct suitable evidence cells" (p. 30), and that "some layers will contain evidence cells, and some, output cells" (p. 37) and "there is no reason to have evidence cells and output cells particularly near each other" (p. 37) and suggests the perforant path may connect them. Consistent with this, the paper assigns entorhinal cortex and presubiculum to be layer $\mathscr{P}_2$ in his model (Marr, 1971, p. 75) and notes that "star cells or small pyramids … are codon cells, used only at the first stage of a simple memory" (Marr, 1971, p. 75), and that "Regio Entorhinalis and the Region Presubicularis prepare information from many different sources for its simple representation in the CA and FD" (Marr, 1971, p. 75). Thus, Marr proposed that codon formation occurs within the archicortex, and attributed it to entorhinal cortex.

Several papers in the late 1980s and early 1990s reviewed basic ideas from Marr's paper, and amplified the impact of this paper on the field. One such study was the review by McNaughton and Morris, (1987), which gave a very clear set of mathematical examples of matrix multiplication to explain the theory of pattern completion, and attributed the function to the recurrent collaterals in region CA3. They also reviewed Marr's important proposal that different inhibitory neurons provide subtraction and division operations for setting appropriate thresholds. The paper also described the formation of associations between individual patterns in a sequence. This paper and a chapter by Rolls (1987) provided the start of a series of papers citing pattern completion effects in CA3. Another important early description of Marr's theories was the comprehensive review of Marr's theory by Willshaw and Buckingham (1990).

The McNaughton and Morris paper also cites Marr's codon hypothesis and describes the need to reduce spurious recall by reducing the overlap between stored patterns. In contrast to the Marr paper, the later paper proposes that cortical inputs to the dentate gyrus contact an expanded number of cells, allowing formation of less overlapping representations (McNaughton and Morris, 1987). Thus, this paper gives the first published description of mechanisms for pattern separation and expansion coding in the dentate gyrus. (Note that Table 1 on p. 42 of Marr's paper shows a smaller number of neurons and less sparse activity α in layer $\mathscr{P}_2$ compared to $\mathscr{P}_1$.)

Subsequent papers expanded on the topics of pattern separation in dentate gyrus (McNaughton and Morris, 1987; McNaughton, 1991; O'Reilly and McClelland, 1994; Treves and Rolls, 1994; Hasselmo and Wyble, 1997) and pattern completion by autoassociative memory function in hippocampal region CA3 (McNaughton and Morris, 1987; Treves and Rolls, 1992, 1994; Hasselmo et al., 1995). The principles of pattern separation and pattern completion were also combined in large-scale simulations of the role of the hippocampus in human episodic memory as tested in human verbal memory tasks (Hasselmo and Wyble, 1997). The concept of the collateral effect was extended to address attractor dynamics at excitatory recurrent connections in CA3 (Treves and Rolls, 1992, 1994; Hasselmo et al., 1995). Detailed computational models of the dentate gyrus have focused on the trade-off between pattern separation and pattern completion (O'Reilly and McClelland, 1994; Treves and Rolls, 1994), showing how the expansion from entorhinal cortex to dentate gyrus could reduce overlap between patterns to enhance encoding, but also showing that the process of pattern separation implicitly includes a type of pattern completion phenomenon, because those patterns that are not separated into distinct representations will activate the same unified representation.

It is very interesting that John O'Keefe's seminal first paper on place cells (O'Keefe and Dostrovsky, 1971) appeared in the same year as Marr's model of archicortex. Many subsequent papers used elements of the Marr framework for modeling the formation of associations between spatial representations in the hippocampal formation. For example, many papers used the recurrent connections in region CA3 to store associations between sequentially activated place cells. These included papers predicting effects of trajectory learning on hippocampal dynamics (Abbott and Blum, 1996; Blum and Abbott, 1996; Mehta et al., 2000), and papers modeling the role of hippocampus in guiding spatial behavior (Touretzky and Redish, 1996; Redish and Touretzky, 1997, 1998). Attractor dynamics were used to model place cell firing as a stable bump of activity that would move around based on path integration (Samsonovich and McNaughton, 1997). In more recent work, place cells were combined with grid cells and head direction cells to encode the complex spatiotemporal trajectories of episodic memory in a complex world (Hasselmo, 2009, 2012). The interaction of a broader range of cortical regions including parietal cortex was described in a model of memory, navigation, and imagery (Byrne et al., 2007).

David Marr's ideas had a strong influence on subsequent experimental work. For example, he had proposed the important role of Hebb synapses in the hippocampus for forming associations, and even cites an early paper on long-term potentiation (Lomo, 1971). Marr's proposal was supported by in-vivo work showing Hebbian properties of synapses in the dentate gyrus (McNaughton et al., 1978; Levy and Steward, 1979). This led to the subsequent discovery of the phenomenon later described as spike-timing dependent plasticity that was initially discovered in the dentate gyrus by William B. "Chip" Levy (Levy and Steward, 1983) and modeled extensively by Holmes and Levy (1990). The temporal asymmetry of synaptic modification modeled by Holmes and Levy was incorporated in circuit models (Minai and Levy, 1993; Abbott and Blum, 1996; Blum and Abbott, 1996; Levy, 1996) that focused on the encoding of sequences as previously discussed by McNaughton and Morris (1987). This circuit modeling predicted (Abbott and Blum, 1996) that the potentiation of excitatory connections should cause a backward expansion of hippocampal place fields. Subsequently Mehta and McNaughton presented experimental data showing the predicted backward expansion of the size of place fields of hippocampal place cells (Mehta et al., 2000, 2002). The encoding of sequences was used in models of theta-phase precession discussed in a later section of this review. The notion of sequence encoding and retrieval was also supported by evidence for rapid sequential replay of previously learned place cell sequences on a linear track when the rat was stationary (Lee and Wilson, 2002; Jadhav et al., 2012; Diba and Buzsaki, 2007; Davidson et al., 2009).

The principles of pattern separation and pattern completion that started with Marr's paper continued to have an impact on experimental work over 20 years later. For example, when selective genetic manipulations in mice allowed selective knockout of the NMDA receptor in hippocampal region CA3, these mice were used to demonstrate an impairment of pattern completion based on learning a spatial response in an environment with multiple cues and being tested for their response in an environment with a single cue (Nakazawa et al., 2002). Similar tests were performed with selective expression of tetanus toxin in mouse region CA3 to block synaptic transmission from these neurons and to demonstrate impairment of pattern completion in that task (Nakashiba et al., 2008). In contrast, selective knockout of NMDA receptors in the dentate gyrus caused impairment of responses that required distinguishing two separate but similar contextual environments (McHugh et al., 2007; Nakashiba et al., 2012). In addition, selective lesions of the dentate gyrus impaired the capacity of rats to encode and selectively respond to spatial locations that are close to each other (Gilbert et al., 2001).

Subsequent unit recording studies also analyzed the response properties of the dentate gyrus versus other hippocampal subregions. Neurons in the dentate gyrus showed sparser coding of the environment, with fewer responsive cells and smaller response fields for dentate place cells (Barnes et al., 1990). Minimal changes in the spatial environment can cause distinct responses of dentate gyrus granule cells (Leutgeb et al., 2007). It has been suggested that neurogenesis in the dentate gyrus could reduce overlap between neural representations (Becker, 2005).

Unit recording studies have tested for the effect of partial shifts in the environment on neural responses in region CA3, as a means of testing for pattern completion. In one study, the partial shift caused less change of neural response in CA3 compared to CA1, suggesting pattern competion (Lee et al., 2004), whereas in another study region CA3 responded with distinct representations with partial changes (Leutgeb et al., 2004). These apparently conflicting results were unified by demonstration of a nonlinear transformation in region CA3 (Vazdarjanova and Guzowski, 2004). Inputs that are somewhat similar to each other induce very similar response patterns, whereas patterns that are more different evoke more strongly differentiated patterns of neural activity (Guzowski et al.,

2004; Vazdarjanova and Guzowski, 2004). The phenomenon of pattern completion was shown even more clearly in a more recent unit recording study that allowed direct analysis of completion in CA3 based on recordings of the input activity in the dentate gyrus (Neunuebel and Knierim, 2014).

In his original paper, Marr proposed that patterns stored as simple associations in the hippocampus could later be transferred to the neocortex. This basic idea was extensively elaborated in subsequent models, initially in simulations showing simple transfer of associations from the hippocampus to the neocortex (Alvarez and Squire, 1994; Hasselmo et al., 1996). More extensive analysis (McClelland et al., 1995) showed how this temporary memory store could be essential for allowing training of the neocortex with interleaved patterns, to prevent catastrophic interference that could break down the existing semantic structure of the neocortex with each new association. These models have had a strong effect on guiding subsequent studies on consolidation effects in humans (Dewar et al., 2014; 2012).

Further experimental work has explored Marr's hypotheses using imaging techniques in human subjects. When the technique of positron emission tomography (PET) became available for measuring the activity of brain regions, studies of memory focused on finding activation of the hippocampus. Initial studies analyzed PET activation during verbal memory tasks such as word stem completion based on recall (Buckner et al., 1995), but these studies did not show robust activation of the hippocampal formation. The first demonstration of hippocampal activation using functional magnetic resonance imaging (fMRI) was obtained with a study testing activity during encoding of complex visual scenes for subsequent post-scan recognition (Stern et al., 1996) contrasted with repeated presentation of a single visual scene. Later fMRI techniques measured event-related activity associated with individual stimuli and showed differences in hippocampal and parahippocampal activity associated with stimuli that were later remembered versus those that were forgotten in a subsequent memory task (Brewer et al., 1998; Wagner et al., 1998). Further studies showed that different types of stimuli could activate hippocampal regions, with greater left hippocampal activation for word stimuli versus bilateral coding for pictures (Kirchhoff et al., 2000).

To address encoding and retrieval at a more detailed anatomical resolution, techniques for registration of the fMRI activity onto anatomical scans have allowed more detailed analysis of different subregions activated during behavioral tasks. Using these techniques, Craig Stark and colleagues tested for activity in hippocampal subregions associated with pattern separation versus pattern completion (Bakker et al., 2008). Limitations on imaging resolution forced them to combine the dentate gyrus with region CA3. They tested pattern separation by having participants encode visual stimuli (e.g., a rubber duck), and then presenting test stimuli that were exactly the same or had small differences (a rubber duck with slightly different shape and coloring). Participants were required to correctly identify either an exact match (old) or a similar stimulus. The dentate gyrus and CA3 showed differential activity between the similar conditions (lure, correct rejection) versus the old conditions (exact match, hit), suggesting a selective role of these regions in pattern separation. Thus, almost 40 years after his paper was published, David Marr's theories were being tested in imaging of human subjects.

The dynamics of pattern completion

Marr's paper also had a significant role in the expansion of neural modeling research in the 1970s and 1980s. This research included major streams of theoretical models, including the connectionist models (Rumelhart et al., 1986; McClelland and Rumelhart, 1988) and attractor dynamic models (Amit, 1988; Amit and Treves, 1989) in the 1980s.

Marr's paper influenced research addressing biological mechanisms for associative memory function. The theory of associations has a long history in research on human cognition, dating back to philosophers in past centuries. A review can be found in Schacter (1982). These models received a mathematical treatment in early linear associative memory models (Anderson, 1972; Kohonen, 1972, 1984). In these models, vectors represented patterns of neural activity in the brain. An association was encoded by modification of synapses, represented mathematically by computing the outer product matrix between a presynaptic activity vector and the associated postsynaptic activity vector. Retrieval of the association was performed by allowing the presynaptic activity cue to spread across the modified synapses, represented mathematically by matrix multiplication of the presynaptic vector by the pattern of synaptic connections.

These models did not focus on the role of specific brain structures, so Marr was a pioneer in proposing that the excitatory recurrent connections from hippocampal pyramidal cells could underlie autoassociative memory function (Marr, 1971). As mentioned earlier, this was expanded upon in subsequent papers by hippocampal researchers (McNaughton and Morris, 1987; Rolls, 1987; Willshaw and Buckingham, 1990; Treves and Rolls, 1992, 1994; Hasselmo et al., 1995). Of interest to the modeling of three-layered cortices, later work proposed that the primary olfactory cortex, or piriform cortex, which has a three-layered structure similar to the hippocampus, could also function as an associative memory based on excitatory recurrent collaterals terminating in the layer proximal to the cell bodies similar to the hippocampus (Haberly and Bower, 1989; Hasselmo et al., 1992).

Excitatory recurrent connections will cause an explosion of activity unless the excitatory feedback is limited by the input–output function of individual neurons or by feedback inhibition. A dominant stream of research in the 1980s focused on fixed-point attractor dynamics in associative memory function, in which activity converges to a stable fixed point. Mathematically, Lyapunov functions were used to show the stability of attractor states (Hopfield, 1982, 1984; Cohen and Grossberg, 1983). Many of these studies focused on relatively abstract representations of neurons, and the computation of the storage capacity of attractor networks (Amit, 1988). Despite Marr's earlier work focusing on physiological details of such circuits, many initial models of attractor dynamics were highly unrealistic: for example, they violated Dale's law by having both excitatory and inhibitory connections arise from the same neuron, and driving neurons up to an asymptotic maximum activity. However, later studies addressed making these attractor networks more biologically realistic, for example by modeling neurons with lower firing rates (Amit and Treves, 1989; Amit et al., 1990; Treves and Rolls, 1992, 1994).

Many of the early models used single-neuron models that artificially limited the maximal output of neurons (i.e., using a step function or sigmoid function). This was justified as representing the maximal intrinsic firing rate of a neuron. However, recordings of cortical neurons in vivo almost never go above 100 Hz, whereas the maximal firing rate limited by intrinsic properties is usually higher. The intrinsic frequency–current (f–I) curve of a neuron is more accurately modeled with a threshold linear function. A more realistic way of limiting the maximal firing rate of modeled neurons is by use of feedback inhibition, as initially implemented by Wilson and Cowan (1972, 1973). Later models used threshold linear excitatory and inhibitory neurons in attractor models of the hippocampus (Hasselmo et al., 1995; Kali and Dayan, 2000). These models were a precursor to the current theory of balanced networks (van Vreeswijk and Sompolinsky, 1996) in which chaotic activity involves a balance of excitatory and inhibitory activity.

Early associative memory models all used different dynamics during encoding and retrieval (Anderson, 1972; Kohonen, 1972, 1984; Hopfield, 1982; Amit, 1988). During encoding, activity in the network would be clamped to an external input pattern. The dynamics of retrieval were explicitly ignored during computation of an outer product for encoding of new input patterns. This was essential for the proper function of associative memory models, as retrieval during encoding would cause a build-up of interference between overlapping patterns (Hasselmo et al., 1992; Hasselmo, 2006). However, there was no clear biological mechanism for this difference in dynamics during encoding and retrieval.

The effects of acetylcholine provided a reasonable biological mechanism for the difference in dynamics between encoding and retrieval in associative memory. The effects of acetylcholine are consistent across most cortical structures (Hasselmo, 1999, 2006). In particular, acetylcholine causes an important selective presynaptic inhibition of glutamatergic transmission at excitatory recurrent synapses within cortical structures. For example, activation of muscarinic acetylcholine receptors caused much stronger presynaptic inhibition of glutamate release at excitatory recurrent synapses in piriform cortex layer Ib compared to afferent synapses in layer Ia (Hasselmo and Bower, 1992, 1993). In computational models, interference from previously stored patterns was prevented by cholinergic suppression of synaptic transmission, and the rate of encoding was enhanced by cholinergic depolarization of pyramidal cells and the suppression of spike frequency accommodation (Barkai et al., 1994; Barkai and Hasselmo, 1994).

These findings in the piriform cortex have been shown to generalize to other cortical structures, including subregions of the hippocampal formation. In region CA1 of the hippocampus, muscarinic presynaptic inhibition is stronger at excitatory connections arising from within the hippocampus (in region CA3) and terminating in stratum radiatum of region CA1 compared to afferent input from entorhinal cortex terminating in stratum lacunosum-moleculare (Hasselmo and Schnell, 1994). Similarly, muscarinic presynaptic inhibition is stronger for synapses in stratum radiatum of region CA3 arising from

CA3 pyramidal cells, compared to weaker presynaptic inhibition at afferent synapses in stratum lucidum or region CA3 arising from the dentate gyrus (Hasselmo et al., 1995). This effect was later replicated in comparing stratum radiatum and stratum lucidum (Vogt and Regehr, 2001), and was extended to show less presynaptic inhibition in stratum lacunosum-moleculare of region CA3 (Kremin and Hasselmo, 2007).

This principle of selective cholinergic suppression of excitatory feedback but not afferent input also proves to generalize to neocortical structures (Hasselmo, 1999, 2006). In an early study, connections within somatosensory neocortex showed greater presynaptic inhibition than afferent input arising from the white matter (Hasselmo and Cekic, 1996). This was subsequently confirmed in a study using thalamocortical slice preparations, showing muscarinic presynaptic inhibition of excitatory recurrent connections in neocortex and also showing nicotinic enhancement of afferent input (Gil et al., 1997).

In the visual cortex, optical imaging was used to show cholinergic suppression of the internal spread of activity along excitatory recurrent connections compared to afferent input (Kimura and Baughman, 1997; Kimura, 2000). This indicated that acetylcholine should reduce the functional spread of activity on excitatory recurrent connections in visual cortex. This was supported by in-vivo experimental data showing that iontophoretic application of acetylcholine decreases the extent of spatial integration, assessed by measuring a neuron's length tuning (Roberts et al., 2005). These effects appear to contribute to the influence of top-down attention on the dynamics of visual cortex processing (Herrero et al., 2008). This work has been extended to human subjects in a study showing that the acetylcholinesterase blocker donepezil reduces the extent of the spread of activity in visual cortical areas associated with foveal stimulation (Silver et al., 2008).

The hippocampal data and modeling based on the Marr model generated the prediction that blockade of muscarinic receptors by the muscarinic antagonist scopolamine should enhance proactive interference in a paired associate memory task (Hasselmo and Wyble, 1997; Wyble and Hasselmo, 1997). This was supported by experimental data on scopolamine effects in human subjects (Atri et al., 2004). Enhancement of proactive interference was also shown in studies on discrimination of pairs of odors in rats administered scopolamine (De Rosa and Hasselmo, 2000) or after receiving selective lesions of the cholinergic innervation of the olfactory cortex (De Rosa et al., 2001). In computational models, the build-up of proactive interference causes runaway synaptic modification within cortical networks that can spread from one region to another. This mechanism was proposed to underlie the early appearance of tangles in lateral entorhinal cortex and the progressive spread from lateral entorhinal cortex to other regions (Hasselmo, 1994, 1997). This provides a computational framework that would predict reductions in Alzheimer's pathology with loss of fast hippocampal learning (e.g., in the most extreme case, patient HM would be expected to show absence of Alzheimer's pathology in his remaining temporal lobe structures). This framework could account for the beneficial effects of the NMDA blocker memantine (Reisberg et al., 2003) and supports the use of selective activation of presynaptic muscarinic receptors with M4 agonists in treatment of the disorder (Shirey et al., 2008) as this selective presynaptic inhibition of recurrent glutamatergic synapses could prevent the build-up of intereference between overlapping memories during encoding.

The levels of acetylcholine change dramatically during different stages of waking and sleep (Hasselmo, 1999). Acetylcholine levels are high during active waking, show decreases during quiet waking, and decrease to less than one-third of waking levels during slow-wave sleep (Marrosu et al., 1995). The decrease in acetylcholine levels during slow-wave sleep has been proposed to release the presynaptic inhibition from hippocampus back to neocortex, allowing activity based on recently formed associations in the hippocampus to spread back to the neocortex and drive consolidation of memories in the neocortex (Hasselmo, 1999). This is consistent with the hypothesis of Marr that was simulated in models of hippocampal–cortical interactions (Alvarez and Squire, 1994; McClelland et al., 1995; Hasselmo et al., 1996; Hasselmo, 1999).

This proposal is consistent with the muscarinic cholinergic presynaptic inhibition shown at a number of stages of the feedback connections (Hasselmo, 1999), including the excitatory recurrent connections in region CA3 (Hasselmo et al., 1995; Vogt and Regehr, 2001; Kremin and Hasselmo, 2007), the connections from region CA3 to region CA1 (Hounsgaard, 1978; Valentino and Dingledine, 1981; Hasselmo and Schnell, 1994; de Sevilla et al., 2002), and the feedback connections within neocortical structures (Hasselmo and Cekic, 1996; Gil et al., 1997).

This model of the role of acetylcholine in consolidation led to some functional predictions that have been tested (Hasselmo, 1999). If a reduction in cholinergic presynaptic inhibition enhances consolidation during slow-wave sleep, then an increase in acetylcholine levels during slow-wave sleep should impair consolidation. This was tested in a study in which subjects were administered physostigmine during slow-wave sleep, and showed reductions in subsequent tests of declarative memory consolidation performed after the subjects were awakened (Gais and Born, 2004). On the other hand, the model predicts that reductions in acetylcholine modulation during waking should enhance consolidation. This was shown in a study in which scopolamine was administered to block muscarinic cholinergic receptors after encoding of information, and subjects showed an enhancement of consolidation on a later memory test (Rasch et al., 2006) similar to the effect of a rest period after encoding (Dewar et al., 2012; 2014). Thus, computational modeling has provided an exciting link between cellular mechanisms of muscarinic presynaptic inhibition and behavioral studies in animals and humans.

This framework describes how the transitions between different levels of acetylcholine during waking and sleep can regulate the transition between encoding and consolidation. But this leaves the question of how more rapid transitions between encoding and retrieval could be regulated. Muscarinic presynaptic inhibition cannot change rapidly, as shown by studies in which 100 ms pressure pulse applications of acetylcholine cause changes in presynaptic inhibition that persist for 10–20 seconds (Hasselmo and Fehlau, 2001). In contrast, rapid transitions between encoding and retrieval could be mediated by the change in dynamics during individual cycles of the theta rhythm oscillations in hippocampus (Hasselmo et al., 2002). These dynamical changes could be regulated by postsynaptic $GABA_A$ inhibition (Toth et al., 1997) and presynaptic $GABA_B$ inhibition (Molyneaux and Hasselmo, 2002). Encoding could take place when entorhinal synaptic input is strongest at the trough of the EEG recorded at the hippocampal fissure (Hasselmo et al., 2002), and retrieval could be dominant when region CA3 input is strongest at the peak of fissure theta. The change in relative strength of synaptic input is supported by studies showing phasic changes in strength of evoked synaptic transmission on different pathways at different phases of the theta rhythm oscillation (Wyble et al., 2000; Villarreal et al., 2007). Consistent with the theorized role of these different phases in encoding and retrieval, the human EEG shows reset to different phases of theta rhythm during encoding and retrieval (Rizzuto et al., 2006), and spiking in rat hippocampus appears on different phases of hippocampal theta during match and nonmatch stimuli (Manns et al., 2007). In further support of these theories, gamma coherence with entorhinal cortex versus CA3 has been shown at different phases of theta (Colgin et al., 2009) and activation of inhibition at different phases of the theta cycle has differential effects on encoding and retrieval (Siegle and Wilson, 2014).

Oscillatory dynamics and grid cells

The basic model initially proposed by David Marr provided the groundwork for extension into additional physiological phenomena. In early models, memories were represented by single static input vectors that did not address the continuous dynamics of the hippocampal formation. An important subsequent body of modeling research has focused on the role of oscillations in cortical function, including the role of theta rhythm in hippocampal function.

As mentioned earlier, Marr's collateral effects could mediate encoding of sequences. This modeling appeared relevant to the phenomenon of theta-phase precession that was first discovered by O'Keefe (O'Keefe and Recce, 1993) and then replicated extensively in other studies (Skaggs et al., 1996; Huxter et al., 2003). In theta-phase precession, the spiking response of hippocampal place cells changes relative to theta rhythm oscillations recorded simultaneously in the hippocampal EEG. When a rat first enters the place field of an individual place cell, the spikes occur predominantly at a relatively late phase of the theta rhythm. The spikes shift to progressively earlier phases as the rat traverses the field.

A number of initial models of theta-phase precession used the collateral effect to encode and retrieve sequences of place cells, generating precession based on the timing of retrieval. The experimental replication of phase precession in the McNaughton laboratory was accompanied by a model of phase precession based on slow retrieval of a learned sequence of spatial locations during each theta cycle (Tsodyks et al., 1996). A similar sequence readout model was presented that year by Jensen and Lisman (1996a). In the Jensen and Lisman model, the phase precession during encoding arose from a working memory buffer in which afterdepolarization allowed neurons to be played out in a sequence on each theta cycle (Jensen and Lisman, 1996b). Both of these models required relatively slow readout of the sequence across the full theta cycle, at a rate slower than the time constants of glutamatergic AMPA conductances. The following year a different model was presented (Wallenstein and Hasselmo, 1997) in which readout had the faster time course of AMPA conductances, but the length of the readout would shift across the theta cycle based on level of presynaptic inhibition or the level of postsynaptic depolarization. This model was extended later to include the context-dependent retrieval of sequences, accounting for the reappearance of theta-phase precession over initial trials on each new day (Hasselmo and Eichenbaum, 2005).

However, the readout of sequences based on Hebbian synaptic modification was not the only approach to modeling theta-phase precession. In the original paper describing theta-phase precession, the phenomenon was proposed to arise from a progressive phase shift between the network EEG oscillation frequency and the intrinsic spiking frequency of the neuron which was shown to have a higher frequency based on the autocorrelation of spiking activity (O'Keefe and Recce, 1993). That paper presents a simple figure showing how the interaction of two oscillations of slightly different frequency will cause a precession of the summed oscillation relative to the lower frequency oscillation. This model makes an interesting additional prediction that there should be multiple firing fields, each showing the same precession. Since most place cells had a single firing field, this was perceived as a problem of the model, and later implementations kept the oscillations out of phase with each other until one was shifted to a higher frequency in the firing field (Lengyel et al., 2003). However, the later discovery of grid cells casts a different light on the original model, fulfilling the prediction of the model for multiple firing fields that was initially perceived as a problem of the model. Thus, the model by O'Keefe and Recce essentially predicted the existence of grid cells with multiple firing fields. Another related model generates interference effects using a variant involving inhibitory influences on pyramidal cells (Bose et al., 2000; Bose and Recce, 2001).

Another class of models proposed that phase precession arose from progressive shifts in the postsynaptic depolarization of neurons, causing spikes to occur at different phases relative to network inhibitory oscillations (Kamondi et al., 1998; Magee, 2001; Mehta et al., 2002). These different models have motivated a number of different experimental studies. The sequence retrieval models were supported by an initial study showing that stimulation inducing reset of theta-phase oscllations did not shift phase: spiking after reset would commence at the same phase as before the reset (Zugaro et al., 2005). However, a more recent study strongly supported the oscillatory interference model by showing that intracellularly recorded oscillations in membrane potential also show phase precession relative to network oscillations (Harvey et al., 2009; Schmidt-Hieber and Hausser, 2013), an effect not predicted by the sequence readout model. The postsynaptic depolarization model did not predict this shift in phase of intracellular oscillations (Kamondi et al., 1998). In addition, the postsynaptic depolarization models predicted an asymmetrical sawtooth waveform for a depolarizing shift in the place field, whereas the data showed a symmetrical depolarization in the place field (Harvey et al., 2009).

As noted above, the original presentation of the oscillatory interference model of theta-phase precession predicted the existence of neurons with multiple, regularly spaced firing fields (O'Keefe and Recce, 1993). Though the authors initially saw this as a problem for the model, the generation of multiple firing fields by the model is explicitly shown in Figure 10 of O'Keefe and Recce(1993). This initially undesired prediction of the model was validated by the later discovery of grid cells in the medial entorhinal cortex in the Moser laboratory. In the data from the Moser laboratory, the existence of repeating firing fields was first noted in the dorsal portion of medial entorhinal cortex (Fyhn et al., 2004), and subsequently the regular hexagonal arrangement of firing fields was noted and found to extend to more ventral regions of medial entorhinal cortex with larger spacing between the firing fields (Hafting et al., 2005). The systematic increase in spacing between firing fields for neurons in more ventral locations has been shown in great detail in subsequent papers (Sargolini et al., 2006), including very large and widely spaced firing fields in more ventral medial entorhinal cortex (Brun et al., 2008; Stensola et al., 2012).

When the first paper on grid cells appeared, O'Keefe and Burgess immediately recognized the significance of the repeating nature of grid cell firing, as this had been a strong feature of the theta-phase precession model. They rapidly pointed out how oscillatory interference could underlie the properties of grid cell firing (O'Keefe and Burgess, 2005). At the Computational Cognitive Neuroscience meeting in Washington, DC in 2005, Neil Burgess presented a poster with a detailed model using velocity modulation of firing frequency to generate realistic grid cell firing fields (Burgess et al., 2005, 2007). The oscillatory interference model of grid cells immediately generated a prediction about the mechanism for the difference in spacing of grid cells along the dorsal to ventral axis of medial entorhinal cortex (O'Keefe and Burgess, 2005). To quote that paper directly:

> The increasing spatial scale of the grid-like firing as you move from the postrhinal border of the medial entorhinal cortex would result from a gradually decreasing intrinsic frequency.

This prediction was supported by intracellular whole-cell patch recording from stellate cells in slice preparations of medial entorhinal cortex (Giocomo et al., 2007). These recordings showed a clear difference in the resonant frequency and the frequency of subthreshold membrane potential oscillations (Giocomo et al., 2007), with a gradual decrease in these intrinsic frequencies for slices more ventral relative to the postrhinal border. Thus, the prediction of the model was clearly supported by the data. The data on frequency membrane potential oscillations and resonance has been replicated by other groups (Boehlen et al., 2010; Pastoll et al., 2012) as well as my own (Heys et al., 2010; Shay et al., 2012).

In our initial presentation of the data on differences in intrinsic frequency (Giocomo et al., 2007), we illustrated the functional significance of the data by incorporating the difference in intrinsic frequency into the oscillatory interference model by Burgess (Burgess et al., 2007; Burgess, 2008). Using a multiplicative version of the model, we showed that higher intrinsic frequency in dorsal cells could generate the narrower spacing between firing fields of grid cells recording in dorsal entorhinal cortex, and the lower frequency in ventral cells could generate the wider spacing in more ventral cells. In a later paper, we showed that the data was more consistent with the additive model (Burgess et al., 2007; Burgess, 2008) that could account for very wide spacings by having a shallower slope of change in frequency with velocity (Giocomo and Hasselmo, 2008a).

The dorsal to ventral difference in intrinsic frequency was accompanied by a gradual slowing of the time constant of the depolarizing sag in stellate cells caused by hyperpolarizing current injections activating the h current and causing a depolarizing rebound (Giocomo et al., 2007). This suggested a role for h current in the dorsal to ventral difference in intrinsic frequency, which was supported by voltage clamp data suggesting a difference in the time constant of the h current as well as a trend toward differences in the magnitude of the h current (Giocomo and Hasselmo, 2008b). Testing of intrinsic frequencies in mice with knockout of the h current showed a flattening of the gradients of intrinsic frequencies (Giocomo and Hasselmo, 2009). These results were consistent with recordings in oocytes showing that homomeric h current channels using just the HCN1 subunit had faster time constant than homomeric HCN2 channels, with an intermediate time constant for heteromeric channels combining HCN1 and HCN2 subunits (Chen et al., 2001). Thus, this model provided an exciting link between molecular and cellular properties of neurons in medial entorhinal cortex, and the functional coding of space by the grid cell firing properties of these neurons. However, implementations of entorhinal stellate cell models (Fransén et al., 2004) show that subthreshold oscillations on different dendrites tended to synchronize (Remme et al., 2009; Remme et al., 2010). In addition, analysis of the variability of oscillation period showed that the membrane potential oscillations were too noisy to allow stable coding of location by phase (Giocomo and Hasselmo, 2008a; Zilli et al., 2009). These points argued against a single-cell implementation of the model and argued for a network implementation.

The effect of single-cell resonance on spike timing is a topic of ongoing research. It is clear that resonance does not result in rhythmic spiking only at the resonant frequency, but allows a range of frequencies with only a small deflection at the resonant frequency (Giocomo and Hasselmo, 2008a). In contrast, more robust spiking around theta rhythm could be mediated by rebound spiking in stellate cells (Hasselmo, 2014; Hasselmo and Shay, 2014) or by the intrinsic persistent spiking mechanisms in medial entorhinal pyramidal cells (Egorov et al., 2002; Fransén et al., 2006; Tahvildari et al., 2007). A model of grid cells based on persistent spiking cells can hold a steady baseline frequency. Cells with stable baseline frequencies have been shown in deep layers of medial entorhinal cortex (Egorov et al., 2002; Fransén et al., 2006; Tahvildari et al., 2007), in layer III of lateral entorhinal cortex (Tahvildari et al., 2007) and in the postsubiculum (Yoshida and Hasselmo, 2009). These neurons tend to fire at the same stable baseline frequency regardless of the duration of the stimulation causing persistent spiking (Yoshida and Hasselmo, 2009). A computational model of grid cells based on persistent spiking was developed using grid cells responding to the convergent input from different groups of persistent spiking cells that receive input from different sets of head direction cells (Hasselmo, 2008). This effectively simulated grid cells based on shifts in the frequency of persistent spiking input (Hasselmo, 2008), and effectively simulates theta-phase precession in grid cells consistent with experimental data showing theta-phase precession in grid cells (Hafting et al., 2008).

Persistent spiking also shows variability in firing frequency that could interfere with the stability of phase coding. However, network-level dynamics may overcome this variability, allowing cells that are intrinsically noisy and irregular in their firing to still participate in a network oscillation with frequency and phase sufficiently stable to generate grid cell firing (Zilli and Hasselmo, 2010). This model can respond with different frequencies for different depolarizing inputs depending on the magnitude of the h current in individual neurons, though it is difficult to maintain a linear relationship between depolarizing input and magnitude of frequency change. I have also developed another alternative model in which rebound spiking based on h current properties can regulate the spiking of neurons (Hasselmo, 2014; Hasselmo and Shay, 2014). The further development of such models provides a framework for explaining the relationship between intrinsic resonance and the spacing of grid cell firing fields.

A number of alternate mechanisms have been proposed for the generation of grid cell firing properties, including attractor dynamics due to structured excitatory recurrent connectivity (Fuhs and Touretzky, 2006; McNaughton et al., 2006; Burak and Fiete, 2009) and self-organization of afferent input (Kropff and Treves, 2008). The attractor dynamics models do not account for some data as well as oscillatory interference models, but they are better at accounting for the consistent orientation and spacing of grid cells within local regions of the medial entorhinal cortex (Hafting et al., 2005), and the quantal transitions in the spacing between firing fields (Barry et al., 2007; Stensola et al., 2012).

Most attractor dynamic models do not utilize theta frequency oscillations in spiking activity and do not account for theta-phase precession. However, a recent model used attractor dynamics and simulated grid cell theta-phase precession, while generating differences in spacing based on the time course of medium afterhyperpolarization (Navratilova et al., 2012). The importance of theta rhythm oscillations for grid cell generation has been demonstrated by local infusions into the medial septum that block network theta rhythm oscillations in the entorhinal cortex. Grid cell firing patterns do not appear during pharmacological blockade of theta rhythm oscillations (Brandon et al., 2011; Koenig et al., 2011), whereas head direction responses are spared.

As described here, the discovery of grid cells and their relationship to the intrinsic resonance properties of entorhinal neurons provides fascinating clues to the function of the entorhinal cortex and hippocampus in human episodic memory. A theoretical framework based on the oscillatory interference model and elements of the Marr model can perform the encoding and retrieval of complex trajectories as episodic memories (Hasselmo, 2009; Hasselmo, 2012). The data have not yet converged on a final model of the mechanism for generation of grid cells, but the ongoing interaction of computational modeling guidance and experimental neurophysiology has provided insights beyond any that might have been imagined at the time of Marr's seminal paper.

Evidence for a general theory of cerebral cortex

Though Marr's paper on cerebral cortex (Marr, 1970) is not the primary focus of this chapter, any study of hippocampus and entorhinal cortex raises questions of the function of neocortical regions based on the importance of interactions of these regions with other areas. In particular, the sensory influences of visual stimuli on grid cell firing require processed inputs from visual cortex, whereas navigation mechanisms appear to involve regions of parietal cortex (Byrne et al., 2007), and generation of decisions during behavior appear to involve regions of prefrontal cortex. As proposed in Marr (1970), it is generally accepted that the neocortex is involved in extraction of common features from sensory input, and this capacity appears to be consistent across different neocortical regions resulting in the capacity to respond to rewired input (Roe et al., 1990), or to mediate recovery after cortical damage. But there are more complex cognitive functions of cortex that remain to be accounted for, such as the functions of planning or reasoning. It remains to be shown how these functions can be mediated, but Marr's notion of a theory of cerebral cortex has been echoed in subsequent papers attempting to find regular features of neocortical function (Douglas et al., 1989; Grossberg and Seitz, 2003; Douglas and Martin, 2007; Howard et al., 2014).

Marr presented an overview of the function of local circuits of cerebral cortex with remarkable specificity about the function of individual neuronal subtypes. Though Marr did not have sufficient physiological information, this overall approach has been validated by subsequent studies showing specialized functions of individual interneuron subtypes in hippocampus and neocortex that appear to be consistent across different regions. Neocortical interneurons have specific defining markers that define three nonoverlapping category markers: parvalbumin (PV), somatostatin (SST), and ionotropic serotonin receptors (5HT3A) (Lee et al., 2010; Rudy et al., 2011). Within the 5HT3A category, there are additional markers including vasoactive intestinal peptide (VIP) and neuropeptide Y (NPY). Recent studies of neocortical circuitry have revealed cortical motifs that appear to be consistent across different regions. In particular, it has been shown that activation of VIP neurons appears to selectively inhibit SST and PV interneurons (Lee et al., 2013; Fu et al., 2014), thereby disinhibiting neocortical pyramidal cells. This appears to underlie the increased activity observed in running mice versus stationary mice (Niell and Stryker, 2010) due to the cholinergic nicotinic activation of VIP interneurons that then inhibit other interneurons as shown in cortical regions including V1 (Fu et al., 2014). This mechanism also appears to underlie effects of reinforcement signals (reward and punishment) on auditory cortex responses, in which activation of VIP neurons inhibits SST and PV cells (Pi et al., 2013), consistent with earlier studies showing disinhibition mediated by layer I interneurons (Letzkus et al., 2011). A similar mechanism appears to mediate increases and decreases in spiking activity during whisker movements due to M1 cortical inputs to VIP interneurons (Lee et al., 2013). Stimulation of the basal forebrain has been shown to activate VIP interneurons but not PV interneurons via nicotinic cholinergic receptors (Alitto and Dan, 2012). Acetylcholine directly depolarizes VIP neurons (Lee et al., 2010) and depolarizes somatostatin but not PV cells (Kawaguchi, 1997). Testing of connectivity patterns between interneuron subtypes using pairwise recordings in slices of visual cortex revealed that VIP interneurons strongly inhibit somatostatin cells, and somatostatin cells inhibit almost all other interneurons including PV cells (Pfeffer et al., 2013), thereby setting up complex dynamics of inhibition or disinhibition that influence pyramidal cells. These studies provide examples of a local functional circuit that appears to be replicated within neocortex. It does not address the complexity of the self-organization properties proposed by Marr, but it shows how research has progressed to provide more detailed circuit-level models that could be incorporated in future models.

The need for more people like Marr

The influence of Marr's paper arises not only from the importance of the ideas he expressed but also from his unique talents as a mathematician who was willing and able to delve into the detailed neurophysiological connectivity of the structures that he modeled. The field needs more geniuses of this caliber who are willing to devote the time to studying the detailed information available about hippocampal and cortical circuits. Marr accomplished a lot with incomplete data. With the dramatically enhanced experimental data available today on both an anatomical and a physiological level, the field is ripe for a sophisticated breakthrough model of this type.

There have been many theoretical advances since the time of Marr's paper. However, most of these have tended to tap into an existing framework of mathematical theory that was not initially generated to understand brain circuits. This is understandable because the work of most mathematicians and physicists is still being evaluated by other mathematicians or physicists within their own departments, or at least by what they consider their peer groups. In order to maintain what they see as an appropriate level of rigor, they will stay within existing mathematical frameworks. For example, much current theoretical work on brain function uses the framework of Bayesian theory (Chikkerur et al., 2010; Gershman et al., 2012), or the framework of reinforcement learning theory (Sutton and Barto, 1998) which draws on the mathematics of dynamic programming. Both of these have been very useful approaches, but these mathematical frameworks do not directly focus on relating function to the detailed dynamics of neural circuitry.

On the level of neural circuitry, considerable research has used the framework of dynamical systems for describing network dynamics, including the use of attractor dynamics for describing pattern completion, and the use of phase response curves for analyzing the phase relationships of oscillations. These techniques have been very useful for addressing the local dynamics of neuronal membrane potentials as well as rhythmic circuits and field potential oscillations in cortical structures. This forms the foundation for creating overarching models that link these circuit-level dynamics to the larger-scale network dynamics within cortical structures.

As reviewed in the introductory section of this chapter, there are many outstanding researchers who have presented theories of hippocampal and cortical function that have been influential in the manner of Marr's work. However, we have not yet seen a breakthrough on a scale that would achieve consensus in the field around a single theory. Marr did not achieve such a consensus with his model, despite its subsequent influence. If we take physics as a model for neuroscience, then the true judge of a breakthrough model will be its adoption by the majority of researchers, in the way that Newtonian mechanics was adopted, or Maxwell's equations for electromagnetism. An essential feature of such an adoption is that the theory should be widely useful for simulating and predicting quantitative data, in the nature of previous successful theories in the field of physics.

What would be the characteristics of a future David Marr? Such a person would likely be trained as a mathematician or physicist, to have the necessary theoretical skills for describing the model in concise mathematical form, but they would also have a deep immersion in the experimental data on the anatomy, physiology, and behavioral function of the hippocampal formation. Above all, they should have the talent and focus to bring together these diverse concepts and unify them in a coherent mathematical framework that can account for the existing data and correctly predict future experimental tests of the theory.

What would an effective theory look like? A possible form of an effective theory would be a wave-based model representing propagation of rhythmic neural activity within multiple dimensions of cortical representation. During encoding, the activity in hippocampus and entorhinal cortex would code the complex spatiotemporal trajectory of self-location and time during behavior, and encode associations between different elements of the trajectory. The segments of this complex spatiotemporal trajectory would also be associated with a vector representing the spherical angle and information content of sensory input encountered at specific locations and head directions along the trajectory, via modifications of synaptic connections or intrinsic properties. During replay or recollection, a retrieval cue activating a specific segment of the trajectory would trigger retrieval of other segments and the associated multidimensional information content and spherical angle of sensory input.

This is only a brief sketch of a possible model. One salient difference from the Marr standard model is that a new theory should incorporate the new physiological data on place cells, grid cells, border cells, and head direction cells. In addition, a new model should address the dynamics of hippocampal circuits to account for the theta rhythm oscillations and theta-phase precession as well as the interactions of low and high gamma frequencies with theta rhythm oscillations. These physiological properties should be associated with more complex functional properties for encoding episodes as spatiotemporal trajectories and using the retrieval of these episodes for memory-guided behavior in tasks such as delayed spatial alternation or the Morris water maze. These physiological and behavioral datasets are primarily associated with studies in rats and mice, so it might be necessary to focus the initial hippocampal theory specifically on rat hippocampus. It would be a substantial accomplishment to create a special theory that accounts for anatomy, physiology, and function in the rat hippocampal formation. Subsequently, the theory could be expanded to address what is known about the function of the human hippocampal formation.

Acknowledgments

Research supported by R01 MH60013, R01 MH61492, Silvio O. Conte Center P50 MH094263, NSF EAGER grant PHY144389, and the Office of Naval Research MURI grant N00014-10-1-0936.

References

Abbott LF, Blum KI. (1996). Functional significance of long-term potentiation for sequence learning and prediction. Cereb Cortex. **6**:406–416.

Alitto HJ, Dan Y. (2012). Cell-type-specific modulation of neocortical activity by basal forebrain input. Front Syst Neurosci. **6**:79.

Alvarez P, Squire LR. (1994). Memory consolidation and the medial temporal lobe: a simple network model. Proc Natl Acad Sci U S A. **91**:7041–7045.

Amit DJ. (1988). Modeling Brain Function: The World of Attractor Neural Networks. Cambridge: Cambridge University Press.

Amit DJ, Evans MR, Abeles M. (1990). Attractor neural networks with biological probe records. Network. **1**:381–405.

Amit DJ, Treves A. (1989). Associative memory neural networks with low temporal spiking rates. Proc Natl Acad Sci U S A. **86**:7671–7673.

Anderson JA. (1972). A simple neural network generating an interactive memory. Math Biosci. **14**:197–220.

Atri A, Sherman S, Norman KA, Kirchhoff BA, Nicolas MM, Greicius MD, et al. (2004). Blockade of central cholinergic receptors impairs new learning and increases proactive interference in a word paired-associate memory task. Behav Neurosci. **118**:223–236.

Bakker A, Kirwan CB, Miller M, Stark CE. (2008). Pattern separation in the human hippocampal CA3 and dentate gyrus. Science. **319**:1640–1642.

Barkai E, Bergman RE, Horwitz G, Hasselmo ME. (1994). Modulation of associative memory function in a biophysical simulation of rat piriform cortex. J Neurophysiol. **72**:659–677.

Barkai E, Hasselmo ME. (1994). Modulation of the input/output function of rat piriform cortex pyramidal cells. J Neurophysiol. **72**:644–658.

Barnes CA, McNaughton BL, Mizumori SJ, Leonard BW, Lin LH. (1990). Comparison of spatial and temporal characteristics of neuronal activity in sequential stages of hippocampal processing. Prog Brain Res. **83**:287–300.

Barry C, Hayman R, Burgess N, Jeffery KJ. (2007). Experience-dependent rescaling of entorhinal grids. Nat Neurosci. **10**:682–684.

Becker S. (2005). A computational principle for hippocampal learning and neurogenesis. Hippocampus. **15**:722–738.

Blum KI, Abbott LF. (1996). A model of spatial map formation in the hippocampus of the rat. Neural Comput. **8**:85–93.

Boehlen A, Heinemann U, Erchova I. (2010). The range of intrinsic frequencies represented by medial entorhinal cortex stellate cells extends with age. J Neurosci. **30**:4585–4589.

Bose A, Booth V, Recce M. (2000). A temporal mechanism for generating the phase precession of hippocampal place cells. J Comput Neurosci. **9**:5–30.

Bose A, Recce M. (2001). Phase precession and phase-locking of hippocampal pyramidal cells. Hippocampus. **11**:204–215.

Brandon MP, Bogaard AR, Libby CP, Connerney MA, Gupta K, Hasselmo ME. (2011). Reduction of theta rhythm dissociates grid cell spatial periodicity from directional tuning. Science. **332**:595–599.

Brewer JB, Zhao Z, Desmond JE, Glover GH, Gabrieli JD. (1998). Making memories: brain activity that predicts how well visual experience will be remembered. Science. **281**:1185–1187.

Brun VH, Solstad T, Kjelstrup KB, Fyhn M, Witter MP, Moser EI, Moser MB. (2008). Progressive increase in grid scale from dorsal to ventral medial entorhinal cortex. Hippocampus. **18**:1200–1212.

Buckner RL, Petersen SE, Ojemann JG, Miezin FM, Squire LR, Raichle ME. (1995). Functional anatomical studies of explicit and implicit memory retrieval tasks. J Neurosci. **15**(1 Pt 1):12–29.

Burak Y, Fiete IR. (2009). Accurate path integration in continuous attractor network models of grid cells. PLoS Comput Biol **5**:e1000291.

Burgess N, Barry C, Jeffery KJ, O'Keefe J. (2005). A grid and place cell model of path integration utilizing phase precession versus theta. Computational Cognitive Neuroscience Conference Poster; Washington DC. http://posters.f1000.com/PosterList.

Burgess N, Barry C, O'Keefe J. (2007). An oscillatory interference model of grid cell firing. Hippocampus. **17**:801–812.

Byrne P, Becker S, Burgess N. (2007). Remembering the past and imagining the future: a neural model of spatial memory and imagery. Psychol Rev. **114**:340–375.

Chen S, Wang J, Siegelbaum SA. (2001). Properties of hyperpolarization-activated pacemaker current defined by coassembly of HCN1 and HCN2 subunits and basal modulation by cyclic nucleotide. J Gen Physiol. **117**:491–504.

Chikkerur S, Serre T, Tan C, Poggio T. (2010). What and where: a Bayesian inference theory of attention. Vision Res. **50**:2233–(2247).

Cohen MA, Grossberg S. (1983). Absolute stability of global pattern formation and parallel memory storage by competitive neural networks. IEEE Trans Syst Man Cybern. **13**:815–826.

Colgin LL, Denninger T, Fyhn M, Hafting T, Bonnevie T, Jensen O, et al. (2009). Frequency of gamma oscillations routes flow of information in the hippocampus. Nature. **462**:353–357.

Davidson TJ, Kloosterman F, Wilson MA. (2009) Hippocampal replay of extended experience. Neuron **63**:497–507.

De Rosa E, Hasselmo ME. (2000). Muscarinic cholinergic neuromodulation reduces proactive interference between stored odor memories during associative learning in rats. Behav Neurosci. **114**:32–41.

De Rosa E, Hasselmo ME, Baxter MG. (2001). Contribution of the cholinergic basal forebrain to proactive interference from stored odor memories during associative learning in rats. Behav Neurosci. **115**:314–327.

de Sevilla DF, Cabezas C, de Prada AN, Sanchez-Jimenez A, Buno W. (2002). Selective muscarinic regulation of functional glutamatergic Schaffer collateral synapses in rat CA1 pyramidal neurons. J Physiol **545**(Pt 1):51–63.

Dewar M, Alber J, Butler C, Cowan N, Della Sala S. (2012). Brief wakeful resting boosts new memories over the long term. Psychol Sci. **23**:955–60.

Dewar M, Alber J, Cowan N, Della Sala S. (2014). Boosting long-term memory via wakeful rest: intentional rehearsal is not necessary, consolidation is sufficient. PLoS ONE **9**:e109542.

Diba K, Buzsaki G (2007) Forward and reverse hippocampal place-cell sequences during ripples. Nat. Neurosci. **10**:1241–1242.

Douglas RJ, Martin KA. (2007). Mapping the matrix: the ways of neocortex. Neuron. **56**:226–238.

Douglas RJ, Martin KA, Witteridge D. (1989). A canonical microcircuit for neocortex. Neural Comput. **1**:480–488.

Egorov AV, Hamam BN, Fransen E, Hasselmo ME, Alonso AA. (2002). Graded persistent activity in entorhinal cortex neurons. Nature. **420**:173–178.

Fransen E, Alonso AA, Dickson CT, Magistretti J, Hasselmo ME. (2004). Ionic mechanisms in the generation of subthreshold oscillations and action potential clustering in entorhinal layer II stellate neurons. Hippocampus. **14**:368–384.

Fransén E, Tahvildari B, Egorov AV, Hasselmo ME, Alonso AA. (2006). Mechanism of graded persistent cellular activity of entorhinal cortex layer v neurons. Neuron. 49:735–746.

Fu Y, Tucciarone JM, Espinosa JS, Sheng N, Darcy DP, Nicoll RA, et al. (2014). A cortical circuit for gain control by behavioral state. Cell. 156:1139–1152.

Fuhs MC, Touretzky DS. (2006). A spin glass model of path integration in rat medial entorhinal cortex. J Neurosci. 26:4266–4276.

Fyhn M, Molden S, Witter MP, Moser EI, Moser MB. (2004). Spatial representation in the entorhinal cortex. Science. 305:1258–1264.

Gais S, Born J. (2004). Low acetylcholine during slow-wave sleep is critical for declarative memory consolidation. Proc Natl Acad Sci U S A. 101:2140–2144.

Gershman SJ, Vul E, Tenenbaum JB. (2012). Multistability and perceptual inference. Neural Comput. 24:1–24.

Gil Z, Conners BW, Amitai Y. (1997). Differential regulation of neocortical synapses by neuromodulators and activity. Neuron. 19:679–686.

Gilbert PE, Kesner RP, Lee I. (2001). Dissociating hippocampal subregions: double dissociation between dentate gyrus and CA1. Hippocampus. 11:626–636.

Giocomo LM, Hasselmo ME. (2008a). Computation by oscillations: implications of experimental data for theoretical models of grid cells. Hippocampus. 18:1186–1199.

Giocomo LM, Hasselmo ME. (2008b). Time constants of h current in layer II stellate cells differ along the dorsal to ventral axis of medial entorhinal cortex. J Neurosci. 28:9414–9425.

Giocomo LM, Hasselmo ME. (2009). Knock-out of HCN1 subunit flattens dorsal-ventral frequency gradient of medial entorhinal neurons in adult mice. J Neurosci. 29:7625–7630.

Giocomo LM, Zilli EA, Fransen E, Hasselmo ME. (2007). Temporal frequency of subthreshold oscillations scales with entorhinal grid cell field spacing. Science. 315:1719–1722.

Grossberg S, Seitz A. (2003). Laminar development of receptive fields, maps and columns in visual cortex: the coordinating role of the subplate. Cereb Cortex. 13:852–863.

Guzowski JF, Knierim JJ, Moser EI. (2004). Ensemble dynamics of hippocampal regions CA3 and CA1. Neuron. 44:581–584.

Haberly LB, Bower JM. (1989). Olfactory cortex: Model circuit for study of associative memory? Trends Neurosci. 12:258–264.

Hafting T, Fyhn M, Bonnevie T, Moser MB, Moser EI. (2008). Hippocampus-independent phase precession in entorhinal grid cells. Nature. 453:1248–1252.

Hafting T, Fyhn M, Molden S, Moser MB, Moser EI. (2005). Microstructure of a spatial map in the entorhinal cortex. Nature. 436:801–806.

Harvey CD, Collman F, Dombeck DA, Tank DW. (2009). Intracellular dynamics of hippocampal place cells during virtual navigation. Nature. 461:941–946.

Hasselmo ME. (1994). Runaway synaptic modification in models of cortex: Implications for Alzheimer's disease. Neural Netw. 7:13–40.

Hasselmo ME. (1997). A computational model of the progression of Alzheimer's disease. MD Comput. 14:181–191.

Hasselmo ME. (1999). Neuromodulation: acetylcholine and memory consolidation. Trends Cogn Sci. 3:351–359.

Hasselmo ME. (2006). The role of acetylcholine in learning and memory. Curr Opin Neurobiol. 16: 710–715.

Hasselmo ME. (2008). Grid cell mechanisms and function: contributions of entorhinal persistent spiking and phase resetting. Hippocampus. 18:1213–1229.

Hasselmo ME. (2009). A model of episodic memory: mental time travel along encoded trajectories using grid cells. Neurobiol Learn Mem. 92:559–573.

Hasselmo ME. (2012). How We Remember: Brain Mechanisms of Episodic Memory. Cambridge, MA: MIT Press.

Hasselmo ME. (2014). Neuronal rebound spiking, resonance frequency and theta cycle skipping may contribute to grid cell firing in medial entorhinal cortex. Philos Trans R Soc Lond B Biol Sci. 369:20120523.

Hasselmo ME, Anderson BP, Bower JM. (1992). Cholinergic modulation of cortical associative memory function. J. Neurophysiol. **67**:1230–1246.

Hasselmo ME, Bodelon C, Wyble BP. (2002). A proposed function for hippocampal theta rhythm: separate phases of encoding and retrieval enhance reversal of prior learning. Neural Comput. **14**:793–817.

Hasselmo ME, Bower JM. (1992). Cholinergic suppression specific to intrinsic not afferent fiber synapses in rat piriform (olfactory) cortex. J Neurophysiol. **67**:1222–1229.

Hasselmo ME, Bower JM. (1993). Acetylcholine and memory. Trends Neurosci. **16**:218–222.

Hasselmo ME, Cekic M. (1996). Suppression of synaptic transmission may allow combination of associative feedback and self-organizing feedforward connections in the neocortex. Behav Brain Res **79**:153–161.

Hasselmo ME, Eichenbaum H. (2005). Hippocampal mechanisms for the context-dependent retrieval of episodes. Neural Netw. **18**:1172–1190.

Hasselmo ME, Fehlau BP. (2001). Differences in time course of ACh and GABA modulation of excitatory synaptic potentials in slices of rat hippocampus. J Neurophysiol. **86**:1792–1802.

Hasselmo ME, Schnell E. (1994). Laminar selectivity of the cholinergic suppression of synaptic transmission in rat hippocampal region CA1: computational modeling and brain slice physiology. J Neurosci. **14**:3898–3914.

Hasselmo ME, Schnell E, Barkai E. (1995). Dynamics of learning and recall at excitatory recurrent synapses and cholinergic modulation in rat hippocampal region CA3. J Neurosci **15**(7 Pt 2):5249–5262.

Hasselmo ME, Shay CF. (2014). Grid cell firing patterns may arise from feedback interaction between intrinsic rebound spiking and transverse traveling waves with multiple heading angles. Front Syst Neurosci. **8**:201.

Hasselmo ME, Stern CE. (2014). Theta rhythm and the encoding and retrieval of space and time. Neuroimage **85**: 656–666.

Hasselmo ME, Wyble BP. (1997). Free recall and recognition in a network model of the hippocampus: simulating effects of scopolamine on human memory function. Behav Brain Res **89**:1–34.

Hasselmo ME, Wyble BP, Wallenstein GV. (1996). Encoding and retrieval of episodic memories: role of cholinergic and GABAergic modulation in the hippocampus. Hippocampus. **6**:693–708.

Herrero JL, Roberts MJ, Delicato LS, Gieselmann MA, Dayan P, Thiele A. (2008). Acetylcholine contributes through muscarinic receptors to attentional modulation in V1. Nature. **454**:1110–1114.

Heys JG, Giocomo LM, Hasselmo ME. (2010). Cholinergic modulation of the resonance properties of stellate cells in layer II of medial entorhinal cortex. J Neurophysiol. **104**:258–270.

Holmes WR, Levy WB. (1990). Insights into associative long-term potentiation from computational models of NMDA receptor-mediated calcium influx and intracellular calcium concentration changes. J Neurophysiol. **63**:1148–1168.

Hopfield JJ. (1982). Neural networks and physical systems with emergent selective computational abilities. Proc Natl Acad Sci U S A. **79**:2554–2559.

Hopfield JJ. (1984). Neurons with graded response have collective computational properties like those of two-state neurons. Proc Natl Acad Sci U S A **81**:3088–3092.

Hounsgaard J. (1978). Presynaptic inhibitory action of acetylcholine in area CA1 of the hippocampus. Exp Neurol. **62**:787–797.

Howard MW, MacDonald CJ, Tiganj Z, Shankar KH, Du Q, Hasselmo ME, Eichenbaum H. (2014). A unified mathematical framework for coding time, space, and sequences in the hippocampal region. J Neurosci. **34**:4692–4707.

Huxter J, Burgess N, O'Keefe J. (2003). Independent rate and temporal coding in hippocampal pyramidal cells. Nature. **425**:828–832.

Jadhav SP, Kemere C, German PW, Frank LM. (2012) Awake hippocampal sharp-wave ripples support spatial memory. Science 336: 1454–1458.

Jensen O, Lisman JE. 1996a. Hippocampal CA3 region predicts memory sequences: accounting for the phase precession of place cells. Learn Mem. **3**:279–287.

Jensen O, Lisman JE. 1996b. Novel lists of 7 ± 2 known items can be reliably stored in an oscillatory short-term memory network: interaction with long-term memory. Learn Mem. **3**:257–263.

Kali S, Dayan P. (2000). The involvement of recurrent connections in area CA3 in establishing the properties of place fields: a model. J Neurosci. **20**:7463–7477.

Kamondi A, Acsady L, Wang XJ, Buzsaki G. (1998). Theta oscillations in somata and dendrites of hippocampal pyramidal cells in vivo: activity-dependent phase-precession of action potentials. Hippocampus. **8**:244–261.

Kawaguchi Y. (1997). Selective cholinergic modulation of cortical GABAergic cell subtypes. J Neurophysiol. **78**:1743–1747.

Kimura F. (2000). Cholinergic modulation of cortical function: a hypothetical role in shifting the dynamics in cortical network. Neurosci Res. **38**:19–26.

Kimura F, Baughman RW. (1997). Distinct muscarinic receptor subtypes suppress excitatory and inhibitory synaptic responses in cortical neurons. J Neurophysiol. **77**:709–716.

Kirchhoff BA, Wagner AD, Maril A, Stern CE. (2000). Prefrontal-temporal circuitry for episodic encoding and subsequent memory. J Neurosci. **20**:6173–6180.

Koenig J, Linder AN, Leutgeb JK, Leutgeb S. (2011). The spatial periodicity of grid cells is not sustained during reduced theta oscillations. Science. **332**:592–595.

Kohonen T. (1972). Correlation matrix memories. IEEE Trans. Computers. **C-21**:353–359.

Kohonen T. (1984). Self-organization and Associative Memory. Berlin: Springer-Verlag.

Kremin T, Hasselmo ME. (2007). Cholinergic suppression of glutamatergic synaptic transmission in hippocampal region CA3 exhibits laminar selectivity: Implication for hippocampal network dynamics. Neuroscience. **149**:760–767.

Kropff E, Treves A. (2008). The emergence of grid cells: Intelligent design or just adaptation? Hippocampus. **18**:1256–1269.

Lee AK, Wilson MA. (2002) Memory of sequential experience in the hippocampus during slow wave sleep. Neuron. 36:1183–1194.

Lee I, Yoganarasimha D, Rao G, Knierim JJ. (2004). Comparison of population coherence of place cells in hippocampal subfields CA1 and CA3. Nature. **430**:456–459.

Lee S, Hjerling-Leffler J, Zagha E, Fishell G, Rudy B. (2010). The largest group of superficial neocortical GABAergic interneurons expresses ionotropic serotonin receptors. J Neurosci. **30**:16796–16808.

Lee S, Kruglikov I, Huang ZJ, Fishell G, Rudy B. (2013). A disinhibitory circuit mediates motor integration in the somatosensory cortex. Nat Neurosci. **16**:1662–1670.

Lengyel M, Szatmary Z, Erdi P. (2003). Dynamically detuned oscillations account for the coupled rate and temporal code of place cell firing. Hippocampus. **13**:700–714.

Letzkus JJ, Wolff SB, Meyer EM, Tovote P, Courtin J, Herry C, Luthi A. (2011). A disinhibitory microcircuit for associative fear learning in the auditory cortex. Nature. **480**:331–335.

Leutgeb JK, Leutgeb S, Moser MB, Moser EI. (2007). Pattern separation in the dentate gyrus and CA3 of the hippocampus. Science. **315**:961–966.

Leutgeb S, Leutgeb JK, Treves A, Moser MB, Moser EI. (2004). Distinct ensemble codes in hippocampal areas CA3 and CA1. Science. **305**:1295–1298.

Levy WB. (1996). A sequence predicting CA3 is a flexible associator that learns and uses context to solve hippocampal-like tasks. Hippocampus. **6**:579–590.

Levy WB, Steward O. (1979). Synapses as associative memory elements in the hippocampal formation. Brain Res. **175**:233–245.

Levy WB, Steward O. (1983). Temporal contiguity requirements for long-term associative potentiation/depression in the hippocampus. Neuroscience. **8**:791–797.

Lomo T. (1971). Potentiation of monosynaptic EPSP's in the perforant path–dentate granule cell synapse. Exp Brain Res. **12**:46–63.

Magee JC. (2001). Dendritic mechanisms of phase precession in hippocampal CA1 pyramidal neurons. J Neurophysiol. **86**:528–532.

Manns JR, Zilli EA, Ong KC, Hasselmo ME, Eichenbaum H. (2007). Hippocampal CA1 spiking during encoding and retrieval: relation to theta phase. Neurobiol Learn Mem. **87**:9–20.

Marr D. (1969). A theory of cerebellar cortex. J Physiol. **202**:437–470.

Marr D. (1970). A theory of cerebral cortex. Proc R Soc Lond B Biol Sci. **176**:161–234.

Marr D. (1971). Simple memory: A theory for archicortex. Philos Trans R Soc Lond B Biol Sci. **262**:23–81.

Marrosu F, Portas C, Mascia MS, Casu MA, Fa M, Giagheddu M, et al. (1995). Microdialysis measurement of cortical and hippocampal acetylcholine release during sleep-wake cycle in freely moving cats. Brain Res. **671**:329–332.

McClelland JL, McNaughton BL, O'Reilly RC. (1995). Why there are complementary learning systems in the hippocampus and neocortex: insights from the successes and failures of connectionist models of learning and memory. Psychol Rev. **102**:419–457.

McClelland JL, Rumelhart DE. (1988). Explorations in Parallel Distributed Processing. Cambridge, MA: MIT Press.

McHugh TJ, Jones MW, Quinn JJ, Balthasar N, Coppari R, Elmquist JK, Lowell BB, Fanselow MS, Wilson MA, Tonegawa S. (2007). Dentate gyrus NMDA receptors mediate rapid pattern separation in the hippocampal network. Science. **317**:94–99.

McNaughton BL. (1991). Associative pattern completion in hippocampal circuits: New evidence and new questions. Brain Res Rev. **16**:193–220.

McNaughton BL, Battaglia FP, Jensen O, Moser EI, Moser MB. (2006). Path integration and the neural basis of the "cognitive map." Nat Rev Neurosci. **7**:663–678.

McNaughton BL, Douglas RM, Goddard GV. (1978). Synaptic enhancement in fascia dentata: Cooperativity among coactive afferents. Brain Res. **157**:277–293.

McNaughton BL, Morris RGM. (1987). Hippocampal synaptic enhancement and information storage within a distributed memory system. Trends Neurosci. **10**:408–415.

Mehta MR, Lee AK, Wilson MA. (2002). Role of experience and oscillations in transforming a rate code into a temporal code. Nature. **417**:741–746.

Mehta MR, Quirk MC, Wilson MA. (2000). Experience-dependent asymmetric shape of hippocampal receptive fields. Neuron. **25**:707–715.

Minai AA, Levy WB. (1993). Sequence learning in a single trial. In: Proceedings of the World Congress on Neural Networks. **2**:505–508.

Molyneaux BJ, Hasselmo ME. (2002). GABA(B) presynaptic inhibition has an in vivo time constant sufficiently rapid to allow modulation at theta frequency. J Neurophysiol. 87:1196–1205.

Nakashiba T, Cushman JD, Pelkey KA, Renaudineau S, Buhl DL, McHugh TJ, et al. (2012). Young dentate granule cells mediate pattern separation, whereas old granule cells facilitate pattern completion. Cell. 149:188–201.

Nakashiba T, Young JZ, McHugh TJ, Buhl DL, Tonegawa S. (2008). Transgenic inhibition of synaptic transmission reveals role of CA3 output in hippocampal learning. Science. 319:1260–1264.

Nakazawa K, Quirk MC, Chitwood RA, Watanabe M, Yeckel MF, Sun LD, et al. (2002). Requirement for hippocampal CA3 NMDA receptors in associative memory recall. Science. 297:211–218.

Navratilova Z, Giocomo LM, Fellous JM, Hasselmo ME, McNaughton BL. (2012). Phase precession and variable spatial scaling in a periodic attractor map model of medial entorhinal grid cells with realistic after-spike dynamics. Hippocampus. 22:772–789.

Neunuebel JP, Knierim JJ. (2014). CA3 retrieves coherent representations from degraded input: direct evidence for CA3 pattern completion and dentate gyrus pattern separation. Neuron. 81:416–427.

Niell CM, Stryker MP. (2010). Modulation of visual responses by behavioral state in mouse visual cortex. Neuron. 65:472–479.

O'Keefe J, Burgess N. (2005). Dual phase and rate coding in hippocampal place cells: theoretical significance and relationship to entorhinal grid cells. Hippocampus. 15:853–866.

O'Keefe J, Dostrovsky J. (1971). The hippocampus as a spatial map. Preliminary evidence from unit activity in the freely-moving rat. Brain Res. 34:171–175.

O'Keefe J, Recce ML. (1993). Phase relationship between hippocampal place units and the EEG theta rhythm. Hippocampus. 3:317–330.

O'Reilly RC, McClelland JL. (1994). Hippocampal conjunctive encoding, storage, and recall: avoiding a trade-off. Hippocampus. 4:661–682.

Pastoll H, Ramsden HL, Nolan MF. (2012). Intrinsic electrophysiological properties of entorhinal cortex stellate cells and their contribution to grid cell firing fields. Front Neural Circuits. 6:17.

Pfeffer CK, Xue M, He M, Huang ZJ, Scanziani M. (2013). Inhibition of inhibition in visual cortex: the logic of connections between molecularly distinct interneurons. Nat Neurosci. 16:1068–1076.

Pi HJ, Hangya B, Kvitsiani D, Sanders JI, Huang ZJ, Kepecs A. (2013). Cortical interneurons that specialize in disinhibitory control. Nature. 503:521–524.

Rasch BH, Born J, Gais S. (2006). Combined blockade of cholinergic receptors shifts the brain from stimulus encoding to memory consolidation. J Cogn Neurosci. 18:793–802.

Redish AD, Touretzky DS. (1997). Cognitive maps beyond the hippocampus. Hippocampus. 7:15–35.

Redish AD, Touretzky DS. (1998). The role of the hippocampus in solving the Morris water maze. Neural Comput. 10:73–111.

Reisberg B, Doody R, Stoffler A, Schmitt F, Ferris S, Mobius HJ. (2003). Memantine in moderate-to-severe Alzheimer's disease. N Engl J Med. 348:1333–1341.

Remme MW, Lengyel M, Gutkin BS. (2009). The role of ongoing dendritic oscillations in single-neuron dynamics. PLoS Comput Biol 5:e1000493.

Remme MW, Lengyel M, Gutkin BS. (2010). Democracy-independence trade-off in oscillating dendrites and its implications for grid cells. Neuron. 66:429–437.

Rizzuto DS, Madsen JR, Bromfield EB, Schulze-Bonhage A, Kahana MJ. (2006). Human neocortical oscillations exhibit theta phase differences between encoding and retrieval. Neuroimage. 31:1352–1358.

Roberts MJ, Zinke W, Guo K, Robertson R, McDonald JS, Thiele A. (2005). Acetylcholine dynamically controls spatial integration in marmoset primary visual cortex. J Neurophysiol. **93**:2062–2072.

Roe AW, Pallas SL, Hahm JO, Sur M. (1990). A map of visual space induced in primary auditory cortex. Science. **250**:818–820.

Rolls ET. (1987). Information representation, processing and storage in the brain: analysis at the single neuron level. In: The Neural and Molecular Bases of Learning (**Changeux JP, Konishi M**, eds), pp. 503–540. Chichester: Wiley.

Rudy B, Fishell G, Lee S, Hjerling-Leffler J. (2011). Three groups of interneurons account for nearly 100% of neocortical GABAergic neurons. Dev Neurobiol. **71**:45–61.

Rumelhart RE, Hinton GE, Williams RJ. (1986). Learning representations by back-propagating errors. Nature. **323**:533–536.

Samsonovich A, McNaughton BL. (1997). Path integration and cognitive mapping in a continuous attractor neural network model. J. Neurosci. **17**:5900–5920.

Sargolini F, Fyhn M, Hafting T, McNaughton BL, Witter MP, Moser MB, Moser EI. (2006). Conjunctive representation of position, direction, and velocity in entorhinal cortex. Science. **312**:758–762.

Schacter D. (1982). Stranger Behind the Engram: Theories of Memory and the Psychology of Science. Hillsdale, NJ: Lawrence Erlbaum Associates.

Schmidt-Hieber C, Hausser M. (2013). Cellular mechanisms of spatial navigation in the medial entorhinal cortex. Nat Neurosci. **16**:325–331.

Shay CF, Boardman IS, James NM, Hasselmo ME. (2012). Voltage dependence of subthreshold resonance frequency in layer II of medial entorhinal cortex. Hippocampus. **22**:1733–1749.

Shirey JK, Xiang Z, Orton D, et al. (2008). An allosteric potentiator of M4 mAChR modulates hippocampal synaptic transmission. Nat Chem Biol. **4**:42–50.

Siegle JH, Wilson MA. (2014). Enhancement of encoding and retrieval functions through theta phase-specific manipulation of hippocampus. ELife **3**:e03061.

Silver MA, Shenhav A, D'Esposito M. (2008). Cholinergic enhancement reduces spatial spread of visual responses in human early visual cortex. Neuron. **60**:904–914.

Skaggs WE, McNaughton BL, Wilson MA, Barnes CA. (1996). Theta phase precession in hippocampal neuronal populations and the compression of temporal sequences. Hippocampus. **6**:149–172.

Stensola H, Stensola T, Solstad T, Froland K, Moser MB, Moser EI. (2012). The entorhinal grid map is discretized. Nature. **492**:72–78.

Stern CE, Corkin S, Gonzalez RG, Guimaraes AR, Baker JR, Jennings PJ, et al. (1996). The hippocampal formation participates in novel picture encoding: evidence from functional magnetic resonance imaging. Proc Natl Acad Sci U S A. **93**:8660–8665.

Sutton RS, Barto AG. (1998). Reinforcement Learning: An Introduction (Adaptive Computation and Machine Learning). Cambridge, MA: MIT Press.

Tahvildari B, Fransen E, Alonso AA, Hasselmo ME. (2007). Switching between "On" and "Off" states of persistent activity in lateral entorhinal layer III neurons. Hippocampus. **17**:257–263.

Toth K, Freund TF, Miles R. (1997). Disinhibition of rat hippocampal pyramidal cells by GABAergic afferent from the septum. J Physiol. **500**:463–474.

Touretzky DS, Redish AD. (1996). Theory of rodent navigation based on interacting representations of space. Hippocampus. **6**:247–270.

Treves A, Rolls ET. (1992). Computational constraints suggest the need for two distinct input systems to the hippocampal CA3 network. Hippocampus. **2**:189–199.

Treves A, Rolls ET. (1994). Computational analysis of the role of the hippocampus in memory. Hippocampus. 4:374–391.

Tsodyks MV, Skaggs WE, Sejnowski TJ, McNaughton BL. (1996). Population dynamics and theta rhythm phase precession of hippocampal place cell firing: a spiking neuron model. Hippocampus. 6:271–280.

Valentino RJ, Dingledine R. (1981). Presynaptic inhibitory effect of acetylcholine in the hippocampus. J Neurosci. 1:784–792.

van Vreeswijk C, Sompolinsky H. (1996). Chaos in neuronal networks with balanced excitatory and inhibitory activity. Science. 274:1724–1726.

Vazdarjanova A, Guzowski JF. (2004). Differences in hippocampal neuronal population responses to modifications of an environmental context: evidence for distinct, yet complementary, functions of CA3 and CA1 ensembles. J Neurosci. 24:6489–6496.

Villarreal DM, Gross AL, Derrick BE. (2007). Modulation of CA3 afferent inputs by novelty and theta rhythm. J Neurosci. 27:13457–13467.

Vogt KE, Regehr WG. (2001). Cholinergic modulation of excitatory synaptic transmission in the CA3 area of the hippocampus. J Neurosci. 21:75–83.

Wagner AD, Schacter DL, Rotte M, Koutstaal W, Maril A, Dale AM, et al. (1998). Building memories: remembering and forgetting of verbal experiences as predicted by brain activity. Science. 281:1188–1191.

Wallenstein GV, Hasselmo ME. (1997). GABAergic modulation of hippocampal population activity: sequence learning, place field development, and the phase precession effect. J Neurophysiol. 78:393–408.

Willshaw DJ, Buckingham JT. (1990). An assessment of Marr's theory of the hippocampus as a temporary memory store. Philos Trans R Soc Lond B Biol Sci. 329:205–215.

Willshaw DJ, Dayan P, Morris RG. (2015). Memory, modelling and Marr: a commentary on Marr, 1971, "Simple memory: a theory of archicortex". Philos Trans R Soc Lond B Biol Sci 370:1666.

Wilson HR, Cowan JD. (1972). Excitatory and inhibitory interactions in localized populations of model neurons. Biophys J. 12:1–24.

Wilson HR, Cowan JD. (1973). A mathematical theory of the functional dynamics of cortical and thalamic nervous tissue. Kybernetik. 1973:2.

Wyble BP, Hasselmo ME. (1997). A model of the effects of scopolamine on human memory performance. In: Computational Neuroscience: Trends in Research 1997 (Bower JM, ed.), pp. 891–896. New York: Plenum Press.

Wyble BP, Linster C, Hasselmo ME. (2000). Size of CA1-evoked synaptic potentials is related to theta rhythm phase in rat hippocampus. J Neurophysiol. 83:2138–2144.

Yoshida M, Hasselmo ME. (2009). Persistent firing supported by an intrinsic cellular mechanism in a component of the head direction system. J Neurosci. 29:4945–4952.

Zilli EA, Hasselmo ME. (2010). Coupled noisy spiking neurons as velocity-controlled oscillators in a model of grid cell spatial firing. J Neurosci. 30:13850–13860.

Zilli EA, Yoshida M, Tahvildari B, Giocomo LM, Hasselmo ME. (2009). Evaluation of the oscillatory interference model of grid cell firing through analysis and measured period variance of some biological oscillators. PLoS Comput Biol. 5:e1000573.

Zugaro MB, Monconduit L, Buzsaki G. (2005). Spike phase precession persists after transient intrahippocampal perturbation. Nat Neurosci. 8:67–71.

Chapter 7

Marr's theory of the hippocampus as a simple memory: Decades of subsequent research suggest it is not that simple

Suzanna Becker

Marr's simple memory theory of archicortex

In 1971, Marr published his highly influential theory of the hippocampus. By making several assumptions about the hippocampal circuit, Marr derived constraints on the type of neural computations performed by this structure. Although today the entire model could be simulated feasibly on modern-day computers, in Marr's time, it could only be evaluated as a theoretical exercise. Even so, Marr's ideas have been tremendously influential, and permeate virtually every modern theory of hippocampal function. Given the influence Marr has had over current thinking, it is worth looking back at his key ideas, which aspects of the theory have been supported by subsequent empirical investigations, which have not, and how the field should move forward in light of more recent discoveries.

Key assumptions

Marr's hippocampal theory was derived out of necessity for the proper functioning of his neocortical model. Marr argued that the neocortex necessarily required an associative memory that could memorize a series of events rapidly, and retrieve an event quite accurately when cued with a subset of its elements. This memorizing device would relieve the neocortex of the burden of having to learn associations among different categorical inputs rapidly, as it was simultaneously attempting to learn the categories. Later, some of this associative knowledge could be transferred to the neocortex in the form of new categories, once it had been determined which aspects of the event were most critical to be retained. Importantly, Marr assumed that the hippocampus formed a temporary store, recording about one day's worth of memories. At the end of each day, probably during sleep, some or all aspects of those memories would be transferred to neocortex.

According to Marr, the basic requirements of the hippocampal memory system were to store approximately 10^5 complex events, the number of events that would be encountered at a rate of about one per second in a single day. Further, when cued with a partial version of an event, an associative retrieval process should recover the entirety of the original event. Associative retrieval had to be completed within the hippocampus, before the pattern was returned to the neocortex in its original form. Therefore, Marr argued that the job of the hippocampus was to form what he called "simple representations." Rather than performing classification of the input, a simple representation should retain sufficient information to allow the original input event to be reconstructed from a subevent. In Marr's framework, a simple representation acts as a template for each event, and involves relatively few cells. Marr argued that the lower the activity level, the more accurately could different events be encoded. These simple representations were contrasted with the type of representations learned by neocortical pyramidal cells. In the neocortex, but not in the hippocampus, the goal of learning was to discover relevant sets of co-occurring features and perform classification.

Given assumptions about the number of available coding cells and synaptic connections available in neocortical versus hippocampal neurons, Marr calculated the activity level within the hippocampus that would achieve the required capacity of 10^5 memorized events. This resulted in an estimated sparseness level of about 0.001. It was assumed that the inhibitory interneurons performed both subtractive and divisive inhibition to keep activity levels normalized to within this target level of activation.

If an incoming pattern of activity from the neocortex had a number of active units above some threshold level, the pattern would be treated as novel and would be stored in the associative memory. Otherwise, a cued recall process would be triggered. Pattern completion[1] had to take place within the hippocampal memory system, and should be complete by the time the event was projected back to the neocortex, so as to require as few neocortical synapses as possible. Thus, the return projections to neocortex were presumed to be used only for indexing the original event, rather than performing an additional associative memory function.

Having worked out the broad computational constraints of an associative memory, Marr then fleshed it out as a simple neural circuit model of the hippocampus. He first considered a two-layered structure, consisting of an input layer and a second layer that combined the functions of sparse coding and associative retrieval into a single stage. This earlier model was rejected in favor of a three-layered structure that separated the functions of coding and associative retrieval into successive stages. Marr argued that storage and recall must be handled separately. He suggested that if an input pattern consists of a small subset (as few as one-third) of the features of a previously stored event, recall will be initiated; otherwise the event will be stored as a new event. Thus, the switch between storage and recall was governed by whether the number of active features in the input was greater than some threshold.

The main elements of Marr's simple memory circuit are shown in Figure 7.1.

---

[1] Pattern completion is the process of recalling the entirety of a stored event when cued with a subset of the elements of an event.

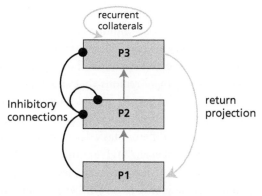

Figure 7.1 The three-layer circuit Marr favored for his simple memory theory of the hippocampus. Dark grey arrows: feedfoward excitatory pathways. Light grey arrows: recurrent and feedback excitatory pathways. Black lines with filled circle endings: inhibitory pathways.

Marr suggested neuroanatomical correlates for each of the three layers shown in Figure 7.1. He associated the input layer P1 with the neocortex, the middle layer P2 with the entorhinal cortex and presubiculum, and the output layer P3 with the dentate gyrus (DG) and CA (cornu ammonis) pyramidal regions (the latter combining the CA3 and CA1 subfields). Interestingly, Marr argued on the one hand that the DG shared many architecture features of the CA pyramidal regions and should be considered to perform the same basic operations. On the other hand, he acknowledged the unique aspects of the DG: the lack of recurrent excitatory collateral connections seen in CA3, and the very sparse but large mossy fiber connections projecting from DG to CA3, suggesting to Marr that the DG code should be even sparser than that of the CA regions.

Empirical support

The three-layer circuit proposed by Marr has been reinterpreted by subsequent modelers as mapping nicely onto known properties of the trisynaptic circuit in the hippocampus. The cortical input in most subsequent hippocampal models is assumed to be the entorhinal cortex. A second stage of sparse coding could be achieved by the granule cells of the DG (although in Marr's model the P2 and P3 layers were actually smaller and less sparse than the cortical input layer P1), while the associative retrieval function could be performed plausibly by CA3 pyramidal cells via their dense set of recurrent collaterals.

Sparse coding in the DG is supported by converging evidence from a wide range of experimental methods. Unit recordings of ongoing neuronal activity and immediate early gene (IEG) markers of recent neuronal activity in the DG in rodents consistently indicate that only 2–4% of dentate granule cells are active in any given environment (Jung and McNaughton, 1993; Gothard et al., 2001; Chawla et al., 2005; Leutgeb et al., 2007; Marrone et al., 2011; Satvat et al., 2011). Moreover, distinct subsets of dentate granule cells responded to similar contexts when small changes were made to the environment (Leutgeb et al., 2007). Remarkably, IEG labeling revealed that even a subtle change in task demands, while holding the spatiotemporal context constant, resulted in distinct populations of DG cells being activated in the two conditions (Satvat et al., 2011). Evidence from functional meagnetic resonance imaging (fMRI) in humans indicates that the DG/CA3 area shows greater differences in response to patterns that are highly similar to previously seen items, relative to other hippocampal regions that show less difference in response (Bakker et al., 2008). Importantly, however, a large subset (about 30%) of granule cells are jointly recruited when an animal is exposed to two different contexts or environments, or even the same environment under different task demands (Alme et al., 2010; Leutgeb et al., 2007; Marrone et al., 2011; Satvat et al., 2011; Schmidt et al., 2012). While these data broadly support the idea that the DG generates sparse, less overlapping codes, the question remains, do these codes have anything to do with event memories? Liu et al. (2012) addressed this question by using optogenetic techniques to label a population of neurons that were involved in encoding a contextual fear memory, and then optically reactivating the same population of neurons. The light stimulation induced increased freezing in the mice, indicating that reactivation of the same neurons induced fear memory recall. Taken together, these data are consistent with the idea that the DG performs pattern separation,[2] generating distinctive neural codes for event memories, even when the original events are highly overlapping.

Marr's conjecture that associative retrieval processes take place in the CA3 region is also supported by a broad range of empirical data. For example, knockout mice lacking NMDA receptors in CA3 show normal acquisition and normal place fields in the Morris water maze task, but a loss of spatial selectivity in both areas CA3 and CA1 after visual cue removal (Nakazawa et al., 2002). Moreover, human volumetric MRI shows that the size of area CA3, but not of other hippocampal subregions, predicts how much retrieval confusion people experience between previously stored episodic memories (Chadwick et al., 2014). If CA3 neurons are performing pattern completion, many models predict that attractor dynamics should be observed. Thus, when presented with an ambiguous pattern that is similar to two or more stored memories, the nearest stored pattern should be retrieved, rather than a blend of two or more patterns. To some degree, this prediction has been borne out. When CA3 place cell recordings were made in familiar circular and square activity boxes, distinct CA3 cell ensembles fired within each box (Wills et al., 2005). On the other hand, when the box was gradually morphed from being circular to being square, or vice versa, many (but not all) place cells abruptly remapped at some point in the transition from circular to square, broadly consistent with the idea that the CA3 recurrent collaterals are used for associative retrieval of the nearest stored pattern.

Whereas Marr's assumptions about coding and associative retrieval are broadly supported by a wealth of data, his assumption about the temporary nature of the hippocampal

---

[2] Pattern separation is a property of sparse distributed neural coding, such that the sets of output neurons activated by different input patterns have very little overlap, even when the input patterns are highly similar. This is desirable if the organism must respond differentially to very similar inputs.

memory trace is more controversial. Evidence in support of this assumption comes mainly from rodent studies where hippocampal lesions were made at varying intervals after learning. For some (but not all) hippocampal-dependent tasks, lesions made 1 day after learning cause severe memory deficits, while hippocampal lesions made weeks after learning do not (for a review, see e.g., Nadel and Moscovitch, 1997). This is consistent with Marr's assumption that memories are temporarily stored in the hippocampus, but are eventually consolidated elsewhere. We return to this issue later in the chapter where we consider evidence against the assumption that the hippocampus acts as a temporary memory store.

Regardless of whether memories in the hippocampus remain hippocampally dependent or can be consolidated elsewhere and become hippocampally independent, there is now ample evidence for Marr's conjecture that memories for recently experienced events are replayed during sleep. For example, when rats navigated through a maze, sequential patterns of hippocampal place cell activation were recorded; later, similar patterns of sequential activation were recorded from the rat hippocampi during slow-wave sleep (Wilson and McNaughton, 1994). Moreover, simultaneous recordings in the hippocampus and parietal cortex indicated that the hippocampal–neocortical circuits were jointly re-replaying recent patterns of activation during sleep (Qin et al., 1997). Interestingly, such reactivation patterns have been recorded in all regions of the hippocampus including the DG (Shen et al., 1998), suggesting that the entire hippocampal circuit may be involved in associative retrieval. This finding necessitates a re-evaluation of Marr's assumption that the hippocampus strictly separates the functions of sparse coding and associative recall into separate hippocampal regions, but still fits within the spirit of his original theory of archicortex (this is phylogenetically the oldest part of the brain, and includes the hippocampus and DG).

Data that challenge Marr's assumptions

While there has been considerable empirical support for Marr's model, as discussed above, some of its underlying assumptions are overly simplifying. By relaxing these assumptions and incorporating additional details of the hippocampal circuitry, subsequent theorists have been able to extend the model to account for a broader range of data.

Three-layered circuit structure

Marr's simple memory theory of the hippocampus was strongly constrained by the anatomical data available at the time. While little was known about the activity levels of each hippocampal subregion, gross connectivity patterns and morphology of different cell types had been studied across many mammalian species. However, even relative to what was known at the time, Marr's model was highly simplified in terms of its layering and connectivity. The architecture of the rat hippocampus, based on more recent data, is shown in Figure 7.2.

While simplification is intrinsic to modeling, the modeler aims to retain the critical features of the thing being modeled, so as to provide insight into the underlying mechanisms.

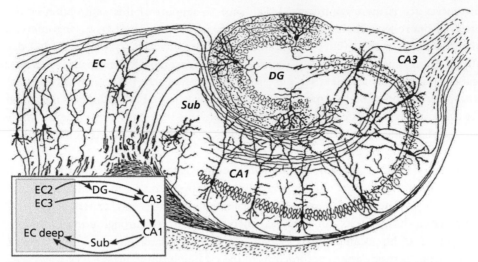

Figure 7.2 The neural circuitry of the hippocampus, modified from a drawing by Santiago Ramón y Cajal. (1911).

This figure was created by Martin Pyka and Stefanie Bothe. It has not been modified from its original form and is publically available at https://github.com/MartinPyka/NueroSVG under the terms of the Creative Commons Attribution 4.0 International License http://creativecommons.org/licenses/by/4.0/.

The risk is always that the modeler may omit some critical aspects of the circuitry that are essential for understanding the functions of the circuit being modeled.

Marr first considered a simpler two-layer model but rejected this on the grounds that it could not achieve adequate storage capacity, and therefore adopted the three-layer model. Interestingly, however, using Marr's computational constraints on memory capacity, sparseness, input layer size, and connectivity, Willshaw and Buckingham (1990) demonstrated in computer simulations that the two-layer and three-layer models described by Marr achieved similar performance. Why then does the hippocampus require the extra layers?

Subsequent to Marr's 1971 paper, other modelers elaborated on Marr's theory by incorporating additional physiological and anatomical features of the hippocampus. The direct versus indirect pathways through the hippocampal circuit have been hypothesized to play distinct roles in memory storage versus recall. The CA3 and CA1 regions receive both direct input from the entorhinal cortex (EC) via the perforant path, and indirect input through the trisynaptic circuit via the DG. The DG granule cells project to the CA3 field via mossy fiber synapses, which are few in number but are among the largest in the brain, such that only a few mossy fiber synapses may be sufficient to activate a CA3 pyramidal cell (Brown and Johnston, 1983). It has therefore been suggested that these terminals act as "detonator synapses," so that during encoding, a sparse pattern of activation in the DG mandatorily causes a postsynaptic CA3 cell to fire (McNaughton and Morris, 1987; Treves and Rolls, 1992). On the other hand, during retrieval, the CA3 recurrent collaterals and CA3-to-CA1 Shaffer collaterals may dominate in driving CA3 and CA1 cells to perform associative recall (Treves and Rolls, 1992; Hasselmo and Schnell, 1994; Hasselmo et al.,

1996). The switch between storage and retrieval dynamics may be controlled by levels of the neuromodulator acetylcholine (Hasselmo et al., 1995; Hasselmo, 1999; Hasselmo and McGaughy, 2004). For a more detailed discussion of this, see Hasselmo's Chapter 6 in this volume. There also exist back-projections from the CA3 to the DG that have both excitatory and inhibitory effects (Scharfman, 2007). These connections have been ignored by virtually all modelers from Marr's time to the present, but could also have important implications for neural coding and/or retrieval.

Time and memory

Marr sidestepped the thorny issue of time in memory, but acknowledged that events are not typically isolated at specific time points. Instead, events continuously unfold over time. The importance of the hippocampus for temporal associative memory has long been supported by results from lesion studies. For example, rodents with CA1 lesions were impaired at forming associations between items separated by a 10 second delay (Kesner et al., 2005) and on tasks that required judgments of temporal order (Farovik et al., 2009). Similarly, human patients with medial temporal lobe (MTL) amnesia are impaired on memory for temporal order (Downes et al., 2002). The MTL includes the hippocampus proper (DG and CA regions), entorhinal, perirhinal, and parahippocampal cortices.

Consideration of how the brain represents time raises many questions, for example: How are temporally discontiguous events integrated into a single episode? How are different episodes parsed into separate events? While answers to these questions remain elusive, some progress has been made.

One way in which the hippocampus may contribute to temporal coding is by representing a gradually evolving temporal context signal (Manns et al., 2007), as predicted by the Temporal Context Model (TCM) of memory (Howard and Kahana, 2002; Howard et al., 2005) and supported by neuroimaging data (Staresina and Davachi, 2009). Such a mechanism could allow the hippocampus to create a representational bridge that spans time delays. Further, the hippocampus may be important for forming predictions of future events, a topic that we return to in the final section of this chapter ("The future of hippocampal modeling"). Data from human neuroimaging studies supports this hypothesis (see e.g. Bornstein and Daw, 2012; Buckner, 2010; Davachi and Dubrow, 2015). For example, when participants read narratives that contained event boundaries, activation in the MTL, prefrontal cortex, and caudate ramped up as successive words of a sentence were read, but dropped suddenly at event boundaries (Ezzyat and Davachi, 2011). If the hippocampus is forming a temporal predictive model of its inputs, then a sudden violation in its prediction could trigger a reset of its temporal context and the formation of a new episodic trace.

Game-changing discoveries

The data reviewed in the previous section challenge some of the core assumptions of Marr's hippocampal theory. However, these challenges do not necessarily indicate that the theory is fatally flawed and should be rejected. Others have extended and further advanced Marr's model to address the finer nuances of recall and retrieval dynamics and temporal coding. On the other hand, there have been several fundamental discoveries in the last few decades that have been truly "game changers" for many hippocampal theorists.

Memory versus perception

A central tenet of Marr's theories was the sharp divide between the functions of the hippocampal system/archicortex and neocortex:

> Archicortex is essentially *memorizing cortex*, in the sense that a given area of archicortex is likely to contain one or more layers of a simple memory ... Neocortex, on the other hand, although undoubtedly used a great deal for simple associational storage, can probably be regarded as *classifying cortex*" (Marr, 1971).

Broadly speaking, this divide between memorizing and classifying cortex is supported by data from individuals with damage to the MTL versus the neocortex. A hallmark feature of MTL amnesia is a deficit in memory for complex associations. Such deficits were first documented in great detail for the famous patient HM (Scoville and Milner, 1957). HM, after undergoing bilateral hippocampal transections to treat his intractable epilepsy, was severely impaired in his ability to form new memories for people, places, and events. This type of memory is known as autobiographical or episodic memory. Although HM's memory for events that happened in the distant past seemed to be intact, he also exhibited retrograde amnesia for the events in the months leading up to his surgery. Similar patterns of deficits have since been observed in many other MTL patients. On the other hand, patients with neocortical damage that spares the MTL appear to have intact episodic memory, but impaired domain-specific knowledge or abilities; the specific domain of the knowledge impairment, e.g., perceptual, procedural, emotional, or semantic, depends on the locus of the damage (for a review, see Squire, 2004). The wide range of specific deficits associated with damage to different areas of the brain has led to the broadening of the "dual memory systems" view into a "multiple memory systems" perspective (Squire, 2004).

In contrast to the trend to divide the cortex into ever more fine-grained memory systems, there has been an opposing trend toward a more unifying perspective. In particular, the boundary between perceptual and memory systems has been called into question. A core issue in this debate is whether the MTL memory system is merely retrieving and remembering information, or is also involved in the ongoing classification and perception of stimuli. The divide between perceptual versus memory systems is broadly analogous to Marr's distinction between the classifying versus memorizing functions of neocortex and allocortex respectively. Marr argued that the sole job of the hippocampus was memorization, for the purpose of subsequent recoding and storage in neocortex. According to this view, the hippocampus should *not* be required for ongoing perceptual decisions. However, it appears that under some circumstances it *is*.

A prime example is the coding of space. In rodents, hippocampal "place cells" reflect the animal's current location in space and are critical for navigation (e.g., O'Keefe, 1976). O'Keefe and Nadel (1978) argued that this collection of neurons forms the basis of a cognitive map and provides the rat's internal allocentric representation of the environment.

The same appears to be true in humans; many hippocampal neurons recorded during a virtual navigation task reflected the person's current location in the virtual town (Ekstrom et al., 2003).

The importance of the MTL for representing perceptual information also extends to nonspatial perceptual judgments. A growing body of evidence from both lesion and neuroimaging studies points to a central role for the hippocampus in representing higher-order perceptual features and making complex perceptual decisions (for a review, see Lee, Yeung and Barense, 2012). For example, patients with selective hippocampal lesions were impaired at deciding which of a pair of altered scenes was closer to a previously viewed target scene; importantly, the same deficit was observed when the two test scenes were viewed simultaneously with the target scene, eliminating the memory component from the task (Lee et al., 2005). Moreover, healthy individuals exhibited increased activation in the hippocampus and perirhinal cortex when discriminating meaningful faces and objects relative to novel stimuli, even when those faces and objects were not subsequently well remembered (Barense et al., 2011). These findings point to a key role for the hippocampus and surrounding MTL structures in perceptual matching and classification. Such a role is difficult to reconcile with Marr's view that the hippocampus is purely for memorization and not classification.

Recall versus imagination and future thinking

Marr's view of the hippocampus was that it acts as a memorization device. This implies that the main goal of memory retrieval is to reconstruct the original event as precisely as possible. This too has been called into question. Instead, a large body of evidence suggests that the hippocampal "memory system" is as much involved in imagining and predicting the future as it is in remembering the past. Patients with MTL damage not only show autobiographical memory retrieval deficits; they also have great difficulty imagining future scenarios (e.g., Tulving, 1985; Hassabis et al., 2007; Rosenbaum et al., 2009; Andelman et al., 2010). The future scenarios that they attempt to imagine, like the past events that they attempt to remember, are notably lacking in episodic detail. These data imply that the same neural systems subserving recollection of past events are engaged in imagining future events.

Neuroimaging studies in healthy individuals lend further support to this notion. When asked to imagine a future event, people activate the same neural structures, including the hippocampus, parahippocampal regions, retrosplenial cortex, and posterior parietal areas, as during autobiographical memory retrieval tasks (e.g., Okuda et al., 2003; Addis et al., 2007; Szpunar et al., 2007). Moreover, those amnesic patients who do have the ability to construct fictitious or real future events may rely on residual functions in these same brain regions (Mullally et al., 2012).

The fact that the hippocampal system is involved in imagery and predicting the future is inconsistent with the notion that its chief function is exact memorization. Instead, it may play a central role in planning for the future and selecting the most appropriate response option in the current context. This makes sense from an adaptive perspective.

There is obvious utility in being able to recognize the similarities between one's present circumstances and past contexts that have been experienced, in order to make the best future choices. However, the current context is never precisely identical to a previously experienced event. Thus, one needs the capacity to flexibly retrieve one or more relevant contexts in order to predict a future scenario that may involve a novel combination of one or more past events.

Few if any computational models have addressed the complex operations implied above, namely, using past remembered episodes to imagine and plan for the future. The "BBB" model (Byrne and Becker, 2004; Byrne, Becker, and Burgess, 2007) proposed a parietal–frontal–hippocampal neural circuit by which a single remembered event could be transformed from an allocentric representation in long-term memory into an egocentric mental image. Moreover, this mental image could be translated and rotated, to generate imagined navigation sequences. Such a model, with the ability to generate a mental image of one's remembered past, could form the basis for a planning and spatial navigation system. While the BBB model is highly simplified, it sets the stage for future model developments that may explain how we are able to imagine never before experienced future scenarios as novel combinations of past memories.

A temporary memory system?

Marr's justification for a "simple memory system" residing in the hippocampus was grounded in memory capacity calculations. He argued that the pyramidal cells of the neocortex required all of their available synaptic connections to learn the appropriate combinations of input features for classification. These pyramidal cells did not have enough interconnectivity to also support associative learning. Therefore, a memorizing device was required that could quickly lay down a trace of each event encountered throughout the day, without the need to recode or classify the information. This system could itself run into capacity issues, however, if it were not a temporary memory store. Thus, Marr further assumed that the hippocampus is only temporarily involved in memory formation. Once the neocortex has had time to work out which aspects of a memory are relevant and commit them to long-term storage, the contents of the hippocampal memory trace could safely be discarded. This view of memories temporarily being laid down in the hippocampus and gradually being consolidated in neocortex has come to be known as the "systems consolidation" hypothesis.

There is support for the systems consolidation hypothesis from studies of both nonhuman animals with hippocampal lesions and humans with MTL damage. For example, rats who were given hippocampal lesions 1 day after a contextual fear-conditioning paradigm lost the contextual specificity of their conditioned fear response; on the other hand, when rats were lesioned 28 days after the conditioning, their contextual fear memory was intact (Kim and Fanselow, 1992). Moreover, when rats were given tone-shock pairings in one context, further tone-shock pairings 50 days later in a second context, followed by hippocampal lesions 1 day later, their remote memory for the initial contextual fear association was intact whereas their memory for the more recent contextual fear event was impaired (Anagnostaras et al., 1999). These data suggest a time-limited role for the hippocampus in contextual fear memory, after which time the memory is consolidated elsewhere (presumably in neocortex) in a more permanent form. Further, the rodents' retrograde amnesia was graded, with remote memories being relatively spared. Similar findings have been reported in humans. Patient HM, who had extensive bilateral hippocampal damage, showed a graded retrograde amnesia, with remote memories for events that occurred long ago being spared relative to memories for more recent events that occurred just prior to HM's surgery (Scoville and Milner, 1957). McClelland, McNaughton and O'Reilly (1995) fleshed out and extended Marr's ideas about the complementary roles of the hippocampus versus the neocortex. Their highly influential model laid out why it is computationally advantageous to have both fast and slow learning systems, with the former hippocampal system being optimal for learning of exceptional or novel information, and the latter neocortical system being optimal for gradual learning of general statistical regularities. A single system that attempted to do both would suffer from "catastrophic interference," with new knowledge overwriting old knowledge.

Although the cases in the literature of graded retrograde amnesia after MTL damage seem to support the systems consolidation hypothesis, when one looks more closely at the data there are problems with this interpretation. A meta-analysis of many such studies indicates that the temporal extent of the retrograde memory loss can vary widely from one patient to the next, spanning months to years to many decades (Nadel and Moscovitch, 1997). There are even patients who exhibit a flat gradient, with virtually no ability to recall any specific life events, in spite of intact knowledge of skills and perceptual and semantic information (Nadel and Moscovitch, 1997). Moreover, many nonhuman animal studies of retrograde amnesia also show a flat gradient, with equal deficits when hippocampal lesions are made 1 day versus several weeks after the learning (Nadel and Moscovitch, 1997). Such findings of retrograde amnesia spanning weeks to years do not accord with Marr's view of the hippocampus. Marr's calculations of the capacity, sparsity, and connectivity of the hippocampus were based on the assumption that the hippocampus would need to store approximately 1 day's worth of memories. He envisioned a consolidation process that would take on the order of days, not weeks and certainly not years. Thus, a retrograde memory loss spanning many decades is not consistent with Marr's notion of the hippocampus as a temporary memory store. Moreover, as Nadel and Moscovitch (1997) aptly put it, "It is difficult to conceive of an adaptive basis for a consolidation process that is almost as long as the average human lifespan throughout much of history". While not all types of memory were equally affected by MTL lesions, memories for personal autobiographical events were universally and devastatingly affected. Therefore, they concluded that autobiographical episodic memory must always be dependent upon the integrity of the hippocampus.

As an alternative to the systems consolidation theory, Nadel and Moscovitch (1997) put forward the Multiple Trace Theory (MTT). MTT builds on many of Marr's ideas, but with some important differences. Consistent with Marr's and related models, MTT postulates that the hippocampus rapidly lays down memory traces of events using sparse distributed codes. However, the entire hippocampal–neocortical ensemble in MTT constitutes the memory trace for an episode. Moreover, each time a memory trace is reactivated, it is laid down with slightly different subsets of neurons participating in the ensemble. Thus an event that has been re-experienced or remembered often will be supported by many variable memory traces. This explains why certain remote memories—those that are highly salient and likely to have been remembered often—should be more robust to partial damage. Furthermore, the neocortical component of a memory trace of an event will be a generalized version, lacking the original episodic details that are encoded in the hippocampal component of the trace. Thus, in the absence of hippocampal input, a retrieved neocortical memory trace will be more schematized. This accords with studies of remote memory in MTL amnesics. For example, patient KC, who had extensive bilateral hippocampal damage, exhibited deficits in both remote autobiographical and spatial memories although he was able to recognize highly salient landmarks from remotely learned neighborhoods (Rosenbaum et al., 2000).

Neurogenesis in the adult hippocampus

If the hippocampus is not in fact a temporary memory store, and yet it maintains a very high level of plasticity, then a dilemma arises. How does the hippocampus overcome interference between successively stored memories? Sparse coding can help to reduce collisions between similar memories and increase pattern separation, as demonstrated in computer simulations by O'Reilly and McClelland (1994). Further, it is now well established that there is ongoing generation of new neurons throughout the lifespan in the DG of the hippocampus. Adult hippocampal neurogenesis was first discovered in the guinea pig in the 1960s (Altman and Das, 1965) and has since been found in a wide range of mammalian species including humans (Eriksson et al., 1998; Knoth et al., 2010; Spalding et al., 2013).

The ongoing neurogenesis in the hippocampus has profound implications for neural coding. Whereas mature dentate granule cells fire very sparsely, as they are under tight control by inhibitory interneurons, the newly generated neurons have very different properties. When they reach about 3–4 weeks of age, they are able to fire action potentials, and yet they are much more plastic (Schmidt-Hieber et al., 2004) and more highly excitable (Mongiat et al., 2009). Over the next several weeks, the young neurons mature and become progressively more like adult DG granule cells. How would this varying population of dentate granule cells affect learning and memory? Simulations of a multilevel computational model of the hippocampus, including the EC, DG, CA3, and CA1 regions, suggest that the incorporation of neurogenesis in the dentate layer protected the hippocampus from interference (Becker, 2005). In Becker's model, shown in Figure 7.3, the increased levels of excitability and plasticity in the simulated younger population of neurons caused the younger neurons to be preferentially recruited into novel memory formation, thereby protecting older memories from interference. The incorporation of neurogenesis was particularly crucial when the model was challenged to store a set of

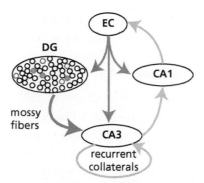

Figure 7.3 Becker's model of the hippocampus, including neurogenesis in the dentate gyrus (DG). Young neurons are show as grey circles; a subset of these are active, shown as filled circles. The input layer to the model represents the entorhinal cortex (EC). Dark grey arrows: during encoding, activation flows from the input via the trisynaptic circuit through the DG, as well as via direct projections monosynaptic connections from the EC, to the CA3 and CA1. Light grey arrows: during retrieval, activation flows in the reverse direction from the CA3 and CA1 back to the EC.

highly overlapping memories. The predictions from Becker's model that neurogenesis helps to mitigate against both proactive and retroactive interference have been tested and validated experimentally. Rodents with suppressed neurogenesis were less able to overcome the proactive interference induced when they were challenged to learn to discriminate olfactory odor pairs that overlapped with previously learned pairs (Luu et al., 2012). Additionally, rodents with reduced neurogenesis were more susceptible to the retroactive interference induced by a secondary learning task involving a similar visual discrimination task; on subsequent probe trials, animals with reduced neurogenesis showed greater forgetting of the previously learned visual discrimination (Winocur et al., 2012).

Manipulations that suppress neurogenesis have also been shown to impact performance on a wide range of other hippocampal-dependent tasks, including distinguishing between similar contexts, environments, objects, and spatial locations (Saxe et al., 2006; Winocur et al., 2006; Warner-Schmidt, Madsen and Duman, 2008; Wojtowicz et al., 2008; Hernandez-Rabaza et al., 2009; Kitamura et al., 2009; Ko et al., 2009; Creer et al., 2010; Guo et al., 2011; Sahay et al., 2011; Pan et al., 2012a; Kohman et al., 2012; Nakashiba et al., 2012). Neurogenesis has also been implicated in the long-term retention of memories (Snyder et al., 2005; Deng et al., 2009; Jessberger et al., 2009; Pan et al., 2012b, 2013) and in tasks that require forgetting or overcoming previously learned task demands in order to respond effectively to new ones (Saxe et al., 2007; Pan et al., 2012a). All of these neurogenesis-dependent memory tasks have a high interference component. In addition to mitigating interference, it has been proposed also that neurogenesis contributes to the formation of temporal associations (Aimone et al., 2006; Becker and Wojtowicz, 2007) and remote memories (Snyder et al., 2005; Déry, Goldstein and Becker, 2015), and to the clearance of old memories from the hippocampus (Feng et al., 2001; Weisz and

Argibay, 2012; Frankland et al., 2013). Future theoretical developments are needed to reconcile the role of the hippocampus, including neurogenesis, in these various functions.

Future of hippocampal modeling: A hierarchy of memory systems

In light of the empirical findings and further modeling developments in the 45 years since Marr published his model of the hippocampus, two things are clear. First, Marr's ideas have had a tremendous impact on our thinking about the functions computed by the hippocampus, and have infiltrated virtually every subsequent model of hippocampal coding. Second, many of Marr's core assumptions were incorrect. The hippocampus is not just a memorization device; it is also important for perception and classification of stimuli. The hippocampus is not a temporary memory store. At least when it comes to richly detailed episodic memories, the hippocampus may always be required to retrieve such memories. It is also not a static neural circuit; rather, it supports ongoing neurogenesis throughout the lifespan. The range of properties in younger versus more mature dentate granule cells may facilitate the encoding of novel information while preserving memories for stable properties of the environment. The hippocampus does not merely encode a static series of snapshot memories, but rather, it is integrally involved in encoding temporal sequences and temporal context. It is also very likely involved in predictive coding. This fits well with findings suggesting that the hippocampus is as important for imaging future scenarios as it is for remembering past events.

It is clear that a new kind of model of the hippocampus is called for. The basic functions of the hippocampus must be rethought. The hippocampus operates integrally with the neocortex to encode, retrieve, and predict information. As a first step in this direction, Kali and Dayan (2004) proposed a hierarchical model of the cortex, with the hippocampus at the top of the hierarchy. They proposed that replay of recently stored events serves to maintain the correspondence between neocortical and hippocampal representations, as both may be evolving over time. Future developments of this sort of model could potentially account for a wide range of the data reviewed here.

References

Addis DR, Wong AT, Schacter DL. (2007). Remembering the past and imagining the future: common and distinct neural substrates during event construction and elaboration. Neuropsychologia. 45:1363–1377.

Aimone JB, Wiles J, Gage FH. (2006). Potential role for adult neurogenesis in the encoding of time in new memories. Nat Neurosci 9:723–727.

Alme CB, Buzzetti RA, Marrone DF, et al. (2010). Hippocampal granule cells opt for early retirement. Hippocampus. 20:1109–1123.

Altman J, Das GD. (1965). Autoradiographic and histological evidence of postnatal hippocampal neurogenesis in rats. J Comp Neurol. 124:319–335.

Anagnostaras SG, Maren S, Fanselow MS. (1999). Temporally graded retrograde amnesia of contextual fear after hippocampal damage in rats: Within-subjectsexamination. J Neurosci. 19:1106–1114.

Andelman F, Hoofien D, Goldberg I, Aizenstein O, Neufeld MY. (2010). Bilateral hippocampal lesion and a selective impairment of the ability for mental time travel. Neurocase. 16:426–435.

Bakker A, Kirwan CB, Miller M, Stark CEL. (2008). Pattern separation in the human hippocampal CA3 and dentate gyrus. Science. 319:1640–1642.

Barense MD, Henson, RNA, Graham KS. (2011). Perception and conception: Temporal lobe activity during complex discriminations of familiar and novel faces and objects. J Cogn Neurosci. 23:3052–3067.

Becker S. (2005). A computational principle for hippocampal learning and neurogenesis. Hippocampus. 15:722–738.

Becker S, Wojtowicz JM. (2007). A model of hippocampal neurogenesis in memory and mood disorders. Trends Cogn Sci. 11:70–76.

Bornstein AM, Daw ND. (2012). Dissociating hippocampal and striatal contributions to sequential prediction learning. Eur J Neurosci. 35:1011–1023.

Brown T, Johnston D. (1983). Voltage-clamp analysis of mossy fiber synaptic input to hippocampal neurons. J Neurophysiol. 50:487–507.

Buckner RL. (2010). The role of the hippocampus in prediction and imagination. Annual Review of Psychology. 61:27–48.

Byrne P, Becker, S. (2004). Modeling mental navigation in scenes with multiple objects. Neural Comput. 16:1851–1872.

Byrne P, Becker S, Burgess N. (2007). Remembering the past and imagining the future: a neural model of spatial memory and imagery. Pyschol Rev. 114:340–375.

Chadwick MJ, Bonnici HM, Maguire EA. (2014). CA3 size predicts the precision of memory recall. Proc Natl Acad Sci U S A. 111:10720–10725.

Chawla MK, Guzowski JF, Ramirez-Amaya V, Lipa P, Hoffman KL, Marriott LK, et al. (2005). Sparse, environmentally selective expression of Arc RNA in the upper blade of the rodent fascia dentata by brief spatial experience. Hippocampus. 15:579–586.

Creer DJ, Romberg C, Saksida LM, van Praag H, Bussey TJ. (2010). Running enhances spatial pattern separation in mice. Proc Natl Acad Sci U S A. 107:2367–2372.

Davachi L and Dubrow S. (2015). How the hippocampus preserves order: the role of prediction and context. Trends Cogn Sci. 19:92–99.

Deng W, Saxe MD, Gallina IS, Gage FH. (2009). Adult-born hippocampal dentate granule cells undergoing maturation modulate learning and memory in the brain. J Neurosci 29: 13532–13542.

Déry N, Goldstein A, Becker S. (2015). A role for adult hippocampal neurogenesis at multiple time scales: A study of recent and remote memory in humans. Behav Neurosci. 129:435–449.

Downes JJ, Mayes AR, MacDonald C, Hunkin NM. (2002). Temporal order memory in patients with Korsakoff's syndrome and medial temporal amnesia. Neuropsychologia. 40:853–861.

Ekstrom A, Kahana M, Caplan J, Fields T, Isham E, Newman E, Fried I. (2003). Cellular networks underlying human spatial navigation. Nature. 425:184–187.

Eriksson PS, Perfilieva E, Björk-Eriksson T, Alborn AM, Nordborg C, Peterson DA, Gage FH. (1998). Neurogenesis in the adult human hippocampus. Nat Med. 4:1313–1317.

Ezzyat Y, Davachi L. (2011). What constitutes an episode in episodic memory? Psychol Sci. 22:243–252.

Farovik A, Dupont LM, Eichenbaum H. (2009). Distinct roles for dorsal CA3 and CA1 in memory for sequential nonspatial events. Learn Mem. 17:12–17.

Feng R, Rampon C, Tang YP, Shrom D, Jin J, Kyin M, et al. (2001). Deficient neurogenesis in forebrain-specific presenilin-1 knockout mice is associated with reduced clearance of hippocampal memory traces. Neuron. 32:911–26.

Frankland PW, Kohler S, Josselyn SA. (2013). Hippocampal neurogenesis and forgetting. Trends Neurosci. 36:497–503.

Gothard KM, Hoffman KL, Battaglia FP, McNaughton BL. (2001). Dentate gyrus and CA1 ensemble activity during spatial reference frame shifts in the presence and absence of visual input. J Neurosci. 21:7284–7292.

Guo W, Allan AM, Zong R, Zhang L, Johnson EB, Schaller EG, et al. (2011). Ablation of Fmrp in adult neural stem cells disrupts hippocampus-dependent learning. Nat Med. 17:559–565.

Hassabis D, Kumaran D, Vann SD, Maguire EA. (2007). Patients with hippocampal amnesia cannot imagine new experiences. Proc Natl Acad Sci U S A. 104:1726–1731.

Hasselmo M. (1999). Neuromodulation: acetylcholine and memory consolidation. Trends Cogn Sci. 9:351–359.

Hasselmo M, McGaughy J. (2004). High acetylcholine levels set circuit dynamics for attention and encoding and low acetylcholine levels set dynamics for consolidation. Prog Brain Res. 145:207–231.

Hasselmo M, Schnell E. (1994). Laminar selectivity of the cholinergic suppression of synaptic transmission in rat hippocampal region CA1: computational modeling and brain slice physiology. J Neurosci. 14:3898–3914.

Hasselmo M, Schnell E, Barkai E. (1995). Dynamics of learning and recall at excitatory recurrent synapses and cholinergic modulation in rat hippocampal region CA3. J Neurosci. 15:5249–5262.

Hasselmo M, Wyble B, Wallenstein G. (1996). Encoding and retrieval of episodic memories: role of cholinergic and gabaergic modulation in the hippocampus. Hippocampus. 6:693–708.

Hernandez-Rabaza V, Llorens-Martin M, Velazquez-Sanchez C, Ferragud A, Arcusa A, Gumus HG, et al. (2009). Inhibition of adult hippocampal neurogenesis disrupts contextual learning but spares spatial working memory, long-term conditional rule retention and spatial reversal. Neuroscience. 159:59–68.

Howard MW, Kahana MJ. (2002). A distributed representation of temporal context. J Math Psychol. 46:269–299.

Howard MW, Fotedar MS, Datey AV, Hasselmo ME. (2005). The temporal context model in spatial navigation and relational learning: Toward a common explanation of medial temporal lobe function across domains. Psych Rev. 112:75–116.

Jessberger S, Clark RE, Broadbent NJ, ClemensonJr GD , Consiglio A, Lie DC, et al. (2009). Dentate gyrus-specific knockdown of adult neurogenesis impairs spatial and object recognition memory in adult rats. Learn Mem. 16:147–154.

Jung MW, McNaughton BL. (1993). Spatial selectivity of unit activity in the hippocampal granular layer. Hippocampus. 3:165–182.

Kesner RP, Hunsaker MR, Gilbert PE. (2005). The role of CA1 in the acquisition of an object-trace-odor paired associate task. Behav Neurosci. 119:781–786.

Kim JJ, Fanselow MS. (1992). Modality-specific retrograde amnesia of fear. Science. 256:675–677.

Kitamura T, Saitoh Y, Takashima N, Murayama A, Niibori Y, Ageta H, et al. (2009). Adult neurogenesis modulates the hippocampus-dependent period of associative fear memory. Cell. 139:814–827.

Knoth R, Singec I, Ditter M, Pantazis G, Capetian P, Meyer RP, et al. (2010). Murine features of neurogenesis in the human hippocampus across the lifespan from 0 to 100 years. PLoS ONE 5:e8809.

Ko HG, Jang DJ, Son J, Kwak C, Choi JH, Ji YH, et al. (2009). Effect of ablated hippocampal neurogenesis on the formation and extinction of contextual fear memory. Mol Brain. 2:1–10.

Kohman RA, Clark PJ, Deyoung EK, Bhattacharya TK, Venghaus CE, Rhodes JS. (2012). Voluntary wheel running enhances contextual but not trace fear conditioning. Behav Brain Res. 226:1–7.

Lee ACH, Bussey TJ, Murray EA, Saksida LM, Epstein RA, Kapur N, et al. (2005). Perceptual deficits in amnesia: challenging the medial temporal lobe "mnemonic" view. Neuropsychologia. 43:1–11.

Lee ACH, Yeung LK, Barense, MD. (2012). The hippocampus and visual perception. Front Hum Neurosci. **6**:91.

Leutgeb S, Leutgeb JK, Moser MB, Moser EI. (2007). Pattern separation in the dentate gyrus and CA3 of the hippocampus. Science. **315**:961–966.

Liu X, Ramirez S, Pang PT, Puryear CB, Govindarajan A, Deisseroth K, Tonegawa S. (2012). Optogenetic stimulation of a hippocampal engram activates fear memory recall. Nature. **484**:381–385.

Luu P, Sill OC, Gao L, Becker S, Wojtowicz JM, Smith DM. (2012). The role of adult hippocampal neurogenesis in reducing interference. Behav Neurosci. **126**:381–391.

Manns JR, Howard MW, Eichenbaum H. (2007). Gradual changes in hippocampal activity support remembering the order of events. Neuron. **56**:530–540.

Marr D. (1971). Simple memory: a theory for archicortex. Philos Trans R Soc Lond B Biol Sci. **262**:23–81.

Marrone DF, Adams AA, Satvat E. (2011). Increased pattern separation in the aged fascia dentata. Neurobiol Aging. **32**: 2317.e23–2317.e32.

McClelland JL, McNaughton BL, O'Reilly RC. (1995). Why there are complementary learning systems in the hippocampus and neocortex: insights from the successes and failures of connectionist models of learning and memory. Psychol Rev. **102**:419–457.

McNaughton BL, Morris RGM. (1987). Hippocampal synaptic enhancement and information storage within a distributed memory systems. Trends Neurosci. **10**:408–415.

Mongiat LA, Espósito MS, Lombardi G, Schinder AF. (2009). Reliable activation of immature neurons in the adult hippocampus. PLoS ONE. **4**:e5320.

Mullally S, Hassabis D, Maguire E. (2012). Scene construction in amnesia: An fMRI study. J Neurosci. **32**:5646–5653.

Nadel L, Moscovitch M. (1997). Memory consolidation, retrograde amnesia and the hippocampal complex. Curr Opin Neurobiol. **7**:217–227.

Nakashiba T, Cushman JD, Pelkey KA, Renaudineau D, Buhl DL, McHugh TJ, et al. (2012). Young dentate granule cells mediate pattern separation, whereas old granule cells facilitate pattern completion. Cell. **149**:188–201.

Nakazawa K, Quirk M, Chitwood R, Watanabe M, Yeckel M, Sun L, et al. (2002). Requirement for hippocampal CA3 NMDA receptors in associative memory recall. Science. **297**:211–218.

O'Keefe J. (1976). Place units in the hippocampus of the freely moving rat. Exp Neurol. **51**:78–109.

O'Keefe J, Nadel L. (1978). The Hippocampus as a Cognitive Map. Oxford: Oxford University Press.

Okuda J, Fujii T, Ohtake H, Tsukiura T, Tanji K, Suzuki K, et al. (2003). Thinking of the future and past: the roles of the frontal pole and the medial temporal lobes. Neuroimage. **19**:1369–1380.

O'Reilly RC, McClelland JL. (1994). Hippocampal conjunctive encoding, storage, and recall: avoiding a tradeoff. Hippocampus. **4**:661–682.

Pan Y-W, Chan GCK, Kuo CT, Storm DR, Xia Z. (2012a). Inhibition of adult neurogenesis by inducible and targeted deletion of ERK5 mitogen-activated protein kinase specifically in adult neurogenic regions impairs contextual fear extinction and remote fear memory. J Neurosci. **32**:6444–6455.

Pan Y-W, Storm DR, Xia Z. (2012b). The maintenance of established remote contextual fear memory requires ERK5 MAP kinase and ongoing adult neurogenesis in the hippocampus. PLoS ONE. **7**:e50455.

Pan Y-W, Storm DR, Xia Z. (2013). Role of adult neurogenesis in hippocampus-dependent memory, contextual fear extinction and remote contextual memory: New insights from ERK5 MAP kinase. Neurobio Learn Mem. **105**:81–92.

Qin YL, McNaughton BL, Skaggs WE, Barnes CA. (1997). Memory reprocessing in corticocortical and hippocampocortical neuronal ensembles. Philos Trans R Soc Lond B Biol Sci. 352:1525–1533.

Ramón y Cajal S. (1911/1955). Histologie du système nerveux de l'homme et des vertébrés. Paris: A. Maloine/Madrid: Consejo Superior De Investigation Cientificas

Rosenbaum RS, Gilboa A, Levine B, Winocur G, Moscovitch M. (2009). Amnesia as an impairment of detail generation and binding: evidence from personal, fictional, and semantic narratives in K.C. Neuropsychologia. 47:2181–2187.

Rosenbaum RS, Priselac S, Köhler S, Black SE, Gao F, Nadel L, Moscovitch M. (2000) Remote spatial memory in an amnesic person with extensive bilateral hippocampal lesions. Nat Neurosci. 3:1044–1048.

Sahay A, Wilson DA, Hen R. (2011). Pattern separation: A common function for new neurons in hippocampus and olfactory bulb. Neuron. 70:582–588.

Satvat E, Schmidt B, Argraves M, Marrone DF, Markus EJ. (2011). Changes in task demands alter the pattern of zif268 expression in the dentate gyrus. J Neurosci. 31:7163–7167.

Saxe MD, Battaglia F, Wang JW, Malleret G, David DJ, Monckton JE, et al. (2006). Ablation of hippocampal neurogenesis impairs contextual fear conditioning and synaptic plasticity in the dentate gyrus. Proc Natl Acad Sci U S A. 103:17501–17506.

Saxe MD, Malleret G, Vronskaya S, Mendez I, Garcia AD, Sofroniew MV, et al. (2007). Paradoxical influence of hippocampal neurogenesis on working memory. Proc Natl Acad Sci U S A. 104:4642–4646.

Scharfman HE. (2007). The CA3 "backprojection" to the dentate gyrus. Prog Brain Res. 163: 627–637.

Schmidt-Hieber C, Jonas P, Bischofberger J. (2004). Enhanced synaptic plasticity in newly generated granule cells of the adult hippocampus. Nature. 429:184–187.

Scoville WB, Milner B. (1957). Loss of recent memory after bilateral hippocampal lesions. J Neurol Neurosurg Psychiat. 20:11–12.

Schmidt B, Marrone DF, Markus EJ. (2012). Disambiguating the similar: The dentate gyrus and pattern separation. Behav Brain Res. 226:56–65.

Shen, JM, Kudrimoti, HS, McNaughton, BL, Barnes, CA. (1998). Reactivation of neuronal ensembles in hippocampal dentate gyrus during sleep after spatial experience. J Sleep Res. 7:6–16.

Snyder J, Hong NS, McDonald RJ, Wojtowicz JM. (2005). A role for adult neurogenesis in spatial long-term memory. Neuroscience. 130:843–852.

Spalding KL, Bergmann O, Alkass K, Bernard S, Salehpour M, Huttner HB, et al. (2013). Dynamics of hippocampal neurogenesis in adult humans. Cell. 153:1219–1227.

Squire LR. (2004). Memory systems of the brain: A brief history and current perspective. Neurobiol Learn Mem. 82:171–177.

Staresina BP, Davachi L. (2009). Mind the gap: Binding experiences across space and time in the human hippocampus. Neuron. 63:267–276.

Szpunar KK, Watson JM, McDermott KB. (2007). Neural substrates of envisioning the future. Proc Natl Acad Sci U S A. 104:642–647.

Treves A, Rolls ET. (1992). Computational constraints suggest the need for two distinct input systems to the hippocampal CA3 network. Hippocampus. 2:189–200.

Tulving E. (1985). Memory and consciousness. Can Psychol. 26:1–12.

Warner-Schmidt JL, Madsen TM, Duman RS. (2008). Electroconvulsive seizure restores neurogenesis and hippocampus-dependent fear memory after disruption by irradiation. Eur J Neurosci. 27:1485–1493.

Weisz VI, Argibay PF. (2012). Neurogenesis interferes with the retrieval of remote memories: forgetting in neurocomputational terms. Cognition. 125:13–25.

Wills TJ, Lever C, Cacucci E, Burgess N, O'Keefe J (2005). Attractor dynamics in the hippocampal representation of the local environment. Science. **308**:873–876.

Willshaw DJ, Buckingham JT. (1990). An assessment of Marr's theory of the hippocampus as a temporary memory store. Philos Trans R Soc Lond B Biol Sci. **329**:205–215.

Wilson MA, McNaughton BL. (1994). Reactivation of hippocampal ensemble memories during sleep. Science. **265**:676–679.

Winocur G, Wojtowicz JM, Sekeres M, Snyder JS, Wang S. (2006). Inhibition of neurogenesis interferes with hippocampus-dependent memory function. Hippocampus. **16**:296–304.

Winocur G, Becker S, Luu P, Rosenzweig S, Wojtowicz JM. (2012). Adult hippocampal neurogenesis and memory interference. Behav Brain Res. **227**:464–469.

Wojtowicz JM, Askew ML, Winocur G. (2008). The effects of running and of inhibiting adult neurogenesis on learning and memory in rats. Eur J Neurosci. **27**:1494–1502.

A theory of neocortex

Chapter 8

Visions of the neocortex

Rodney J. Douglas and Kevan A. C. Martin

Introduction to Marr's approach

David Marr made substantial contributions to the foundations of computational neuroscience, first through his analyses of the operations of the key brain regions of the cerebellum, hippocampus, and neocortex; and later through his syntheses of biological vision and machine vision. While a mathematics undergraduate at Trinity College, Cambridge (where he graduated with first-class honors in 1966) he was allowed to attend the Physiology and Psychology courses of Part 2 of the Natural Sciences Tripos. The Department of Physiology was then populated with luminaries such as Alan Hodgkin, Bryan Matthews, Horace Barlow, Fergus Campbell, William Rushton, and John Robson. It was in the Department of Physiology that Marr encountered the brilliant eccentric Giles Brindley, who was interested in vision and synaptic physiology and network modeling, and who became his PhD advisor. In Psychology he might have heard Larry Weiskrantz lecture on learning and memory. Sydney Brenner and Francis Crick had a growing interest in nervous systems and gave Marr a job in their lab, "simply because he was working on something interesting" (Brenner, 2001). Brenner had been taught mathematics by Seymour Papert, a close friend, when they were colleagues in South Africa, so it was natural that later Brenner would encourage Marr to do his postdoc at MIT, where Papert and Marvin Minsky of "Perceptrons" fame, had developed a lively community in the Artificial Intelligence Laboratory.

In the wider world outside Cambridge, the results of David Hubel and Torsten Wiesel (Hubel and Wiesel, 1962, 1965) were still piping hot from their laboratory, Walter Rosenblith had edited an influential multi-author book called *Sensory Communication* (Rosenblith 1961) that was on most people's desks, and Jack Eccles, Janos Szentágothai, and Masao Ito had just published their opus *Cerebellum as a Neuronal Machine* (Eccles et al., 1967). And of course Claude Shannon's information theory (Shannon, 1949) pervaded thinking about how the brain might deal with information and redundancy, a topic that fascinated Horace Barlow and Fred Attneave in particular (Barlow, 1974).

It was in this heady atmosphere that Marr developed his trilogy. To understand the key aspects of his theory of neocortex, we follow the thread of his early thinking and its embedding. We then review how far we have come in understanding the structure of cortical circuits and their computational functions in the 45 years since his paper appeared in the *Proceedings of the Royal Society* (Marr, 1970). One immediately impressive aspect of

Marr's thinking is his attempt to develop a rational framework and approach for the new field he and others were pioneering, and it is thus with some perambular philosophical reflections that we begin.

Metatheoretical approach

In negotiating the philosophical and practical challenges of the new domain of natural computation, Marr faced the ongoing neuroscientific problem of how to resolve various levels of description, from detailed neuronal mechanisms to abstract purpose. During his early work on neural networks he considered four levels of description: physical, computational primitive, algorithmic, and computational (Marr and Poggio, 1976). Later (Marr, 1982) he collapsed the physical and computational primitives into a single level, resulting in the three levels for which he has been frequently cited. Although these levels are usually described in a top-down sequence, Marr's own scientific development follows a bottom-up sequence. The lowest (earliest) of his three levels describes how a processing system is realized physically. For the brain, this level describes the structural and functional organization of the neural circuits that support the processes underlying a function such as vision. The intermediate algorithmic level describes the functional organization of the process. It describes the representations that are processed, how they arise, and how they are transformed. Finally, the computational level describes the abstract task that the algorithm satisfies.

In attempting to resolve the different resolution and intent of explanation at these three levels, Marr was confronting again the age-old epistemological distinctions of Aristotle and Plato. Both those ancient philosophers sought to understand the universal nature of objects, but they arrived at distinctly different points of view. Both argued for an ideal abstraction that captures the universality of classes of physical objects. Aristotle argues that these higher universal forms are the essence of particular instantiated objects: thus the universal can be reached through bottom-up observation and knowledge of the essence of things. By contrast, the universal prototype is the prior for Plato, and understanding of particular objects can be deduced from these prior universal forms. Thus Aristotle argues for induction from instances toward the class, and its type, whereas Plato argues for deduction from the type toward the class and its instances.

Marr's early work is cast at the level of neuronal circuitry, and considers how neural circuits come to identify classes. His approach to this problem, however, is Platonic: he argues from functional necessities of an abstract computation down toward circuit implementation. He begins by first establishing the mathematical principles that should be respected by subcircuits of neurons, and then he moves downward to identify which neuronal type could possibly fulfill the desired computational role. His later work focuses on algorithms that satisfy some aspects of higher tasks of biological computation. This search was only partially successful in identifying the set of computational priors that support the overall cognition and behavior of intelligent systems, but by this late stage he had taken the position that the actual implementation of the algorithms was a mere detail (see Marr 1982, p. 337). His closing position is essentially that as yet incompletely identified Platonic computational principles unfold onto the algorithms of intelligence. It is very unfortunate that Marr did not have the opportunity to resolve his later ideas in the light of his earlier more biologically inclined work, because that work contained some intriguing functional concepts that were embodied in particular neuronal circuits.

Marr's concept of neuronal computation

Marr's early works (Marr, 1969, 1970, 1971) focus on the overall computational goals that neural networks should express, and the possible neural mechanisms that could support them. The basic concept envisages systematic learning of a very large set of behaviorally relevant information by means of an associative memory that both encodes past data and is also able to use these existing encodings to bootstrap new relevant associations from sparse input data.

In Marr's neocortical model, events arising in the world are transduced by peripheral sense organs to generate the signals that input cells transmit to the associative circuit. The axons of these input cells ramify over a very large field and connect to "codon cells" that detect the subpatterns ("codons") contained in the overall input. The goal of this codon stage is to project the world events into a high-dimensional unorthogonalized space of codons. Marr offers only a sketchy outline how the inputs to the codon cells may be configured initially, and then modified through experience (see Willshaw and Dayan, Chapter 9, for a discussion of codon formation.) The codon cells then project onto a field of output cells that must learn which groups of codons are likely to occur together. Once learned, these output cells should report the presence of codon groups (contexts) even when only some members are actually present in the input. In this way an output cell is expected to detect, e.g., the presence of an occluded object (some of whose codons are absent). The projection of codon cells onto the output cells is learned with the support of a teacher signal supplied to the output cell. This signal is derived from within the network itself, and so the learning process is a kind of bootstrap.

Marr applied these basic principles to three major brain structures—the cerebellum, hippocampus, and neocortex. Unsurprisingly, his models bear a close family resemblance in the organization and function of their synapses, and differ principally in whether they act as a memory or a classifier.

Initially (Marr, 1969) Marr proposed how the cerebellum might use this basic scheme to construct context-dependent sequences of simple movements and postures. Here the input to be interpreted is provided by the mossy fibers carrying data from cerebral cortex, brainstem, and spinal cord. The individual neurons of the olivary nucleus encode motor states. The climbing fibers of these cells gate the learning of motor sensory contexts by Purkinje cells. The activity of the climbing fibers drives the postsynaptic component of Hebbian/Brindley learning (A Brindley synapse is a type of Hebb synapse that contains an unmodifiable excitatory component, whereas the Hebb synapse can have a zero weight.) The motor sensory contexts are represented by the granular cell codons, which suitably encode the more general motor world input events. The notion is that the training of the Purkinje cells by the climbing fibers is eventually replaced by the successive (learned) motor contexts now driving the Purkinje cells without climbing fiber support.

Thus, Marr's network has two components: a forward processing subcircuit that performs recall based on its current configuration, and a learning component that steers the progressive configuration, of the recall circuit. The learning mechanisms are crucial to the recoding process, but in all the neuronal papers, Marr focuses only on learning at the output cell synapses. He assumes that the codon wiring configurations are given, and does not confront the important problem of learning a suitable feature set. The details of the learning method itself are beyond the scope of this paper, which focuses on network structure and dynamics (see Willshaw et al., 1997 for a concise description of Marr's approach to synaptic learning at the output cells.)

In his later neocortical work (Marr, 1970), Marr extended the basic cerebellar scheme toward general concept formation rather than the encoding of motor states and their sequences. In their neocortical incarnation, the codons are more general features of world events, and the contexts (groups of codons) are recoded onto pyramidal output cells. By analogy with the cerebellar circuit, the cortical neural networks recode the uninterpreted sensory events of the world into a representation of relevant elementary features. These features are then combined associatively into behaviorally meaningful clusters (objects) by output cells. These cells are then able to report the presence of meaningful objects. Particular cortical cells, the output cell selectors, provide the teacher signal necessary to train other output cells. These selectors receive nonspecific afferents, and so report the presence of a very active region of input space. Their output climbing fibers then prime nearby output cells to be responsive to learning new associations. The configuration of these privileged cells is assumed to be given.

In general, Marr argues that large distributed architectures composed of his fundamental circuit can support sophisticated associative coding and learning. For example, he proposes that the neural circuits of the neocortex implement only a few fundamental methods for organizing information and that these circuits are distributed uniformly across the cortical gray matter (Marr, 1970). The neocortex is able to learn many different kinds of task using this generic architecture. He argues that such a generic principle is possible because the world contains a generic form of redundancy. It is a crucial action of the nervous system to reduce a particular source of redundancy (a certain collection of features commonly co-occur), and to recode these collections by a new and separate entity (represented by an output cell) that is then added to the vocabulary of concepts with which the brain records and interprets experience.

The ability of this architecture to encode the world effectively rests in the ordered structure of the world that Marr outlines in his crucial "Fundamental Hypothesis." This hypothesis asserts that if instances can be characterized by a particular collection of properties already known (their intrinsic properties), and if these properties tend to group in such a way that if some are present, then most are present; then other as yet unknown properties (extrinsic properties) are then also likely to exist that generalize over these instances. It is this principle of feature nesting that leads Marr to propose that new, extrinsic properties can be recognized from sparse input data on the basis of properly structured knowledge of intrinsic properties.

Marr's Fundamental Hypothesis requires the neocortical circuits to solve three different problems. Firstly, they should discover collections of frequent, closely similar subevents (codons). Secondly, they should transform these collections of subevents into new symbolic types that are represented as output cells. These codons and their learned generalization over types constitute the intrinsic knowledge of the circuits. Finally, the cortical circuits should use this intrinsic knowledge to "diagnose" whether a novel event belongs to a particular class (type). This induction of extrinsic from intrinsic properties is the most important aspect of Marr's processing concept.

Marr's is an analytical consideration of cortical function. He did not validate his model through simulation. Fortunately, part of this important task has been performed by Willshaw et al. (1997) who examined particularly Marr's codon to output cell learning model, and also extended his analysis. They reported successful simulations of self-organizing networks of this kind. However, analysis and modeling of Marr's less well-specified concepts of codon learning (see Chapter 9) require further attention.

Marr's computational model implemented as a neural circuit

Given his later disinterest in particular physical implementations, it is interesting to note how carefully Marr maps his early computational approach onto a neural implementation. He proposes that the various types of neocortical cells (as recognized at that time) have a natural interpretation in terms of his model. To see his argument we need to follow fairly carefully also the details of his model.

External events E impinge on a large set of input axons A. An event activates some individual fibers a_i by $E(a_i)$, thereby assigning binary values to a_i at discrete time-steps, $a_i(t)$. Importantly, Marr considers that the a_i represent features that are obtained by a preprocessing stage and that this preprocessing is assumed as given. E is also more loosely used to denote the set of a_j that are activated by E.

The E are drawn from an extremely large event space. Consequently the set of patterns of activation of A are so large that any particular pattern in A occurs rarely. Therefore A projects into a field of codon cells C that provides an infrastructure for detection and measurement of similarity between patterns in A This network can be used for classification of events as well as for inference on incomplete events. To do this, the codon cells recode the input A into more convenient or relevant subsets.

A codon cell is essentially a threshold logic unit. Its binary output c_i indicates the presence of some subset of activity in input A. The codon may be an R-codon, indicating that all R of its a_i inputs are satisfied; or an (R, Θ)-codon, indicating that at least Θ of its R inputs are satisfied. Thus the size of a codon that will activate a codon cell will depend on the cell's threshold. Marr proposed that codon cells of the cerebellum are the granule cells, while those of the cortex are a population of excitatory neurons composed of 'granule' (stellate) cells and Martinotti cells (see Figure 8.1).

Input events may be incomplete and so the total number of active codons Σc_i must be matched to the total number of active fibers Σa_i in the input field. This matching is achieved by a single population of inhibitory neurons G that sample the activity of input

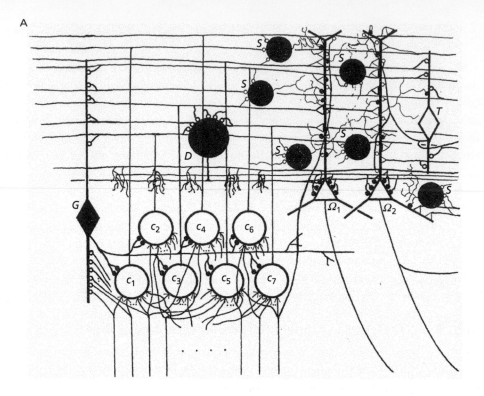

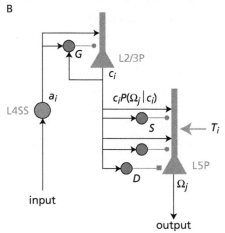

Figure 8.1 David Marr's neocortical circuit. (A) Marr's vision of the possible neuronal implementation of his computational principles for the neocortex. Excitatory cells, white; inhibitory cells, black. Afferent axons, a_i, excite codon cells, c_i. Sparsely active codon cells drive pyramidal output cells, Ω_j via synapses that encode $P(\Omega_j | c_i = 1)$, the probability that the current input event is of class Ω_j, if codon c_i is activated by that event. Overall codon cell population activity is held constant by inhibitory cell G. Inhibitory cells s offset the condon inputs to the output pyramidal, and inhibitory cell D scales its output, so that the pyramid is able to evaluate $P(\Omega_j | E)$. This is an estimate of the probability that the current input event, E, as reported by active codons, is of class Ω_j. The pyramids learn the class they should report through the supervision of climbing fibers from a proposed cell type, T (Marr, 1970) (B) Circuit A transposed into a more recent, and more appropriate, cortical anatomical setting. Excitatory cells, blue; inhibitory cells, red; L4SS, layer 4 spiny stellate cell; L2/3P, superficial pyramidal cell; L5P, layer 5 pyramidal cell.

A: David Marr, "A theory for cerebral neocortex," Proceedings of the Royal Society of London. Series B, 1970, vol 176, pp. 161–234, by permission of the Royal Society.

fibers as well as the codon cells and then apply subtractive inhibition to the dendrites of codon cells (see Figure 8.1). This inhibition provides both feedforward and feedback control of global codon activity by dynamically adjusting their individual thresholds. The inhibition maintains the number of active codon cells at an approximately constant level.

Individual codon cells respond to only small subsets of the input A, and so are expected to be sparsely active. Moreover, the larger R, required to reach threshold the more specific the codon cell. Low activity in the input leads to reduction in the codon cell thresholds allowing less specific codons to be processed by the downstream pyramidal cells. Thus, in the absence of strong world data, a more relaxed interpretation of the available weak data is permitted.

The codon cells now project onto pyramidal output neurons, Ω, by continuous valued synapses that provide the "evidence" (Marr, 1970) for the hypothesis that event E is of type Ω. The circuit does this by encoding in the codon cell to output cell synaptic weights w_{ij} a value proportional to $P(\Omega_j | c_i = 1)$, the probability that event E, which evokes input feature subset (codon) i, belongs to event class j. The values of these synapses can be learned so that the Ω_j come to report the presence in A of an event belonging to one of the relevant classes of events. Thus Marr's approach focuses on the question of recognition of an input event, $P(\Omega | E)$, rather than the classification of events, $P(E | \Omega)$ (Willshaw et al., 1997).

The recognition process is as follows. An event will elicit positive outputs in k of the codons, and these k estimates of $P(\Omega_j | c_i)$ must be combined by pyramid Ω_j. Marr argues that the most efficient method of combination is by taking the average $\sum^k c_i P(\Omega_j | c_i) / k$ over the k active input codon cells. This is the crucial inductive step of the network. It estimates the probability that an event in the set that jointly activates these particular k codons, belongs to the class Ω_j.

All the active excitatory inputs of the codon cells are summed by the pyramidal cell dendrite. However, the number of active codons, k, will vary according to the particular input E, and so the output should be scaling by $k(E)$. Marr proposes to do this by a feedforward divisive inhibition applied to the result of pyramidal processing at the soma. The divisive inhibitory neuron D cannot explicitly count $k(E)$, but it is able to sample the activities of the codon cell pool incident on pyramid Ω_j, and then scale the pyramids output by applying somatic inhibition proportional to codon cell activity.

Marr's scaling inhibition was an important insight. By dividing the total excitation of the cell by the total number of active codon cells providing input, the inhibitory cell adjusts the threshold of the output in proportion to the amount of evidence available. Thus, even if the amount of evidence is small (few codon cells are active), but this evidence is relatively good ($P(\Omega | c_i = 1)$ is high) then the appropriate Ω_j will be activated. Poor evidence will not succeed in driving an input. And, because the evidence cells report only the presence of subpatterns in the input, a small amount of rather good evidence will be sufficient to make the identification of the class of the input even if some components of the input are missing. Furthermore, false positives can be reduced by adaptive setting of subtractive thresholds on the pyramidal output neurons. Once again this is achieved by inhibitory cells S that sample the activity of the codon cells projecting to a particular pyramidal cell, and apply a subtractive threshold proportional to $\sum_i c_i(E)$ to the dendrites of that pyramidal cell in the vicinity of the matching codon cell inputs, in order to reject inadequate evidence.

Identifying cortical circuits and dynamics

It is widely held that function can be derived from structure. But the inverse mapping of ideal function onto underlying structure, as attempted by Marr, is a delicate task. In (Marr, 1970) he expressed his reluctance to assign cell types to his system: "it is unprofitable to attempt a comprehensive survey of cortical cells at this stage: neither the theory, nor the available facts permit more than the merest sketch." Nevertheless, Marr distinguishes at least the roles of excitatory and inhibitory cells. The processing network contains three layers of excitatory cells: input feature cells, codon cells, pyramidal output cells. Marr proposes that codon cells are stellate cells and Martinotti cells, both of which he presumed were excitatory. In fact, Martinotti cells are now known to be GABAergic inhibitory neurons. Inhibitory cells play a distinct and crucial role in Marr's circuit. They provide the thresholding and normalization of the network computations. Importantly, there are no lateral connections between codon cells, nor between output pyramidal cells, since these would introduce correlations between those cells and so reduce the sparseness of the recoding. The suitable operation (learning and recall) of the recoding circuits is very sensitive to the individual and circuit levels of activation of codon and output cells. Consequently the settings of thresholds, and other inhibitory controls of the circuits, are crucial for reliable operation. Marr was concerned to identify sources of subtractive and divisive inhibition for these roles, and his interest in the neuroanatomy of the various structures was largely to justify the abstract mechanisms that he required for the recoding process. He did offer possible neuronal subcircuits, and reasoned estimates for inhibitory parameters. Although the neo-Golgi period of cortical anatomy in the mid-1970s was just around the corner, there were already considerable advances in the detailing of cortical neurons that were not consistent with his detailed interpretation, although his general principles of what neural operations might be necessary remain interesting (Lund, 1973; Jones, 1975; Szentágothai, 1975; Valverde, 1978).

The neocortex is made up of two fundamental functional classes of neuron. First, the excitatory neurons, most of which have a characteristic pyramidal soma and an apical dendrite. The basal and apical dendrites are covered with spines, which are the sites of most of their excitatory synapses, most of which arise from other spiny neurons in the same cortical area. The second fundamental type is the smooth neuron, which is inhibitory, and forms most of its synapses with spiny neurons. There are a number of varieties of these two classes, which were already classified by Ramón y Cajal and his heirs on the basis of somatic location, dendritic structure, and axonal projection pattern. This classification has been considerably refined in recent years through immunochemistry, physiology, and light and electron microscopic analyses (Peters and Jones, 1984; Kawaguchi and Kubota, 1997; Douglas and Martin, 2004; Brown and Hestrin, 2009; Rudy et al., 2011).

Obviously these two functional classes fulfill the basic requirements of Marr's circuit (Figure 8.1A). It was also straightforward to associate the output cells with pyramidal cells. However, the selection of the all-important codon cells proved to be a problem. Marr choose to assign granule (stellate cells) of layer 4 and the Martinotti cells to this role: the latter because Ramón y Cajal (1911) had reported that their somata were located in the deep cortical layers and their axons projected like climbing fibres along the apical dendrites of the pyramidal cells. Marr assumed that the Martinotti cells were excitatory, whereas now their synapses are known to be inhibitory. Indeed, his circuit would probably have been better satisfied by choosing the numerous superficial pyramidal cells for the role of codons. Unfortunately he was forced to make these structural choices at a time when details for cortical circuitry were making a significant advance from the early literature of Cajal and Szentágothai, from which Marr took his inspiration.

Circuit dynamics

In the midst of the neo-Golgi renaissance of the 1970s there occurred a major advance in the method of staining single neurons when it became possible to identify the detailed axonal projection patterns of individual neurons by intracellular injections of horseradish peroxidase (HRP). Gilbert and Wiesel (Gilbert and Wiesel, 1979) applied this technique to describing the basic connection patterns of the major types of cortical neurons in the cat's visual cortex. In a landmark review, Gilbert offered the possible circuit interactions between cortical neurons (Gilbert, 1983). Correlated light microscopic and electron microscopic studies of that time also provided examples of the detailed synaptic interactions between some cortical neuronal types (Somogyi et al., 1983; Kisvárday et al., 1986). However, these methods were limited to one or a few neurons and their connections and could not provide a more general population-level understanding of the dynamics of the cortical circuits. It was this limitation that brought us onto the path of trying to grasp the nature of cortical processing directly from the behavior of the circuitry, rather than trying to shoehorn computational function into a rather indeterminate structure as Marr was forced to do.

Inspired by the engineering methods of systems identification, we set out to characterize the dynamical behavior of neural circuits in cat visual cortex. To do this we recorded the intracellular "impulse response" of neurons in cat visual cortex in vivo and identified them by injecting them with HRP (Douglas et al., 1989, 1991) (Figure 8.2). An approximation to an impulse was obtained by electrical simulation of the thalamic afferents. In response to this impulse, most neurons exhibited a relatively short (10 ms) early phase of depolarization that was terminated by a longer sustained (100 ms) phase of hyperpolarization. We were able to dissect these processes of excitation followed by inhibition using the ionophoretic application of receptor agonists and antagonists, delivered from a multi-barrel glass pipette that was attached to the intracellular recording pipette. The electrical pulse elicited strong mono- and polysynaptic responses in superficial pyramidal cells, that were terminated by a fast $GABA_A$ receptor-mediated inhibition. Blockade of $GABA_A$ receptors resulted in a dramatic and sustained increase of the excitatory phase, suggesting

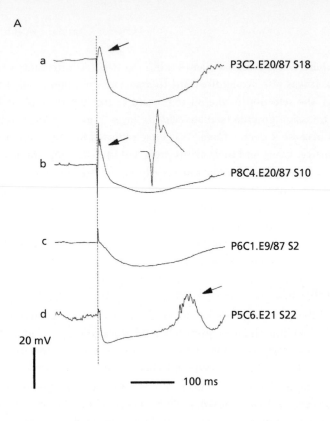

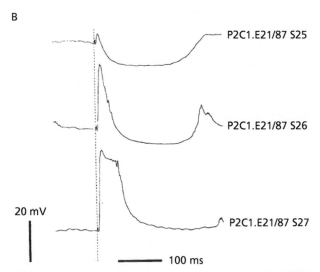

Figure 8.2 Intracellular responses of cortical neurons to afferent pulse stimulation. Averaged responses of representative neurons to electrical pulse stimuli applied to afferent fibers. *In vivo*, cat V1. Controls at left of each trace are at resting level. Superficial cells (a,b) exhibit prominent transient mono- and polysynaptic excitatory wave (arrowed). The transient is less prominent in layer 4 (c), and usually absent in the deep layers (d). Inhibition is sometimes followed by a rebound excitation (d, arrowed). Blockade of GABA$_A$ receptors mediating inhibition is followed by a progressive, florid, prolonged increase in the excitatory phase of the response (three traces at right, same neuron).

Douglas RJ, Martin KA, A functional microcircuit for cat visual cortex, The Journal of Physiology © 1991 John Wiley and Sons with permission from John Wiley and Sons.

that the superficial pyramidal cells are strongly recurrently connected, and that the result-ant feedback excitation is held in check by their GABA$_A$ feedback connections. In the absence of GABA$_A$ control, the exuberant excitatory phase was finally terminated by a sustained GABA$_B$ receptor response.

The pulse responses of deep layer pyramids were markedly different to superficial ones: monosynaptic thalamic excitation was much less prominent, and polysynaptic exci-tation was minimal. Probably because of this lack of polysynaptic excitatory input, the onset of GABA$_A$-mediated hyperpolarizing inhibition was much faster than in superficial layer neurons. As in the superficial neurons, the GABA$_B$ response evolved later than the GABA$_A$ response and was equally deep and sustained. We were able to model these and other observations by the simple neural circuit shown in Figure 8.3. This circuit captured the typical dynamics observed across the population of neurons that we observed, which contained examples of the various neuronal types that had been reported in the anatomi-cal studies of Gilbert and Wiesel and others. In this sense the circuit was "canonical", and we proposed that the organization and dynamics of this canonical circuit could be char-acteristic of all cortical areas (Douglas and Martin, 1991, 2004).

In short, the canonical circuit explains the intracellular responses to pulse stimulation in terms of the dynamical interactions between three basic populations of neurons, which were necessary and sufficient to account for the observed data. The circuit reveals that the following features of cortical processing are important to computational theories of neo-cortex (Douglas et al., 1989). First, inhibition and excitation are not separable processes. Activation of the cortex inevitably sets in motion a sequence of excitation and inhibition in every neuron. Second, subcortical thalamic input does not provide the major excitation

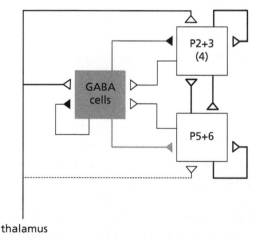

thalamus

Figure 8.3 Canonical cortical circuit. Simple circuit whose interactions are sufficient to model (for suitable connection weights) the dynamics elicited in cortical neurons by pulse stimulation. The strength of the superficial recurrent connection is larger than that of the deep layers.

Douglas, Martin and Whitteridge, "A Canonical Microcircuit for Neocortex," Neural Computation, 1:4 (Winter, 1989), pp. 480–488. ©1989 by the Massachusetts Institute of Technology, published by the MIT Press.

arriving at any neuron. Instead, the intracortical excitatory connections provide most of the excitation, probably through their recurrent connections. Third, the temporal evolution of excitation and inhibition is far longer than the synaptic delays of the circuits involved. This is due to polysynaptic activation as well as the long time constants of neurotransmitter effects, particularly of at GABA$_B$ receptors.

Our data and those of others, showed that the cortical circuits can be understood in terms of the laminar distribution of relatively few (between say 10–100) types of excitatory and inhibitory neurons (Gilbert, 1983; Gilbert and Wiesel, 1983). However, the degree of connectivity between the different cell types was unknown. We considered that a connection matrix of cortical connectivity would be a cornerstone for investigating cortical processing, and so we set about obtaining suitable quantitative data. During the 1990s we were able to improve our simplified model of the cortical connectivity by quantitative analyses of detailed reconstructions of individual neurons obtained by in-vivo intracellular labeling with HRP. These reconstructed neurons from cat V1 served as representatives of the different types and provided morphometrical data about the laminar distribution of the dendritic trees and synaptic boutons and the number of synapses formed by a given type of neuron. We obtained estimates of numbers of the different neuronal types and their distribution across the cortical layers from the literature, and used our reconstructed neurons to provide estimates of the spatial distribution of dendrites and boutons for the various neuron types. Then we assumed a modified form of Peters' rule (Braitenberg and Schüz, 1998), which holds that the synapses between different cell types are formed in proportion to the boutons and dendrites that those cell types contribute to the neuropil in a given layer. Thus, the laminar projection patterns of the source neurons, compared to the laminar distribution of the target dendritic tree, provides an estimate of the profile of average excitatory input across the dendritic tree. With the modification, known as 'White's exceptions' (Braitenberg and Schüz, 1998), that some known neurons like the chandelier cells make very specific connections that violate Peters' rule, we were able to estimate the probable source and number of synapses made onto and between neurons in the six layers (Binzegger et al., 2004) (Figure 8.4).

The resulting quantitative connection matrix confirmed that the majority of cortical excitatory synapses and almost all inhibitory synapses originate from neurons within cortex (Braitenberg and Schüz, 1998). However, the connection matrix has only a few strong excitatory projections (Figure 8.5). The most prominent connection is from superficial layer (layers 2 and 3) pyramidal cells onto cells of their own type. Indeed, the weight matrix indicates that 70% of a superficial layer pyramidal cell's excitatory input is derived from cells of its own class, suggesting that first-order recurrent connections between these superficial cells are relatively common compared to all other layers. There is also a strong feedforward projection from the superficial pyramids onto the pyramidal cells of layer 5. However, the superficial pyramids do not form an unusually large number of synapses in layer 5. Instead the large effect arises because there are many more superficial pyramids than deep ones, at least in this cortical area. Although excitatory neurons in other layers,

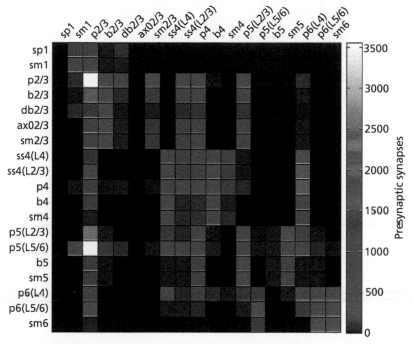

Figure 8.4 Quantitative description of the circuit of cat area 17. Colour bar is indicated at right for the relative number of synapses made by all presynaptic neurons onto a target postsynaptic cell type. Neuron types: b2/3, b4, b5 denote basket cells in layer 2/3, 4, and 5; db2/3, double bouquet cell in layer 2/3; p2/3, p4, p5, p6, pyramidal cells in layer 2/3, 4, 5, and 6; ss4, spiny stellate cells in layer 4. Spiny stellate cells and pyramidal cells in layer 5 and 6 can be further distinguished by the preferred layer of the axonal innervation (ss4(L4) (not shown), ss4(L2/3), p5(L2/3), p5(L5/6), p6(L4), and p6(L5/6)).

Reprinted from Neural Networks, Vol 22, Binzegger T, Douglas RJ, Martin KA, Topology and dynamics of the canonical circuit of cat V1, pp 8441–8453 © 2009, with permission from Elsevier.

such as the spiny stellate neurons of layer 4, or the pyramids of layer 5, also receive input from their neighbors, it is only the superficial layer pyramidal cells that make such extensive connections with each other. In addition to these few "strong" connections, there are many "weak" excitatory projections, each of which may involve only a few percent of the total complement of excitatory synapses of a single neuron.

The anatomical connection matrix is consistent with the features of the canonical microcircuit that we had derived from dynamical data, for example the strong recurrence observed in the superficial layers. It is also consistent with physiological connections (Thomson et al., 2002), and anatomical connections observed in rat cortices in vivo (Oberlaender et al., 2012; Narayanan et al., 2015) and in vitro (Hill et al., 2012). These functional and other quantitative anatomical circuit data reveal a number of intriguing circuit features that challenge accepted neuronal models of cortical processing. For example, the cortical circuits are not immediately recognizable in terms of the typical theoretical models of neural networks. They are neither purely feedforward, nor recurrent. In

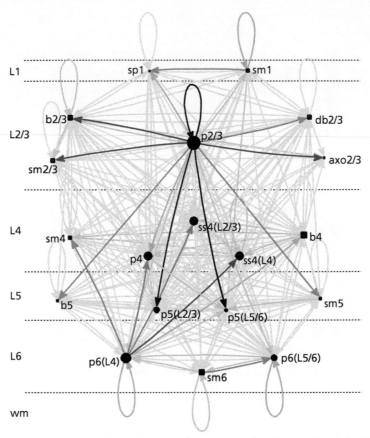

Figure 8.5 Graph of projections between cortical neuronal types. The graph is drawn in relation to the cortical layers based on Figure 8.4. The number of synapses the neuron of each cell type forms with an individual neuron of another cell type is coded by the gray level of the arrow: white, zero synapses; black, maximum possible synapses. Excitatory cell types, circular nodes. Inhibitory cell types, square nodes. The size of each node is proportional to the number of neurons belonging to the class. The largest node (p2/3, the pyramidal cells of layers 2 and 3) contains 8.2×10^6 neurons. Layer borders, dotted horizontal lines. wm, white matter.

Reprinted from Neural Networks, Vol 22, Binzegger T, Douglas RJ, Martin KA, Topology and dynamics of the canonical circuit of cat V1, pp 8441–8453 © 2009, with permission from Elsevier

particular, these data do not support the circuit model of Marr, with its lack of excitatory interaction between codons and between output pyramidal cells.

Functional motifs of the cortical circuit

We do not yet understand the full functional implications of the connection matrix. However, some of the connection motifs can be interpreted as computational primitives, the level of description that Marr prematurely dismissed from his original four levels. The actions and interactions of these primitives offer generic processing properties that form a bridge from detailed neuronal implementation toward algorithm, in the spirit of his original suggestions.

Inputs

As envisaged by Marr, the input fibers of cortex sparsely drive a large population of post-synaptic neurons. However, unlike Marr's model, these inputs play into a substantial locally interacting circuit, so that the individual sources of remote input to a given cortical area are very small relative to the large local synaptic load. Even the thalamic afferents, which provide the major subcortical input to the neocortex, account for less than 1% of excitatory synapses in a cortical area (Garey and Powell, 1971; Winfield and Powell, 1983; Ahmed et al., 1994; Latawiec et al., 2000; da Costa and Martin, 2009). Nevertheless these few afferents clearly provide sufficient excitation to drive neurons in the cortex. Similarly small proportions of excitatory synapses are provided by "feedforward" and "feedback" projections from other cortical areas (Anderson and Martin, 2002, 2006; Anderson et al., 1998; Anderson and Martin, 2009; Anderson et al., 2011).

The small number of synapses provided by the afferent projections raise the question of how the local cortical circuits reliably process the seemingly small input signals that arise from thalamus, or within the cortex itself, and how it is that the fidelity of these signals is retained as they are transmitted through the hierarchy of cortical areas. Of course, although the contributions of individual interareal projections are small, their collective contribution may be very significant. Indeed, the total synaptic input from other cortical areas may be fairly large: an estimated 20% of excitatory synapses arise from sources outside a given cortical area.

Despite decades of research, the means whereby cortex transforms its thalamic input into the cortical receptive field has been intensively studied in only a few areas of cortex. The responses to cortical inputs have been less studied, but in vivo recordings have shown that cortical inputs to layer 1 generate direct, rapid excitatory postsynaptic potentials (EPSPs) in the interneurons that sparsely populate layer 1, as well as in apical dendrites of pyramidal neurons whose somata lie in the deep layers (Larkum and Zhu, 2002; Zhu and Zhu, 2004). Thus the inputs from cortical regions drive monosynaptic excitation and disynaptic inhibition in target area pyramidal cells (Chu et al., 2003; Zhu and Zhu, 2004; Wozny and Williams, 2011; Gentet et al., 2012; Palmer et al., 2012). As one might expect, the inputs from remote cortical areas appear to modulate local activity. For example, layer 1 excitation is selectively and markedly enhanced during attentional tasks (Cauller, 1995; Letzkus et al., 2011). The spatiotemporal ordering of the input signals affects the transfer properties of the deep layer output pyramids. For example, near-synchronous layer 1 modulatory and layer 4 sensory inputs can induce complex dendritic spikes and bursts of somatic/axonal action potentials in output pyramidal cells in layer 5 (Larkum et al., 1999; Larkum and Zhu, 2002).

Recurrent excitation

The architecture of Marr's cortical circuit was essentially a feedforward network. In the 1960s the idea that information entering the cortex is processed serially through hierarchies of cortical layers and hierarchies of cortical areas had received a strong con-solidation from the interpretations of Hubel and Wiesel (1962; 1965) of their physiologi-cal and anatomical data. Many years before, however, Lorente de Nó (1949) had proposed that the elementary unit of cortex was a recurrent loop that maintained ongoing reverber-ant activity. This recurrence meant that the effect of nerve impulses entering the cortex from the thalamic afferents depended on the ongoing state of activity.

On the basis of the canonical circuit we proposed that the strong interaction between excitatory neurons in the superficial layers of visual cortex is a source of positive feedback (Douglas et al., 1989; Douglas and Martin, 1991), and that this feedback plays a crucial role in cortical computation by providing gain for active selection and re-combination of the relatively small afferent signals (Nelson et al., 1994; Douglas et al., 1995). This pro-posal was a substantial departure from the essentially feedforward excitatory architecture proposed by Marr for the neocortex, which was no doubt strongly influenced by the serial and hierarchical models of Hubel and Wiesel (1962, 1965).

The relevance of recurrence for computation is that it permits amplification and selec-tive processing of signals. A simplified view of how this recurrence may be organized, at least in the superficial layers of visual cortex, is shown in Figure 8.6. Thalamic and remote intracortical inputs impinge on the spiny stellate cells of layer 4 that relay and preproc-ess input to the pyramidal cells of the superficial layers. Some proportion of the axons of those cells c_i provide recurrent connections. The recurrently connected neurons occur in cliques. Two members of one clique are shown at left, and a one member of another clique is shown at right. The pyramids make recurrent connections of strength α, which for simplicity are indicated as self-connections in Figure 8.6, which are rare in cortex. However, the description that follows can be extended if necessary to more realistic pat-terns of recurrence between groups of interacting neurons (Douglas et al., 1995, 1999). In addition to these recurrent excitatory connections and whatever feedforward connec-tions these neurons may make, members of the pyramidal clique also drive by strength β_2 a common inhibitory neuron that provides strength β_1 inhibition onto each of the pyramids of its clique. Thus, the neurons experience positive feedback, α, and negative feedback, $\beta_2\beta_1$ (Figure 8.6B).

If we assume that the neurons have linear thresholded activation, then the behavior of a single self-connected pyramid is

$$\dot{x}_i + Gx_i = f\left(I_i(t) + \alpha x_i - \beta_1 x_N - T_{exc}\right)$$

where G is a load conductance, x_N is the output of the inhibitory neuron $\dot{x}_n + Gx_N = f\left(\beta_2 \Sigma_{i,\neq N} - T_{inh}\right)$, and f is linear threshold function max(x, 0). With thresh-olds and feedback coefficients all zero, the steady-state feedforward gain of this pyramidal neuron is $g = 1/G$, and its steady-state response to constant input I is $x = I/G$. With $G = 1$ for simplicity, and the feedback loops engaged, the steady-state gain is $g = 1/(1 + \beta_2\beta_1 - \alpha)$ with response $x = I/(1 + \beta_2\beta_1 - \alpha)$ (Rutishauser and Douglas, 2008). More completely,

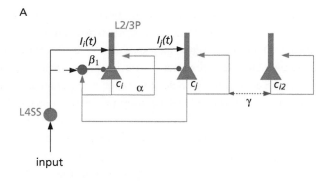

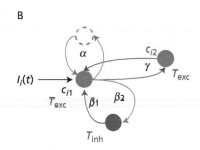

Figure 8.6 Proposed cooperative competitive circuits in L2/3P. (A) Simplified circuit of neuron interactions. Pyramidal neurons c_i, c_j (blue) receive time varying inputs from layer 4 spiny stellate neurons (blue circle), which are in turn driven by thalamic inputs (amongst others). The pyramidal cells are embedded in a recurrent network composed of positive, a, and negative $\beta_1\beta_2$ loops. A population of pyramidal cells individually assert β_2 excitation onto a common inhibitory neuron (red), which in turn asserts competitive β_1 inhibition on the members of its pyramidal population. For suitable values of the parameters a, β this circuit exhibits the signal processing benefits of winner-take-all (WTA) behavior (e.g., multistability, signal restoration). Sparse connections, γ, between pyramids of different WTAs allow the construction of elaborate neuronal state-machines (Rutishauser and Douglas, 2008). (B) Dynamical relationships between neurons of A. Transposition of circuit A, emphasizing the recurrent interactions. WTA cooperative positive feedback a may occur also through other members of its population (blue dashed circle) sharing the same inhibitory cell. The steady-state response of linear thresholded pyramidal neuron i is $c_i = GI_i + GT_{inh}\beta_1 - GT_{exc}$, where G is the circuit induced gain $G = 1/(1 + \beta_1\beta_2 - \alpha - \gamma)$, and T_{exc}, T_{inh} are the thresholds of the excitatory pyramidal, and smooth inhibitory neurons respectively (Rutishauser and Douglas, 2008).

considering also the thresholds of the excitatory and inhibitory cells, $x = gI + g\beta_1 T_{inh} - gT_{exc}$. Note in passing that inhibition of the inhibitory cell by T_{inh} allows a positive offset to the neurons response, above which it will again follow $x = gI$. Such controls may be relevant to the elaborate inhibitory cell interactions now being discovered, and which are discussed below.

The gain equation is rich in implications for circuit performance. Firstly, in the absence of inhibition, positive feedback in the range $0 < \alpha < 1$ provides amplification of the input signal. For example $\alpha = 0.5$ offers a signal gain of about 2, as observed in past cooling, and more recent optogenetic perturbations of the tuning curves of cortical neurons (Ferster et al., 1996; Olsen et al., 2012; Li et al., 2013; Lien and Scanziani, 2013). Secondly, the incorporation of the $\beta_2\beta_1$ negative feedback loop provides a means of also reducing the gain.

Positive feedback may seem inherently dangerous, but neurons subject to positive feedback will be stable while the sum of their input and their positive feedback excitatory currents is less than the total negative current dissipated though their neuronal leak, action potential, and inhibitory conductances. Such circuit-dependent stability surely exists in cortex, because the average discharge rate of active cortical neurons is usually much less than their maximum rate. This means that circuit stability cannot depend on the neurons being driven into discharge saturation as seen artificial recurrent networks with steep sigmoidal activation functions (e.g. Hopfield, 1982, 1984).

Collective processing

Steady-state signal gain is only one advantage offered by positive feedback. Even more significant is the ability of gain-developing circuits to perform useful collective nonlinear processing (Douglas et al., 1989, 1999; Hahnloser et al., 2000; Rutishauser and Douglas, 2008). For example, the high degree of connectivity between neurons of the superficial layers of the cortex, with their recurrent excitation and inhibitory feedback, is consistent with the architecture of cooperative–competitive circuits such as winner-take-all (WTA) (Douglas et al., 1995). WTA circuits offer important computational properties such as selective amplification, signal restoration, and multistability (Ben-Yishai et al., 1995; Douglas et al., 1999; Hahnloser et al., 2000; Pouget et al., 2003).

Signal restoration is a particularly significant property that goes some way toward answering the question of how neural networks are able to avoid signal corruption through their many stages of processing (Von Neumann, 1974). Restoration arises out of the interaction between the feedback excitation, which amplifies the weak external inputs to the network, and the nonlinearity introduced by the inhibitory threshold, which itself depends on the overall network activity. The positive feedback enhances the features of the input that match patterns embedded in the weights of the excitatory feedback connections, while the overall strength of the excitatory response is used to suppress outliers via the dynamical inhibitory threshold imposed by the global inhibitory neuron. In this sense, the network can actively impose, at each processing stage, an interpretation on an incomplete or noisy input signal by restoring it toward some fundamental activity distribution embedded in its excitatory connections.

The principles of computation of these WTA circuits have been described in detail elsewhere (Hahnloser et al., 2000; Rutishauser et al., 2010, 2015). The key principle is that computation is driven by instability. Intuitively, the instability arises because while the network is computing, the recurrent excitation $\alpha > G + \beta_2\beta_1$, and so the activity of the network diverges. It has been shown for these circuits that when a group of active neurons is unstable, the vector of their activities is mixed. That is, there is at least one positive and at least one negative component (Hahnloser et al., 2000; Rutishauser et al., 2015). This means that one neuron will finally be driven beneath threshold. Neurons that are beneath spike threshold do not contribute to the network dynamics. Consequently, the full weight matrix of the WTA clique is replaced by a reduced "effective weight matrix" that is similar to the full matrix, but has the contributions of the silent neurons zeroed out. If this effective matrix is unstable then the current set of active neurons is "forbidden" and the set will finally change when one of its members falls beneath threshold, leading to a new effective matrix. This switching of unstable sets will continue until the network enters a "permitted" set for which the effective weight matrix is stable and the network dynamics converge to solution of the computational problem that is inherent in the inputs and the constraints imposed by the network connectivity (Hahnloser et al., 2000; Rutishauser et al., 2015).

The basic WTA motif can be used to compose more elaborate computing circuits. For example, multistable networks containing a specific number of states can be constructed by cross-coupling individual neurons of two WTAs (γ connections, Figure 8.6) (Rutishauser and Douglas, 2008). These γ connections provide an additional source of positive feedback in the gain equation: $g = 1/(1 + \beta_2\beta_1 - \alpha - \gamma)$. Except for this small number of specific cross-connections necessary to embed the required states, the WTAs have homogeneous locally recurrent connectivity, and so the laminar architecture is essentially uniform. The cross-connections between two WTAs ensure that their winning states are associated and so reinforce one another. If this joint state is chosen, then the activity of those neurons is sustained even after the input that elicited that state is withdrawn. Conditional transitions between such sustained states can be achieved also by sparse connections (Rutishauser and Douglas, 2008). Using these simple rules it is possible to design and construct complex neuronal state machines; and in particular, to configure simple cognitive behaviors based on state machines (Neftci et al., 2013). These principles of rather dense local connections forming the localized WTA, together with sparse longer-range control connections that integrate their collective operation, provide an interesting interpretation of the general topology of cortical neuronal circuits.

The principle whereby instability drives active search for a permitted set of neurons may be more widely applicable than the recurrently connected circuits of the superficial layers. An analysis of our quantitative connection matrix revealed that the distribution of connection strengths, as estimated from synapse numbers, is heavy-tailed (Binzegger et al., 2009). While this distribution reflects only the average static connectivity of the network, by analogy with the more localized WTA that we have investigated, it is easy to conceive how this connection pattern could change dynamically. Consider for example the case where the connection matrix is simply thresholded. When the connection thresholds are so low, the characteristic length and clustering of the cortical network is indistinguishable from a randomly connected network. But as the connection thresholds increase (e.g., through average inhibition) the cortical network becomes significantly more clustered than a random graph, and so more "small-world" in topology (Binzegger et al., 2009). More sophisticated, localized inhibitory control may steer strong positive feedback to configure actively the local networks according to the pattern of thalamic input and the state of the cortex.

Inhibitory specialization

As Marr intuited, the inhibitory neurons play crucial roles in signal normalization and dynamically configuring a circuit. Inhibitory neurons typically have a more localized axonal arborization than the excitatory pyramidal cells, particular laminar distributions, and a few distinct strategies of connection onto their target pyramidal cells. The current view is that, at least for mice, the inhibitory neurons can be completely classified into three types on the basis of their expression of just three intracellular markers: the Ca^{2+}-binding protein parvalbumin (PV), the neuropeptide somatostatin (SST), and the ionotropic serotonin 5HT3a receptor (5HT3aR) (Rudy et al., 2011).

The somata of the PV interneurons (40%) are distributed in both superficial and deep layers. These anatomical "basket cells" have horizontally disposed axonal arborizations that make multiple synaptic contacts on the somata and proximal dendrites of their pyramidal cell targets. The contacts are strategically positioned to quench the total synaptic current being delivered to the central action potential generation region of the cell, and so the basket cells are natural candidates for Marr's divisive feedforward inhibitory neurons, and also for providing the negative feedback required in our WTA model (Douglas et al., 1999)

The SST interneurons (30%) are now assigned to be the "Martinotti cells" whose axons ascend vertically to arborize in the upper superficial layers among the apical tufts of pyramidal cells. They are most prevalent in the deep layers of cortex, but appear in all layers except layer 1. There is a smaller population of SST interneurons that ramify profusely in L4. These neurons are good candidates for thresholding or scaling the input signals from thalamus and more remote cortex (Douglas et al., 1999). The deep-toward-superficial layer polarity of the Martinotti cells suggests that they attenuate or select input signals according to local output conditions. This is obviously a very different role to the climbing fiber-like excitatory function that Marr assigned to them. The third, serotonin-sensitive, group (30%) comprise the "bitufted" and "neurogliaform" types located largely in the superficial layers. They include the vertically ramifying interneuron types, and so they may include those that express the calbindin/calretinin (but unknown as yet). The serotonin-positive interneurons have ionotropic receptors for serotonin and acetylcholine, which are neurotransmitters employed by the modulatory nuclei of the basal forebrain and brainstem. This input suggests that the activity of these inhibitory neurons may implement various cortical operating states(Rudy et al., 2011). The interactions between these distinct classes of interneurons are remarkably differentiated (Pfeffer et al., 2013). For example, the PV interneurons strongly inhibit one another, but provide little inhibition to other populations of smooth cells, whereas the SST interneurons do not inhibit one another, but strongly inhibit the other two populations of smooth cells. Of course, all three types have pyramidal cells as their major target.

Similar morphological types are evident in higher mammals, including macaque monkeys, but less is know about their general classification. Somatostatin is not expressed in their Martinotti neurons. In monkeys the different morphological types correlate broadly with the expression of three types of calcium-binding proteins. The double bouquet cells, bipolar, and Cajal–Retzius neurons are calretinin-positive; large and small basket neurons, and chandelier cells are PV positive; the Martinotti and neurogliaform cells and a subtype of double bouquet cell are calbindin positive (Gabbott and Bacon, 1996a,b; Meskenaite, 1997).

Computational purpose

While it is possible to recognize computational primitives and understand how these might be composed to perform certain tasks, the overall computational purpose (in Marr's sense) of the cortical design remains obscure. We should note, however, that Marr's computational question is posed from the point of view of an observer of the biological system. His top-down emphasis is appropriate in the human-constructed world of theory and implementation of artifactual computation, but it avoids the question of intelligent processing by natural systems that has arisen by evolutionary search and innovation, rather than human intellectual specification. The ability of biology to evolve an elaborate and intelligent neuronal network that can be developed with high fidelity from a single cell suggests that "computational principles" have to do with the structural and functional organization of intelligent networks that are evolutionarily and developmentally attainable. These computational principles, *contra* Marr, are matters of physical implementation. So, for biological systems, Marr's Computational Level is a post-hoc interpretation of processing by self-constructed neuronal circuits. The question to be answered, then, is whether the process of self-construction and constraints on neuronal growth and interaction can cast light on the ability of their circuits to represent and model world processes; and, if so illuminated, how they come to exhibit intelligent economically advantageous behavior. This line of reasoning has led us to reconsider the principles of connectivity and computation brain from the point of view of a self-constructing connectome. The "computational purpose" of a circuit should not be derived from Platonic ideals in the mind of the observer. Instead, its "purpose" is better understood as the range of useful circuits that can be reached through genetic self-construction.

The development of cortex is particularly interesting in this regard, because of the regularities of structure that Marr assumed and are discussed earlier in this chapter raise questions of whether and how apparently complex neuronal connectivity could be established on a basis of relatively simple developmental rules. We have been exploring this problem by a combination of experimental observation and simulation of the development of the neocortical circuitry. In biology the instructions for construction of a target organism are encoded in its DNA and these instructions are selectively decoded by a gene-regulatory network according to prevailing intracellular and extracellular conditions. We approximate this elaborate process with a model that contains

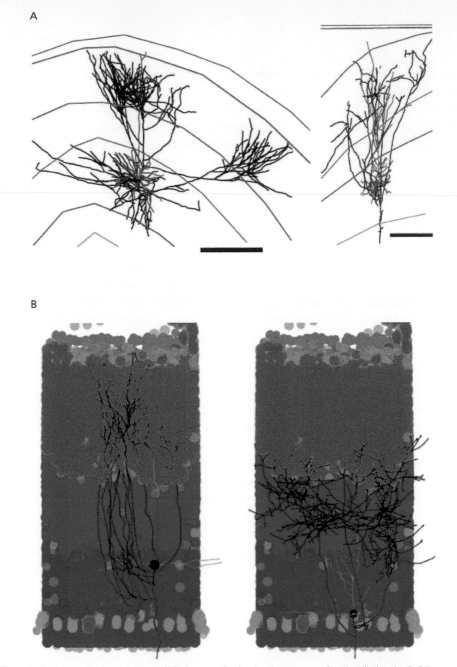

Figure 8.7 Neocortical neurons and their axonal arborizations grown by simulation in Cx3D. (A) Examples of real cortical neurons reconstructed from the cat visual cortex (Binzegger et al., 2004). Left: Pyramidal cell of layer 5. Right: Pyramidal cell of layer 6. Axons black, dendrites blue. Scale bars = 100 μm. (B) Results of simulations of developmental of the necortical lamination (Zubler et al., 2013). Slice views through three-dimensional space exported from the Cx3D simulator. Simulation begins from a layer of a small number of neuroepithelial cells, each of which contains a copy of the same abstract gene-regulatory network. The simulated development unfolds as in biology through mitosis, differentiation, and migration to build a laminated cortex. Layer 1 cells, yellow; layer 2, green; layer 4, red; layer 5, magenta; layer 6, blue. For clarity the subplate cells, though present, are not displayed; and no neurites are shown except for two example cells. The distal axonal outgrowth of these two cells are indicated in black. Layer 5 pyramid (left) and layer 6 pyramid (right), pyramidal neurons. For clarity, the proximal arborizations in the vicinity of the somata are not shown. The layer specificity of the distal axonal projections have similar laminar distributions to the corresponding real neurons of A (layer 3, and layer 4 respectively).

the essential elements of biological self-construction, but is sufficiently tractable to be simulated and analyzed.

We use a simulation framework (Zubler and Douglas, 2009; Zubler et al., 2011) in which cellular mechanisms act in a simulated three-dimensional environment that respects physical forces and diffusion, and allow biological processes such as cellular mitosis, migration, and differentiation to be modeled (Zubler et al., 2013). The cells and their internal mechanisms are autonomous agents that produce and respond to only local forces and molecular signals. There is no global controller. The behaviors of the simulated cells are determined by intracellular molecular-gene-like codes that are expressed according to intracellular or extracellular conditions (Zubler et al., 2011).

Using this framework it has been possible to simulate the overall development of three cortical areas with a surprising degree of verisimilitude (see Figure 8.7). The process begins from a small population of progenitors, each of which contains the same 'genome'. The dynamics of the genomes then control mitosis, migration, and differentiation of individual cells by instantiation of suitable intracellular physical processes. These mechanisms give rise to collective processes of development that result in the formation of some quarter million neurons of different types, distributed according to the observed lamination of cortex and with qualitatively appropriate intra- and interlaminar dendritic and axonal projection patterns. The resulting neurons approximate well the experimentally determined morphology of several cortical cell types including various pyramidal and inhibitory cells. Future work will attempt to bring the connection matrix of the simulated cortex into better agreement with our experimental data, but it is already clear that the basic circuitry of cortex could be accounted for through rather simple genetically encoded rules.

The self-construction approach suggests that fundamental connectivity can be installed through development, and then progressively tuned through electrophysiological signaling. Combining simulations of electrophysiology with neuronal growth is technically difficult because of the large differences in spatiotemporal scales between cellular developmental and electrophysiological signaling processes. Nonetheless, we have have gone some way to combining these processes in a model restricted to development of the superficial layers of the cortex (Bauer et al., 2014). The differentiated, approximately connected neurons adapt their synaptic weights homeostatically to obtain a uniform electrical signaling activity before going on to organize themselves according to the fundamental correlations embedded in a noisy, wave-like input signal. In this way the precursor expands itself through development and unsupervised learning into WTA functionality and orientation selectivity in a biologically plausible manner. Of course, much more work remains to be done, but it is already evident that an understanding of biological self-construction offers a promising avenue for interpreting the final network computation in terms of the developmental process itself: biology can solve computational tasks only through those networks that developmental constraints allow it to build. Thus, for natural computing systems, implementation must be a fundamental consideration for their computation, not a detail of no great consequence, as Marr (1982) held.

Coda

It is interesting to ponder what Marr's position with respect to biological computation would be today. It seems likely that he would hold to the algorithmic level of description, simply because there representations, and the algorithms that operate on them, are inseparable and provide a secure base for the interpretation of neural information processing systems, and for the construction and programming of technological ones. His disinterest in implementation likely reflected his concern that the search for computational understanding in neuroscience might devolve into a relentless reductionism, in which cranking the handle to store zetabytes of detailed data offered an attractive alternative to the difficulties of creative syntheses. On the other hand, increasing understanding of the algorithms of neuronal circuit development, and the ability of biology to install reliably the complex functional circuits that need only be tuned by environmental learning, may have given him new insights into the intrinsic computational nature of biological implementation. These advances would surely have made fine fuel for David Marr's creative mind.

Acknowledgments

We acknowledge the many contributions of our collaborators, with particular thanks to John Anderson, Tom Binzegger, Nuno da Costa, Sabina Pfister, Andreas Hauri, Ueli Rutishauser, and Fred Zubler for their contributions to the data, analyses, simulations, and theories.

References

Ahmed B, Anderson JC, Douglas RJ, Martin KAC, Nelson JC. (1994). Polyneuronal innervation of spiny stellate neurons in cat visual cortex. J Comp Neurol. 341:39–49.

Anderson JC, Binzegger T, Martin KAC, Rockland KS. (1998). The connection from cortical area V1 to V5: a light and electron microscopic study. J Neurosci 18:10525–10540.

Anderson JC, Kennedy H, Martin KAC. (2011). Pathways of attention: synaptic relationships of frontal eye field to V4, lateral intraparietal cortex, and area 46 in macaque monkey. J Neurosci 31:10872–10881.

Anderson JC, Martin KAC. (2009). The synaptic connections between cortical areas V1 and V2 in macaque monkey. J Neurosci. 29:11283–11293.

Anderson JC, Martin KAC. (2002). Connection from cortical area V2 to MT in macaque monkey. J Comp Neurol. 443:56–70.

Anderson JC, Martin KAC. (2006). Synaptic connection from cortical area V4 to V2 in macaque monkey. J Comp Neurol. 495:709–721.

Barlow HB. (1974). Redundancy and perception. In: Physics and Mathematics of the Nervous System (Conrad M, Güttinger W, Cin MD, eds), Lecture Notes in Biomathematics 4, pp. 458–468. Berlin: Springer.

Bauer R, Zubler F, Pfister S, Hauri A, Pfeiffer M, Muir DR, Douglas RJ. (2014). Developmental self-construction and -configuration of functional neocortical neuronal networks. PLoS Comput Biol 10:e1003994.

Ben-Yishai R, Bar-Or RL, Sompolinsky H. (1995). Theory of orientation tuning in visual cortex. Proc Natl Acad Sci U S A. 92:3844–3848.

Binzegger T, Douglas RJ, Martin KAC. (2009). Topology and dynamics of the canonical circuit of cat V1. Neural Netw. **22**:1071–1078.

Binzegger T, Douglas RJ, Martin KAC. (2004). A quantitative map of the circuit of cat primary visual cortex. J Neurosci. **24**:8441–8453.

Braitenberg V, Schüz A. (1998). Cortical architectonics. In: Cortex: Statistics and Geometry of Neuronal Connectivity, pp. 135–137. Berlin: Springer.

Brenner S. (2001). My Life in Science. Biomed Central.

Brown SP, Hestrin S. (2009). Cell-type identity: a key to unlocking the function of neocortical circuits. Curr Opin Neurobiol. **19**:415–421.

Cauller L. (1995). Layer I of primary sensory neocortex: where top-down converges upon bottom-up. Behav Brain Res. **71**:163–170.

Chu Z, Galarreta M, Hestrin S. (2003). Synaptic interactions of late-spiking neocortical neurons in layer 1. J Neurosci. **23**:96–102.

da Costa N, Martin KAC. (2009). The proportion of synapses formed by the axons of the lateral geniculate nucleus in layer 4 of area 17 of the cat. J Comp Neurol. **516**:264–276.

Douglas RJ, Koch C, Mahowald M, Martin KAC, Suarez HH. (1995). Recurrent excitation in neocortical circuits. Science. **269**:981–985.

Douglas RJ, Martin KAC. (1991). A functional microcircuit for cat visual cortex. J Physiol. **440**:735–769.

Douglas RJ, Martin KAC, Whitteridge D. (1991). An intracellular analysis of the visual responses of neurones in cat visual cortex. J Physiol. **440**:659–696.

Douglas R, Koch C, Mahowald M, Martin KAC. (1999). The role of recurrent excitation in neocortical circuits. In: Cerebral Cortex: Models of Cortical Circuits (Ulinski PS, Jones EG, Peters A, eds), pp. 251–282. Berlin: Springer.

Douglas RJ, Martin KAC. (2004). Neuronal circuits of the neocortex. Annu Rev Neurosci. **27**:419–451.

Douglas RJ, Martin KAC, Whitteridge D. (1989). A canonical microcircuit for neocortex. Neural Comput. **1**:480–488.

Eccles JC, Ito M, Szentágothai J. (1967). The Cerebellum as a Neuronal Machine. Berlin: Springer-Verlag.

Ferster D, Chung S, Wheat HS. (1996). Orientation selectivity of thalamic inputs to cat visual cortex. Nature. **380**:249–252.

Gabbott PL, Bacon SJ. (1996a). Local circuit neurons in the medial prefrontal cortex (areas 24a,b,c, 25 and 32) in the monkey: I. Cell morphology and morphometrics. J Comp Neurol. **364**:567–608.

Gabbott PL, Bacon SJ. (1996b). Local circuit neurons in the medial prefrontal cortex (areas 24a,b,c, 25 and 32) in the monkey: II. Quantitative areal and laminar distributions. J Comp Neurol. **364**:609–636.

Garey LJ, Powell TPS. (1971). An experimental study of the termination of the lateral geniculo-cortical pathway in the cat and monkey. Proc R Soc Lond B Biol Sci. **179**:41–63.

Gentet LJ, Kremer Y, Taniguchi H, Huang ZJ, Staiger JF, Petersen CCH. (2012). Unique functional properties of somatostatin-expressing GABAergic neurons in mouse barrel cortex. Nat Neurosci. **15**:607–612.

Gilbert CD, Wiesel TN. (1983). Functional organization of the visual cortex. Progr Brain Res. **58**:209–218.

Gilbert CD. (1983). Microcircuitry of the visual cortex. Annu Rev Neurosci. **6**:217–247.

Gilbert CD, Wiesel TN. (1979). Morphology and intracortical projections of functionally characterised neurones in the cat visual cortex. Nature. **280**:120–125.

Hahnloser RH, Sarpeshkar R, Mahowald MA, Douglas RJ, Seung HS. (2000). Digital selection and analogue amplification coexist in a cortex-inspired silicon circuit. Nature. **405**:947–951.

Hill SL, Wang Y, Riachi I, Schürmann F, Markram H. (2012). Statistical connectivity provides a sufficient foundation for specific functional connectivity in neocortical neural microcircuits. Proc Natl Acad Sci U S A. **109**:E2885–E2894.

Hopfield JJ. (1982). Neural networks and physical systems with emergent collective computational abilities. Proc Natl Acad Sci U S A. **79**:2554–2558.

Hopfield JJ. (1984). Neurons with graded response have collective computational properties like those of two-state neurons. Proc Natl Acad Sci U S A. **81**:3088–3092.

Hubel DH, Wiesel TN. (1962). Receptive fields, binocular interaction and functional architecture in the cat's visual cortex. J Physiol. **160**:106–154.

Hubel DH, Wiesel TN. (1965). Receptive fields and functional architecture in two non-striate visual areas (18 and 19) of the cat. J Neurophysiol. **28**:229–289.

Jones EG. (1975). Varieties and distribution of non-pyramidal cells in the somatic sensory cortex of the squirrel monkey. J Comp Neurol. **160**:205–267.

Kawaguchi Y, Kubota Y. (1997). GABAergic cell subtypes and their synaptic connections in rat frontal cortex. Cereb Cortex. **7**:476–486.

Kisvárday ZF, Martin KAC, Freund TF, Maglóczky Z, Whitteridge D, Somogyi P. (1986). Synaptic targets of HRP-filled layer III pyramidal cells in the cat striate cortex. Exp Brain Res. **64**:541–552.

Larkum ME, Zhu JJ. (2002). Signaling of layer 1 and whisker-evoked Ca^{2+} and Na^+ action potentials in distal and terminal dendrites of rat neocortical pyramidal neurons *in vitro* and *in vivo*. J Neurosci. **22**:6991–7005.

Larkum ME, Zhu JJ, Sakmann B. (1999). A new cellular mechanism for coupling inputs arriving at different cortical layers. Nature. **398**:338–341.

Latawiec D, Martin KAC, Meskenaite V. (2000). Termination of the geniculocortical projection in the striate cortex of macaque monkey: A quantitative immunoelectron microscopic study. J Comp Neurol. **419**:306–319.

Letzkus JJ, Wolff SBE, Meyer EMM, Tovote P, Courtin J, Herry C, Lüthi A. (2011). A disinhibitory microcircuit for associative fear learning in the auditory cortex. Nature. **480**:331–335.

Li Ly, Li Yt, Zhou M, Tao HW, Zhang LI. (2013). Intracortical multiplication of thalamocortical signals in mouse auditory cortex. Nat Neurosci. **16**:1179–1181.

Lien AD, Scanziani M. (2013). Tuned thalamic excitation is amplified by visual cortical circuits. Nat Neurosci. **16**:1315–1323.

Lorente de Nó R. (1949). Cerebral cortex: architecture, intracortical connections, motor projections. In: Physiology of the Nervous System (**Fulton JF**, ed.), pp. 288–313. London: Oxford University Press.

Lund JS. (1973). Organization of neurons in the visual cortex, area 17, of the monkey (*Macaca mulatta*). J Comp Neurol. **147**:455–495.

Marr D. (1969). A theory of cerebellar cortex. J Physiol. **202**:437–470.

Marr D. (1970). A theory for cerebral neocortex. Proc R Soc Lond B Biol Sci. **176**:161–234.

Marr D. (1971). Simple memory: a theory for archicortex. Philos Trans R Soc Lond B Biol Sci. **262**:23–81.

Marr D. (1982). Vision. San Francisco, CA: W. H. Freeman.

Marr D, Poggio T. (1976). From understanding computation to understanding neural circuitry. Neurosciences Research Program Bulletin. **10**/2004:15(3).

Meskenaite V. (1997). Calretinin-immunoreactive local circuit neurons in area 17 of the cynomolgus monkey, *Macaca fascicularis*. J Comp Neurol. **379**:113–132.

Narayanan RT, Egger R, Johnson AS, Mansvelder HD, Sakmann B, de Kock CPJ, Oberlaender M. (2015). Beyond columnar organization: cell type- and target layer-specific principles of horizontal axon projection patterns in rat vibrissal cortex. Cereb Cortex. **25**:4450–4468.

Neftci E, Binas J, Rutishauser U, Chicca E, Indiveri G, Douglas RJ. (2013). Synthesizing cognition in neuromorphic electronic systems. Proc Natl Acad Sci U S A. 110:E3468–3476.

Nelson S, Toth L, Sheth B, Sur M. (1994). Orientation selectivity of cortical neurons during intracellular blockade of inhibition. Science. 265:774–777.

Oberlaender M, de Kock CPJ, Bruno RM, Ramirez A, Meyer HS, Dercksen VJ, et al. (2012). Cell type–specific three-dimensional structure of thalamocortical circuits in a column of rat vibrissal cortex. Cereb Cortex. 22:2375–2391.

Olsen SR, Bortone DS, Adesnik H, Scanziani M. (2012). Gain control by layer six in cortical circuits of vision. Nature. 483:47–52.

Palmer LM, Schulz JM, Murphy SC, Ledergerber D, Murayama M, Larkum ME. (2012). The cellular basis of $GABA_B$-mediated interhemispheric inhibition. Science. 335:989–993.

Peters A, Jones EG. (1984). Classification of cortical neurons. Cereb Cortex. 1:107–121.

Pfeffer CK, Xue M, He M, Huang ZJ, Scanziani M. (2013). Inhibition of inhibition in visual cortex: the logic of connections between molecularly distinct interneurons. Nat Neurosci. 16:1068–1076.

Pouget A, Dayan P, Zemel RS. (2003). Inference and computation with population codes. Annu Rev Neurosci. 26:381–410.

Ramón y Cajal S. (1911/1955). Histologie du système nerveux de l'homme et des vertébrés. Paris: A. Maloine/Madrid: Consejo Superior De Investigation Cientificas.

Rosenblith W. (1961). Sensory communication. In: Contributions to the Symposium on Principles of Sensory Communication, July 19–August 1, 1959. Cambridge, MA: MIT Press.

Rudy B, Fishell G, Lee S, Hjerling-Leffler J. (2011). Three groups of interneurons account for nearly 100% of neocortical GABAergic neurons. Dev Neurobiol. 71:45–61.

Rutishauser U, Douglas RJ. (2008). State-dependent computation using coupled recurrent networks. Neural Comput. 21:478–509.

Rutishauser U, Douglas RJ, Slotine JJ. (2010). Collective stability of networks of winner-take-all circuits. Neural Comput. 23:735–773.

Rutishauser U, Slotine JJ, Douglas R. (2015). Computation in dynamically bounded asymmetric systems. PLoS Comput Biol. 11:e1004039.

Shannon C. (1949). Communication in the presence of noise. Proc IRE. 37:10–21.

Somogyi P, Kisvárday ZF, Martin KAC, Whitteridge D. (1983). Synaptic connections of morphologically identified and physiologically characterized large basket cells in the striate cortex of cat. Neuroscience. 10:261–294.

Szentágothai J. (1975). The "module-concept" in cerebral cortex architecture. Brain Res. 95:475–496.

Thomson AM, West DC, Wang Y, Bannister AP. (2002). Synaptic connections and small circuits involving excitatory and inhibitory neurons in layers 2–5 of adult rat and cat neocortex: triple intracellular recordings and biocytin labelling *in vitro*. Cereb Cortex. 12:936–953.

Valverde F. (1978). The organization of area 18 in the monkey. Anat Embryol. 154:305–334.

Von Neumann J. (1974). The Computer and the Brain. New Haven, CT: Yale University Press.

Willshaw D, Hallam J, Gingell S, Lau S. (1997). Marr's theory of the neocortex as a self-organizing neural network. Neural Comput. 9:911–936.

Winfield DA, Powell TPS. (1983). Laminar cell counts and geniculo-cortical boutons in area 17 of cat and monkey. Brain Res 277:223–229.

Wozny C, Williams SR. (2011). Specificity of synaptic connectivity between layer 1 inhibitory interneurons and layer 2/3 pyramidal neurons in the rat neocortex. Cereb Cortex. 21:1818–1826.

Zhu Y, Zhu JJ. (2004). Rapid arrival and integration of ascending sensory information in layer 1 nonpyramidal neurons and tuft dendrites of layer 5 pyramidal neurons of the neocortex. J Neurosci. 24:1272–1279.

Zubler F, Douglas R. (2009). A framework for modeling the growth and development of neurons and networks. Front Comput Neurosci. 3:25.

Zubler F, Hauri A, Pfister S, Bauer R, Anderson JC, Whatley AM, Douglas RJ. (2013). simulating cortical development as a self constructing process: a novel multi-scale approach combining molecular and physical aspects. PLoS Comput Biol. 9:e1003173.

Zubler F, Hauri A, Pfister S, Whatley AM, Cook M, Douglas R. (2011). An instruction language for self-construction in the context of neural networks. Front Comput Neurosci. 5:57.

Chapter 9

Unsupervised yearning: Marr's theory of the neocortex

Peter Dayan and David Willshaw

Introduction to Marr's theory of the neocortex

David Marr's theory of the neocortex (Marr, 1970) sits proudly between his theories of the cerebellum (Marr, 1969) and the archicortex (hippocampus) (Marr, 1971). It is an attempt to understand this largest and most richly intricate part of the brain, whose elaboration in humans is thought to underlie our extraordinary powers of reasoning, language, and thought. Instead of addressing these highest-level functions, Marr took on the more basic concern of how sensory input is represented and re-represented in neocortex.

Marr proposed that the pyramidal cells of the neocortex extract the structure from the patterns of neural activity impinging on it by learning to identify natural groupings or classes in which these patterns fall. The patterns arise either during observation in the sense organs or alternatively overnight (or during the day in periods of detachment from sensation), from a temporary store in the hippocampus. An intermediate layer of *codon* cells between input and output cells extracts the salient features from the input patterns. With each input pattern represented by a pattern of features in the codon layer, the connections between codon cells and output cells are modified until each output cell comes to respond to, and thus represent, all the patterns from one of the input classes. The output cells are then able to identify further examples of input coming from their particular classes.

The computational problem that Marr considered is what we understand today as unsupervised learning—and indeed, Marr's work can be seen as some of the earliest truly deep investigations of this. He addressed a collection of critical questions, of which the most important is the *goal* of this operation. More specifically, how do the representations learned reflect the *statistical* structure of the overall distribution of sensory input and the fact that this sensory input reflects causes in the world such as objects which present biological (and physical) imperatives? Given the answers to these questions, how can this statistical structure be *discovered* and used to interpret new complete or *partial* inputs?

Marr adopted an unusually heuristic and assumption-rich approach. Although there are alternative answers to the questions he posed, including one family that we explore in some detail to be able to pinpoint Marr's own suggestion, he makes the powerful argument that a completely justifiable treatment is inevitably out of reach.

As he did in his other theories from this era, in answering these questions Marr mixed levels of modeling and computational analysis that later he was to separate more formally (Marr, 1982; Poggio, 2012). He borrowed some of his ideas about neural circuitry from his account of the cerebellum (Marr, 1969), notably the concept of codons (his model for cerebellar granule cells), and the notion that climbing fibers carry a teaching signal. As described in his subsequently appearing theory of the archicortex (Marr, 1971), he also suggested that the hippocampus plays the crucial role of a temporary memory store so that patterns can be presented to the neocortex multiple times as part of the process of the discovery of statistical structure. He also suggested, albeit without exploring the notion further, that the capacity of the hippocampus for autoassociative recall might need to be copied by the neocortex.

The organization of this chapter has parallels with that of Marr's paper. We first consider representational learning in general, contrasting Marr's discrimination-based clustering treatment with an approach based on generative models that subsequently have come to dominate (Hinton and Ghahramani, 1997; Doya, 2007). Our treatment is intended to highlight Marr's and others' answers to the key questions above. We then discuss Marr's own suggestion. We differ from the original paper in not discussing the neuroscientific evidence that Marr hoped to encompass, as this is covered in Chapter 8 of this volume by Rodney Douglas and Kevan Martin. The present chapter amplifies previous analyses (Cowan, 1991; Willshaw et al., 1997).

Unsupervised neocortical learning

Introduction: re-representation and supervision in the neocortex

Sensory processing regions of neocortex comprise successive areas in an apparent hierarchy (Felleman and Van Essen, 1991). Neurons and populations of neurons in higher areas are sensitive to more complex aspects of the input—for the case of vision, for example, going from responding to simple Gabor functions or bars in area V1, to whole faces in fusiform regions of the ventral visual processing stream (Zhaoping, 2014). They are also invariant to (or equivalently generalize over) broader aspects of the input, e.g., maintaining their selectivity in the face of larger changes in the size, position, lighting, occlusion, of the input (DiCarlo and Cox, 2007). This amounts to a progressive re-representation of the sensory input in which potential information (i.e., entropy or variability in the input [Shannon and Weaver, 1949]) is discarded. The basic task for a representational theory of neocortex is to characterize the properties and realization of this re-representation, providing a justification for the choice of information that is jettisoned, together with an account of how it is achieved.

Many, though not all, believe it unlikely that there is enough information available either in the genome ("supervision by survival"; Valiant, personal communication) or through direct specification by an explicit teaching mechanism, to determine this re-representation in detail. The conventional alternative is that genetic information provides a set of rules, embodying prior expectations, according to which the neocortex adapts in the light of its actual sensory input. This adaptation process is probably unsupervised or self-supervised, unlike, for example, for the cerebellar cortex (at least in Marr's (Marr, 1969) and Albus's (Albus, 1971) theories), in which the hard-wired climbing fibers from the inferior olive provide direct, error-reporting, supervisory information. At best, supervision in the neocortex might be able to make minor adjustments once an unsupervised learning scheme has broadly been established.

Many rules for unsupervised learning have been suggested, essentially all of which amount to heuristic guesses about the relationship between two key quantities:

(i) the statistical structure evident in the sensory input that the cortex can directly measure (Marr calls these *intrinsic* properties)

(ii) the functional essence of the input (the *extrinsic* properties that will be diagnosed based on the presence of intrinsic ones, and which are the aspects of the input around which the subject has to organize their inferences and actions).

In one easily understood example (Földiák, 1991; O'Reilly and Johnson, 1994; Wallis and Baddeley, 1997) the environment consists of objects which are the essential elements on which animals must act (ii); and sensory input from such objects is relatively *contiguous* over space and *persistent* over time (i). Thus re-representing the input by recognizing structures in the sensory input that display spatial and temporal contiguity and discarding other sensory information might re-represent the input appropriately. Marr discusses this case early on, ultimately treating it as no more than a source of optimism, apparently because it is tied to a particular sensory modality. Not analyzing this case in detail is perhaps unfortunate, since one of the main conceptual points that Marr makes in the paper is that the computations performed by the neocortex are widely applicable, which should surely include generating this invariant re-representation. Furthermore, the intrinsic statistical properties are systematically different from the cluster-associated properties on which Marr concentrates, in keeping with notions about numerical taxonomy that were prevalent around the time of his work (Sokal and Sneath, 1963; Jardine and Sibson, 1968; Sibson, 1970; Jardine and Sibson, 1971).

Marr is brutally honest that the main conceptual difficulty in schemes of unsupervised learning is justifying any heuristic guess without having to rely on unsatisfactory evolutionary arguments. Marr discussed in some detail his own heuristic, his "fundamental hypothesis" that we consider later, although ultimately this remains as questionable as its more recent alternatives.

Redundancy and distributional models

The first issue in formalizing unsupervised learning is specifying the intrinsic statistical structure that can be measured directly. The most venerable idea is that the distribution $\mathcal{P}(a)$ over sensory input a (like Marr, we ignore the dimension of time) contains *redundancy*; that is, not all conceivable inputs are equally likely. Indeed, the idea of assessing, representing, and reducing redundancy had been central to the neuroscientific application of unsupervised learning (Attneave, 1954; MacKay, 1956; Barlow, 1961, 1989) since the earliest days of the Shannon information theory revolution (Shannon and Weaver, 1949).

Marr starts with the most straightforward application of redundancy reduction in unsupervised learning, which is that commonly thought to occur in the visual system. Here, information from the sensory periphery (e.g., the activity of the $\sim 100 \times 10^6$ photoreceptors in the retina) needs to be conveyed through a limited-capacity, noisy, and energetically expensive channel (the $\sim 1 \times 10^6$ axons in the optic nerve). That the input is redundant implies that this can be done without either as devastating an effect as would otherwise be expected from the dramatic reduction in dimensionality, or undue energetic cost. The way it is done is by recoding, or re-representing, the input ($a \to b(a)$). In the case of the retina, this recoding is evident in the receptive fields of the retinal ganglion cells whose axons form the optic nerve. Marr does not give a detailed or quantitative account of redundancy reduction in the visual system although he did regard Hubel and Wiesel's cortical feature detectors (Hubel and Wiesel, 1962) as representing evidence for successive recodings of visual information. Since Marr's time, theoretically and empirically compelling analyses of this recoding have been performed for the case of early visual processing (Atick and Redlich, 1990, 1992; Linsker, 1990) and are comprehensively reviewed in Zhaoping (2014).

We find it convenient to follow more conventional information theoretic notions in separating the recoding into two separate operations—source and channel coding.

In simple terms, source coding suggests that the number of bits that an optimal code should devote to an input a whose probability is $\mathcal{P}(a)$ is just the information theoretic surprise associated with that pattern, $-\log \mathcal{P}(a)$; note that we follow Marr in generally considering discrete patterns and distributions rather than continuous dimensions and densities. Likely patterns are recoded with few bits; unlikely ones with more. This coding strategy is optimal in terms of minimizing the average length of the code per input pattern, which is then the entropy of the distribution:

$$\mathcal{H}(\mathcal{P}) = -\langle \log \mathcal{P}(a) \rangle = -\sum_a \mathcal{P}(a) \log \mathcal{P}(a)$$

Note that this result directly links optimal recoding to the distribution over the patterns. To put it another way, finding a coding that minimizes the code length of a set $a^1, a^2, \ldots$ of inputs a is equivalent to finding a distribution $\mathcal{P}(a)$, often called a *generative* model, over the inputs that maximizes their probability or likelihood (under the assumption that they are presented independently). The latter process is called *maximum likelihood density estimation*, and underpins major forms of non-Marrian unsupervised learning (Hinton and Ghahramani, 1997). Typically, the generative model $\mathcal{P}(a; \Phi)$ is parameterized, and optimal values of the parameters Φ are sought. This then underpins an optimal recoding $b(a)$ for the inputs, for instance using arithmetic coding (Moffat et al., 1998).

Channel coding takes the optimally recoded inputs $b(a)$ and prepares them for transmission down an imperfect channel. It is one of the glories of information theory (Shannon and Weaver, 1949) that it is possible to exploit a channel efficiently despite its imperfections. Indeed, the theories of retinal coding are based on variants of this (Zhaoping, 2014), including such notions as rate distortion theory, which quantifies the trade-off between the unfaithfulness with which the input can be reconstructed, and the cost of transmission, for example in terms of the number of spikes involved.

However, for all its elegance and importance for bringing information from the sensory periphery to the neocortex, reducing redundancy does not offer a powerful rationale for neocortical recoding (Zhaoping, 2014). For instance, if redundancy reduction is measured in terms of a decrease in the number of neurons required, there is none—in fact, there is a huge expansion in the number of neurons involved. Consistent with this, there are redundant activations in the form of population codes (Oram et al., 1998; Pouget et al., 2003). Simple inputs (e.g., the orientation of a bar of light) are represented by the conjoint activity of very many neurons with overlapping preferences, which must therefore include substantial redundancy.

This is where other heuristic functional or biological constraints come into play. Marr mentions the *implementational* heuristic that redundancy helps robustness in the face of the potential demise of single neurons. However, he does not mention *algorithmic* heuristics associated with the nature of computation—a common currency in computer science, as for instance, the technique of memoization (Michie, 1968). For instance, it turns out that a representation of the orientation of edges can be made by projecting projections onto just two canonical angles, e.g., horizontal and vertical (Simoncelli et al., 1992). Employing this strategy, processing of inputs presented at a canonical orientation would then differ systematically from processing at other orientations. By contrast, a redundant population code with an even representation across orientation could admit homogeneous forms of processing in which operations can be applied to patterns irrespective of their form of presentation. Unfortunately, it is unclear how to quantify the benefit of this against the cost associated with the neural elements and connections.

The heuristics that Marr uses are cut from different cloth, involving making claims about the relationship between the intrinsic and extrinsic properties mentioned earlier. It is to these that we now turn.

Models and mountains

Marr ultimately assumed that the inputs to the neocortex are first of all transformed into patterns of features, the statistical structure of which defines a set of "mountains" of probability over the space of possible inputs. This formulation is somewhat unconventional and involved. We therefore start with a related, but, formally simpler and more conventional, formulation that is rooted in source coding. We then return to Marr's proposal.

Mountains

Consider the case that the pattern elements are binary and are generated as noisy versions of a finite number of exemplars which we write as $a\{1\}, \ldots a\{M\} \in \{0,1\}^N$. Extensions are readily possible to allow for an unbounded number of exemplars, for instance via so-called Bayesian nonparametric models such as Dirichlet process mixtures (Ferguson, 1973).

The probability of selecting $a\{\alpha\}$ to generate the input a is written as $\pi(\alpha)$, with $\sum_{\alpha=1}^{M} \pi(\alpha) = 1$. Then the noise process corrupting $a\{\alpha\}$ is taken to be that of a symmetric binary channel, with the elements of a being set as:

$$a_i = \begin{cases} a_i\{\alpha\} & \text{with probability } 1-p \\ 1-a_i\{\alpha\} & \text{with probability } p \end{cases} \tag{1}$$

where $p \ll \frac{1}{2}$ is the noise probability (which we assume does not depend on α).

These facets jointly determine a generative model over the patterns. According to this model, the overall probability or likelihood $\mathcal{P}(a; \Phi)$ is a finite mixture model (McLachlan and Peel, 2004) that can be written as

$$\mathcal{P}(a; \Phi) = \sum_{\alpha=1}^{M} \pi(\alpha) p^{d(a, a\{\alpha\})} (1-p)^{N-d(a, a\{\alpha\})} \tag{2}$$

where $d(a, a\{\alpha\})$ is the total number of input units at which a and $a\{\alpha\}$ disagree, and $\Phi = \{\{a\{\alpha\}\}, p, \pi\}$ are the *parameters* that define the model. In this likelihood, the exemplars can be seen as defining something that Marr would call probability mountains—if the probability $\mathcal{P}(a; \Phi)$ is high for some input a, implying that the input is near an exemplar, then the probabilities of patterns that are close by (according to the distance defined by $d(\cdot, \cdot)$) are high too, since they can be generated from the same exemplar through the slight distortions of the noise.

Marr's fundamental hypothesis states:

> Where instances of a particular collection of intrinsic properties (i.e., properties already diagnosed from sensory information) tend to be grouped such that if some are present, most are, then other useful properties are likely to exist which generalize over such instances. Further, properties often are grouped in this way.

In our terms, this implies that the mountains that we have identified with exemplars, and have this intrinsic grouping characteristic, are of value in extrinsic terms as information-discarding re-representations of the input.

Making all these assumptions, the entire problem for unsupervised learning and inference can now be laid out. We use Marr's language and his partition of the problem (although, as we discuss later, he eschewed the Bayesian flavor of the treatment that we give):

Spatial recognition

Spatial recognition starts from a whole collection of inputs $\{a^\omega\}$, and finds the parameters Φ, i.e., the exemplars $a\{\alpha\}$ and their frequencies $\pi(\alpha)$ (and potentially their number M), and the corruption probability p. This finds the underlying mountains, identified with their peaks. As mentioned earlier, the conventional way of doing this is by finding parameters Φ^* that maximize the summed log likelihood of the inputs, since this implies that the generative model will best accommodate the whole collection of inputs, according to an information theoretic notion of fitting:

$$\Phi^* = \mathrm{argmax}_\Phi \ \Sigma_\omega \log \mathcal{P}\left(a^\omega; \Phi\right).$$

This mixture model is sometimes called a *latent variable model,* since the exemplar from which inputs were generated is hidden, or latent, when the inputs are presented. There are various ways of finding appropriate parameter values, including the popular expectation-maximization (EM) algorithm, which was gestating around the time of Marr's paper (Baum et al., 1970), and subsequently came into prominence (Dempster et al., 1977). The EM algorithm formalizes the dual observations that (i) if we knew the exemplars, then it would be straightforward to attach inputs to them (according to proximity; this is the so-called E or expectation phase, and is what Marr refers to as diagnosis); and (ii) if we knew which inputs were attached to which exemplars, then it would be straightforward to calculate those exemplars (by averaging; this is the so-called M phase, and embodies spatial recognition along the lines of Marr's §5). EM operates by iterating these two phases until convergence—i.e., until a consistent collection of exemplars and input attachments is found. The optimization problem is not convex, implying that although it may be straightforward for algorithms such as EM (or indeed gradient ascent methods) to find local optima, finding the globally optimal parameters Φ^* can be hard. This places substantial emphasis on the starting values for optimization (which was also a preoccupation of Marr in his §5), or other tricks, such as the inclusion of stochasticity into learning.

Diagnosis

Diagnosis starts from a given input a, and works out the posterior distribution $\mathcal{P}(\alpha | a; \Phi)$ over the exemplars that might have generated a. This is actually the expectation or E step of EM (a coupling between diagnosis and spatial recognition that also arises for Marr's model), and is sometimes referred to as *recognition* (as the statistical inverse of generation). Following Bayes' rule, this is

$$\mathcal{P}\left(\alpha | a; \Phi\right) \propto \mathcal{P}\left(\alpha; \Phi\right) \mathcal{P}\left(a | \alpha; \Phi\right) = \pi(\alpha) p^{d(a, a\{\alpha\})} \left(1 - p\right)^{N - d(a, a\{\alpha\})} \tag{3}$$

Although it is not completely straightforward, the fact that one can write $\log \mathcal{P}(\alpha | a; \Phi)$ as being linearly related to $d(a, a\{\alpha\})$ via the weight $\log(p/(1-p))$ makes it possible to compute this term with simple neural hardware. The normalization necessary for the full posterior distribution can then be achieved, for instance by divisive inhibition (Carandini and Heeger, 2012).

If some more concrete choice of exemplar is required, then Bayesian decision-theoretic considerations become relevant, based on a loss function $\mathcal{L}(\alpha, \beta)$ which indicates the cost of reporting that a comes from exemplar α when it really comes from exemplar β. An important example is $\mathcal{L}(\alpha, \beta) = 1 - \delta_{\alpha\beta}$; this requires diagnosis in terms of the maximum a posteriori (MAP) exemplar $\alpha^{\star}_{\mathrm{MAP}} = \mathrm{argmax}_{\alpha} \mathcal{P}(\alpha \,|\, a; \Phi)$. Note, though, that one of Marr's core, albeit incompletely delivered, intuitions was that diagnosis should include a measure of certainty rather than being all-or-none.

Interpretation

Interpretation is a generalization of diagnosis which applies in the case that only some of the elements of a are observed—what Marr calls a *subevent*. As in Marr's formulation, this is perhaps surprisingly straightforward—in the posterior distribution of equation (3), the discrepancy $d(a, a\{\alpha\})$ is evaluated only over those inputs that are actually observed, and N is replaced by the total number of observed inputs.

To summarize, in this mixture modeling approach, we (i) started from a heuristic (actually Marr's fundamental hypothesis), which is that specific useful combinations of attributes occur often within the population of input patterns and that such intrinsically-defined mountains are extrinsically meaningful; (ii) made a set of substantial structural assumptions underlying the parameterized form of the mixture model in equation (2); (iii) suggested that the parameters Φ within this structure can be fit to observed data a^{ω}; and (iv) showed how recognition, i.e., diagnosis (posterior inference for complete inputs) and interpretation (posterior inference for incomplete inputs) could proceed. The generative model can also be embedded in a richer probabilistic context, for instance with a prior distribution over the parameters Φ, and inference about the posterior distribution over these parameters given the observed data as an alternative to maximum likelihood density estimation. Different structural assumptions, i.e., different forms of generative model, could also have been postulated, as we will see in the discussion.

We suggest that the mixture modeling approach captures a great deal of the intuition articulated by Marr about the goals and modalities of neocortical unsupervised learning, including the mountains. However, Marr made rather different sorts of structural assumptions, focused on the recognition model rather than the generative model. We next describe Marr's treatment, before coming back to a comparison of the two in the discussion.

Marr's model

As mentioned earlier, Marr's essential requirements are to perform spatial recognition, diagnosis, and interpretation. Spatial recognition requires finding the intrinsic statistical structure in the (sensory) inputs, namely the existence of classes $\{\alpha\}$ of inputs in which substantial groups of features are coactive. Diagnosis implies taking a new input and reporting (perhaps probabilistically) the class whence it comes. Interpretation is the same as diagnosis, except for partially specified, rather than complete, input patterns. Marr's probabilistic assumptions are distinctly different, and arguably more heuristic, than those of the mixture model—we now describe the key features.

Marr's model actually involves a conceptually optional, but practically important intermediate, codon, layer between the inputs and the outputs, representing the classes. We first describe the two-layer version of the model, treating the codon cells as if they were the input layer. We then go to show how the extra layer was used by Marr in his model.

Marrian operations in a two-layer network

Mountains

Given the many uncertainties of unsupervised learning mentioned earlier, Marr was generally agnostic about the exact nature of the statistical structure on which he expected the neocortex to work. However, he did provide a concrete characterization in his §5.2.1. This starts from a particular sort of a probability distribution μ_P which assigns a constant probability to each input a for which exactly k input units take the value are 1 out of a support set P of input units (with $k \leq |P| < N$), and with all other input units being 0. Given the constant probability, this is called a plateau distribution. Marr used these to construct what he called probability mountains, which are best seen as ziggurats, i.e., terraced pyramids of successively receding plateaus with nested supports $P_1 \supset P_2 \supset P_3 \supset \ldots$, weights $w_1, w_2, w_3, \ldots$, with $\sum_i w_i = 1$, and resulting distributions $\mu_* = \sum_i w_i \mu_{P_i}$. The supports define the collections of shared inputs; the fundamental hypothesis suggests that finding such mountains defined intrinsically will lead to extrinsically useful structures. Each mountain is identified with a class α.

Diagnosis

It turns out to be simpler to describe diagnosis before, rather than after, spatial recognition (as Marr did), because the latter is defined rather algorithmically in the light of the former, unlike in the mixture model, for which the relationship between the two is computationally crisp.

According to Marr, each activated input line $a_i = 1$ is used to provide an independent estimate of the probability $P(\alpha | a_i = 1)$ that the class of the input as a whole is α. He then argued that the weighted average estimate

$$P(\alpha \mid a) = \frac{\sum_i a_i P(\alpha \mid a_i = 1)}{\sum_i a_i}$$

minimizes the sum over the discrepancies between this net estimate and the individual estimates associated with the inputs. He quantified the discrepancies using a measure, called the Kullback–Leibler divergence, of how different are two probability distributions. This divergence has a venerable association with information theory (and indeed the generative modeling approach to unsupervised learning that we outlined above). The weighted average can be identified with a straightforward network architecture, in which an output neuron representing the class α receives input from the a_i with weights that come, through a plasticity rule, to estimate $P(\alpha | a_i = 1)$. The remaining requirement for normalization could be achieved through inhibition (Carandini and Heeger, 2012).

Spatial recognition

Performing spatial recognition amounts to asking for a self-consistent relationship between the mountain-like input statistical structure that would define $P(\alpha | a_i = 1)$ and the weighted average form of diagnosis (also in the light of inputs arising from all the other, equally unlabelled, mountains). Marr does not quite show that this is possible—and indeed he frequently relies, in an unanalyzed manner, on the use of the temporary storage device which is his model of the hippocampus (Marr, 1971) in order to solve problems of input pattern selection. Nevertheless, he does suggest two important ideas based on an adaptation of cerebellar climbing fibers as an instructive mechanism.

Both of these ideas start from the observation that the notion of coactivated inputs that underlies the mountains implies that a sensible approximation to a class could be obtained from asking when a single input unit (say $i = 1$) associated with this class is active. Suppose that patterns of class α have $a_1 = 1$. According to the first idea, input unit 1 is used as a climbing fiber for the output cell, and thus determines the course of plasticity for the other inputs. Then synapses are gradually strengthened whenever there is conjoint pre- and postsynaptic activity. Marr showed that it is possible for the output to come to specialize on the class for which $a_1 = 1$, while eliminating inputs from, for instance, another class for which $a_1 = 0$. The potential requirement for repeated presentation of the inputs is what makes the hippocampal simple memory so important.

One problem with this scheme is that a whole class, in the sense of the mountain described earlier, is not defined by the activity of just a single input unit $a_1 = 1$. Marr's second idea was therefore that identification of α with $a_1 = 1$ would only be a starting point for adaptation, rather like initialization in the mixture model. He went on to consider the evolution of the synaptic weights once the dominance of the climbing fiber associated with a_1 had ceased. He showed that, for the case of a single binary discrimination, this can lead to a form of mountain climbing, finding higher probability parts of the mountain. Unfortunately, it turns out to be very difficult to derive a statistically compact description for the course of learning.

Interpretation

If the network is presented with a partial, rather than a complete, input pattern, then the weighted averages used for diagnosis can continue to be calculated. The quality of the evidence used would be lower, leading to a less efficient identification of the class.

Codons

We now return to consider Marr's actual model and examine the role that the codon cells have in forming the intermediate layer of a three-layer network. One of the most important differences between Marr's scheme and that of the mixture model lies in the way that the inputs are combined during diagnosis. In the mixture model, the inputs are treated collectively, with their individual deviations from the exemplars being combined multiplicatively. By contrast, in Marr's scheme, each input is treated as a complete estimate in its own right, with the class probabilities which each implies separately being subject to a numerical average. We later consider Marr's objections to the Bayesian basis of mixture model diagnosis. However, Marr's scheme demands higher quality evidence than is typically provided by the basic input units a_i.

He suggested that there was a recoding of the input into the activity of a set of binary codons $c_j(a)$, such that $P(\alpha \mid c_j(a) = 1)$ would offer better evidence about the class α associated with a (or equivalently, a more proficient distance function $d(\cdot,\cdot)$). These codon cells are the direct analogy of the granule cells of his model of the cerebellum, where they also perform a type of information recoding. Indeed, all his three models, of cerebellum, neocortex, and archicortex, had an intermediate (codon) layer between input and output. He might also have been thinking of the contemporary models of brain-like "learning machines" which, like these three models, had a three-layered structure. In addition, with the roots of theoretical neuroscience in models of neuronal networks that carry out logical functions (McCulloch and Pitts, 1943), he would have been aware that any logical function can be realized by a disjunction of conjunctions which can be implemented in a three-layer network.

These patterns of activity in the codons, rather than the raw input patterns, would then become the input to the processes of diagnosis, spatial recognition and interpretation. Mountains in the original inputs a are suggested (albeit without a completely transparent mathematical formulation) to lead to mountains in $c(a)$ that are better separated. To put it another way—following the notion that the mountains are defined by the frequent coactivity of multiple input lines, the idea is that codons report particular subgroups of input neurons that are completely, or almost completely, active in that input. This allows them effectively to multiply individual pieces of evidence from the raw sensory data together— the operation that is achieved in a more sophisticated manner by posterior inference in mixture model diagnosis. Although correlations in the activities of the codons would be induced by their common input, Marr suggested (albeit without proof) that, provided they were largely homogeneous, they would have no significant effect on these operations.

Marr's preferred codons are very like the plateaus of the ziggurats. They are defined on a support set P of input units, and fire if at least a threshold number, θ, of those inputs is active. The greater the size $|P|$ and the threshold, θ, the more specific the codons are to inputs that identify a class, and so the higher the potential quality of the evidence that they provide for that class. However, they would then be less commonly activated in the face of noise or partial inputs. Indeed, for interpretation, Marr suggested reducing the threshold so that the usual number of codon cells are active, allowing the various pieces of evidence still to be averaged. Indeed, Marr considered this particular sort of codon to offer an ideal way of handing variable quality evidence, and interpreted their neural substrate as being tailor-made for this function.

It is worth noting that Minsky and Papert (1969) had provided an elegant analysis of the use of pure AND codons (for which $\theta = |P|$), laying out the qualitatively different types of classifications that can be learned for differing sizes of $|P|$. Marr himself also provides analysis of the utility of these codons in providing appropriate evidence.

The main problem with this feature-detector type of codon is that in order to capture all possibly useful combinations of attributes (i.e., all possible useful collections of sets P), combinatorially many codons may be needed and may need to be specified. Possible ways around these problems are: (i) the wiring being prespecified by evolutionary adaptation; (ii) the feature detectors being wired up at random, which places no burden on the genome; (iii) there could be an initial configuration, perhaps set up at random, which is then modified through exposure to the sensory patterns so that the correct combinations can be recognized. Related to this, authors examining similar types of model had favored solution (ii) (Uttley, 1959; Rosenblatt, 1962) in the light of analysis showing that connectivity in the neocortex can be described probabilistically (Uttley, 1955; Rosenblatt, 1962). Although Marr did hint at the possible genetic origin of the wiring, the method he favored seemed to be (iii), an initial configuration set up randomly which then becomes tuned regularly in response to the statistical structure seen by the network, i.e., another, more limited, form of unsupervised learning. In his conditional probability model that learns to predict the state of some inputs through knowledge of others, (Uttley, 1959) had also mentioned the idea of starting off with an over-exuberance of synapses.

Marr called this method of tuning the initial wiring *codon formation* (§4.3.0). Initially, connections are made at random with each codon cell receiving on average a certain number, R', of connections. In an initial setting-up period, patterns are retrieved from the simple memory (Marr, 1971) to form a continuous stream of input to the neocortex. The value of the threshold, θ, is adjusted through the action of inhibitory interneurons so that the correct number of codon cells fire. At the end of this process, all afferents which have not been active are made ineffective (though not removed), reducing the effective number of afferents to each codon cell to a smaller number. This enables a large number of combinations of attributes to be considered as candidate features with only a smaller number then being used. Codon formation is imagined to re-occur every night, using the 100 000 input patterns which he proposed are stored temporarily in the hippocampus during the previous day. At the start of each setting-up period, the whole set of afferents is considered afresh, including those rendered ineffective during the previous night.

Issues within Marr's model

Setting the parameter values

Compared with Marr's two other papers, the information he gives about his model is remarkably sparse. One significant omission concerns parameter values. He gives some tips about the desired values but does not give possible actual values and how these should be achieved. For example, he gives no hint as to (i) the number of cells in each layer of his model; (ii) the initial number of connections to each codon cell, R'—this is required to be large in order that many combinations of input attributes can be tested, but then there is the danger that not many codon cell afferents will be discarded during codon formation; (iii) the value of the threshold, θ, on codon cell firing, which should ensure that the number of codon cells firing in response to a full input pattern and to a partial pattern should always be the same (unspecified) number, k. It is unfortunate that he did not calculate ranges of possible parameter values as he did in both his cerebellum and his archicortex papers. We can speculate that his lack of certainty as to how the anatomy constrains possible values made it difficult for him to give precise numbers.

The structure of the input patterns

Marr's key assumption required for the functioning of his spatial recognizer effect is that each class of patterns is associated with only a restricted number of codons out of the total that is possible given the number of input lines. This goes back to his assumption about the nature of the natural world generating the sensory patterns which is encapsulated in his fundamental hypothesis. Unlike for the mixture model, the relationship between the ziggurats, the codons, and diagnosis is unclear.

Extension of Marr's model

Marr analyzed the special case of just one output cell performing a binary classification. Willshaw et al. (1997) broadened both this basic model, and his analysis. As the method for computing conditional probabilities in the codon to output cell synapses (which Marr did not give) they adapted an idea due to Minsky and Papert (1969) and found that climbing fibers are not needed.

They extended Marr's analysis to the situation of multiple classes and multiple output cells. In the simplest extension, each codon cell is identified with exactly the same number of classes (as for the binary selection case that Marr analyzed). The number of output cells activated by a particular class of pattern can be controlled through adjusting the threshold, θ, on the summed activity to each output cell. Competition was imposed on the output cells, the strongest firing output cell being deemed to be the winner. When there were as many output cells as classes, Willshaw et al. (1997) calculated the value of the fixed threshold that causes each output cell specializing onto a different class and verified this result by simulation. The limit on the number of classes that can be discriminated correctly is determined by the sensitivity with which the threshold can be adjusted.

When each codon cell was assigned to a class at random, so that different codon cells became associated with different numbers of classes, more than one output cell came to respond to a given pattern, the same combination of output cells being responsive to patterns from the same class. The responses from these cells could be brought together in a further layer of cells to enable individual classes to be recognized. However, this possibility was not considered by Willshaw et al. (1997).

This last point illustrates the main defect in Marr's analysis, namely that it relies heavily on an idealized pattern of encoding within the codon layer.

Discussion

In this chapter, we have described Marr's philosophy of unsupervised learning, given a modern rendition of probabilistic clustering, and discussed Marr's own treatment. We first discuss the relationship between the last two, and then conclude with a more general perspective on unsupervised learning.

Mixtures and Marr: a comparison

Perhaps the starkest contrast between Marr's view and the density estimation approach comes in section §2.1 of his paper, where it is argued that Bayesian reasoning is not an appropriate method for performing diagnosis. As we have seen, instead of using Bayesian inference to calculate the posterior distribution $\mathcal{P}(\alpha \,|\, a; \Phi)$ (equation 3) associated with input a, Marr calculates a weighted average of probabilities $\mathcal{P}(a\{\alpha\} \,|\, a_i)$ associated with each input line i, based on an analysis drawn from numerical taxonomy.

Marr offers two reasons why the Bayesian approach might not be suitable. The first is that the likelihoods $\mathcal{P}(a \,|\, a\{\alpha\})$ have to be assessed for inputs a that the subject might never have seen before in its lifetime. The second is that whether an input belongs to a particular cluster should depend on similarity rather than frequency; to employ Marr's dogged analogies, we can be absolutely sure that a prize poodle, as a poodle *par excellence*, belongs to the poodle exemplar; however, such perfect specimens are extremely rare, whereas their imperfect cousins are common. Marr maintains that our certainty about any given pattern of type "poodle" should be based on the similarity between the paradisiacal and the suboptimal poodle and should not depend on any claim about the relative frequencies of either. We see here his interest in numerical taxonomy where at that time methods were being developed to define class membership by the similarity between individual objects in a class rather than an assessment of their individual properties (Sokal and Sneath, 1963; Jardine & Sibson, 1968).

A good way of resolving these issues is to examine the probability distribution associated with the mountain. As a counter to Marr's first objection, from equation (1), the probability that an input a is generated from an exemplar decreases as the input moves away from the exemplar, i.e., gets less similar. The value of the corruption probability p can be learned from the patterns that are presented, enabling generalization to completely novel patterns. Perhaps somewhat inconsistently, in sections §1.6.1 and §5.2.1, Marr himself provides generalizing definitions of the probability distributions associated with exemplars—i.e., the ziggurats. These directly imply the equivalent of likelihoods for patterns that have never been experienced.

One way to see the second objection is that Marr is suggesting that the probability associated with the exemplar itself could be *lower* than its neighbors—i.e., the mountain might look more like the peak of a volcano. However, it is notable that Marr's own mountain distributions described in sections §1.6.1 and §5.2.1 do have central peaks, or at least plateaux, a property that he requires for his idea for tuning the connection strengths through mountain climbing, his spatial recognition effect (§5.2.4). It would be perfectly possible to parameterize volcanic distributions and proceed with density estimation. Furthermore, although the exemplar itself might indeed have a higher probability than any *particular* deficient version, there are so many possible deficiencies that, taken together, their total probability vastly outweighs any relatively modest probability advantage possessed by the exemplar itself.

In the density estimation approach, the generative model (e.g., equation 2) determines recognition, and so the structural assumptions that underlie it are inherited by the recognition process. A different way to put Marr's second objection is that structural assumptions are needed about the recognition model too. Recognition can be considered to be a process of (perhaps probabilistically) discriminating between different exemplars. In this case, structural assumptions could be made about the discrimination boundaries—how smooth they are, in what directions they prefer to run, etc. Then, one might try and derive clusters whose boundaries have the appropriate form. This distinction is reflected in well-rehearsed statistical debates about directly discriminative versus generative methods for supervised classification. However, such assumptions may not constrain the model of the mountains—perhaps itself an issue when mountains are so central to the notion of clustering. Furthermore, such models are extremely hard to optimize; Marr does not attempt anything along these lines.

There are two other major conceptual differences between Marr's proposal and the simple mixture modeling approach that we have described. First, mixture modeling has to encompass the entire distribution over the inputs a^ω, implying that exemplars (i.e., mountain peaks) must effectively be found for every input. In Marr's spatial recognition process this is not guaranteed; injudicious choices of the persistent (§5.2.3) or transient (§5.2.4) activity of the "climbing fibers" which instruct the output cells can lead to gaps in the overall representation. To put it another way, Marr's mechanism for spatial recognition involves climbing local mountains (in our terms, adjusting a single exemplar to find its nearest peak), whereas density estimation fits the whole geography. Furthermore, unlike EM, in which the generative and recognition models are in perfect harmony, as we have argued, the relationship between Marr's taxonomic recognition model and the collection of mountains is at best obscure. Perhaps reflecting this, Marr recognizes the comparative incompleteness of spatial recognition in his model. Although he suggests that ultimately it will be solved using aspects (notably pattern completion) of his archicortical theory (Marr, 1971), no further paper appeared. We should also note that the case for using climbing fibers in the model is not proven either on anatomical (Douglas and Martin, Chapter 8 of this volume) or computational grounds (Willshaw et al., 1997).

The second major difference is that Marr suggested that inputs a need first to be re-represented by the codons. We argued that this is of particular importance to Marr because in the recognition process that he employed, averaging the individual pieces of evidence is substantially more error-prone than posterior inference in the generative model. By providing information about conjunctions of inputs, an operation close to multiplication for binary valued inputs, use of codons offers the possibility of substantially greater fidelity. However, issues discussed by Marr, such as selecting among the inputs just those that are relevant and reliable to build and exploit the mountains, are clearly important—the noise model in equation (1) unwisely treats all deviations as being of equal significance. It is certainly possible to build a mixture model based on the collection of re-represented inputs $c(a^{\omega})$ rather than that of the direct inputs a^{ω} themselves.

Unsupervised learning

Marr's model, and indeed the probabilistic mixture model that we described, are both based on clustering. However, a wealth of generative models has been suggested that capture more general heuristics about both intrinsic and extrinsic properties. One popular approach is to start from a causal notion about how input is really generated—for the case of vision, from a graphics model rather akin to that of an animation studio. In such a graphics model, input arises from visual objects placed in particular locations, lit in given ways, and observed from a given viewpoint. These higher-level constructs then determine complex statistical relationships among the observed inputs, which unsupervised learning should unearth. For inputs derived in this manner, the equivalent of finding the collection of mountains, and re-representing (diagnosing) an input in terms of the mountains whence it most likely hails is to find the collection of high-level generators, and re-represent each input in terms of the generators responsible for it. The generators are sometimes considered as defining a coordinate system for the lower-dimensional manifold on which the inputs live in the high-dimensional input space; Marr's clustering-based view could be generalized to consider these to be extrinsic properties that lie within the intrinsic statistical structure of the inputs.

Examples include variants of linear and nonlinear factor analysis, directed and undirected sigmoid belief networks, and many more (e.g. Ackley et al., 1985; Hinton and Zemel, 1994; Bell and Sejnowski, 1995; Dayan et al., 1995; Hinton et al., 1995; Olshausen and Field, 1996; Hinton and Ghahramani, 1997; Rao and Ballard, 1997; Oja, 2002; Hyvärinen et al., 2003; Friston and Stephan, 2007; Friston, 2010). These are in turn associated with diverse accounts of recognition, some feedforward, as for Marr (Bell and Sejnowski, 1995; Hinton et al., 1995); others involving richer dynamics, such as interacting bottom-up and top-down streams of information between processing areas (MacKay, 1956; Rao and Ballard, 1997; Dayan, 1999; Friston, 2010); and also ideas about methods for representing the full posterior distributions that are the most complete forms of recognition through deterministic or stochastic methods (Ma et al., 2006; Fiser et al., 2010; Boerlin et al., 2013). Different models have their own learning rules, some more biologically based than others. Many of the more sophisticated generative models are themselves hierarchical, and so generate their own idealized intermediate re-representations that replace Marr's codons. Further, there turns out to be a subtle relationship between these representations and the distance function $d(\cdot,\cdot)$. This is because, as for codons, distances measured in the re-represented space can be very unlike those in the original input space.

Most of these models consider unsupervised learning to occur based on sensory inputs arising directly from the environment. However, following Marr, there have been various suggestions that patterns could indeed be stored temporarily in the hippocampus, and read back to be consolidated into the neocortical representation either during quiet wakefulness or overnight (Alvarez and Squire, 1994; McClelland et al., 1995; Sneve et al., 2015). There is less agreement as to how the importance of these patterns for consolidation is assessed and applied.

Conclusion

In sum, Marr's theory of neocortex is much less complete than his other theories, and arguably has stood the test of time somewhat less well. The form of re-representation that he considered, namely clustering, is not so obviously related to the sorts of cortical population codes that are prevalent in recording studies.

However, the more abstract analysis that Marr offered about the nature and goals of unsupervised learning, and the essential difficulty of providing a clear and compelling rationale that ties intrinsic, statistical, considerations, with extrinsic, biological ones, was very much on target. He clearly presaged many of the difficulties that have afflicted this critical, but underachieving, form of adaptation. For instance, most attempts to use unsupervised learning to elucidate cortical representations beyond early stages of sensory processing have disappointed. Equally, optimism that representations formed through unsupervised learning would actually prove useful for subsequent supervised tasks (Hinton and Salakhutdinov, 2006) seems somewhat to be evaporating in the face of the current juggernauts of purely supervised deep learning approaches.

At the very least, the key questions Marr posed remain embarrassingly unanswered.

Acknowledgments

Our grateful thanks to Jack Cowan, Rodney Douglas, Aapo Hyvärinen, Kevan Martin, Philip Quinlan, Fritz Sommer, Lucia Vaina, and Les Valiant for commenting on an earlier draft of our manuscript. Funding to PD was from the Gatsby Charitable Foundation.

References

Ackley DH, Hinton GE, Sejnowski TJ. (1985). A learning algorithm for Boltzmann machines. Cogn Sci. 9:147–169.

Albus JS. (1971). A theory of cerebellar function. Math Biosci. 10:25–61.

Alvarez P, Squire LR. (1994). Memory consolidation and the medial temporal lobe: a simple network model. Proc Natl Acad Sci U S A. 91:7041–7045.

Atick JJ, Redlich AN. (1990). Towards a theory of early visual processing. Neural Comput. 2:308–320.

Atick JJ, Redlich AN. (1992). What does the retina know about natural scenes? Neural Comput. 4:196–210.

Attneave F. (1954). Some informational aspects of visual perception. Psychol Rev. **61**:183–193.

Barlow HB. (1961). Possible principles underlying the transformation of sensory messages. In: Sensory Communication (**Rosenblith WA**, ed,), p. 217 Cambridge, MA: MIT Press.

Barlow HB. (1989). Unsupervised learning. Neural Comput. **1**:295–311.

Baum LE, Petrie T, Soules G, Weiss N. (1970). A maximization technique occurring in the statistical analysis of probabilistic functions of Markov chains. Ann Math Statist. **41**:164–171.

Bell AJ, Sejnowski TJ. (1995). An information-maximization approach to blind separation and blind deconvolution. Neural Comput. **7**:1129–1159.

Boerlin M, Machens CK, Denève S. (2013). Predictive coding of dynamical variables in balanced spiking networks. PLoS Comput Biol. **9**:e1003258.

Carandini M, Heeger DJ. (2012). Normalization as a canonical neural computation. Nat Rev Neurosci. **13**:51–62.

Cowan JD. (1991). Commentary on a theory for cerebral neocortex. In: From the Retina to Neocortex: Selected Papers of David Marr (Vania LM, ed.), pp. 203–209. Boston, MA: Birkhauser.

Dayan P. (1999). Recurrent sampling models for the Helmholtz machine. Neural Comput. **11**:653–678.

Dayan P, Hinton GE, Neal RM, Zemel RS. (1995). The Helmholtz machine. Neural Comput. **7**:889–904.

Dempster A, Laird N, Rubin D. (1977). Maximum likelihood from incomplete data via the EM algorithm. J R Statist Soc B. **39**:1–38.

DiCarlo JJ, Cox DD. (2007). Untangling invariant object recognition. Trends Cogn Sci. **11**:333–341.

Doya K. (2007). Bayesian Brain: Probilistic Approaches to Neural Coding. Cambridge, MA: MIT Press.

Felleman DJ, Van Essen DC. (1991). Distributed hierarchical processing in the primate cerebral cortex. Cereb Cortex. **1**:1–47.

Ferguson TS. (1973) A Bayesian analysis of some nonparametric problems. Ann Statist. **1**:209–230.

Fiser J, Berkes P, Orban G, Lengyel M. (2010). Statistically optimal perception and learning: from behavior to neural representations. Trends Cogn Sci. **14**:119–130.

Földiák P. (1991). Learning invariance from transformation sequences. Neural Comput. **3**:194–200.

Friston K. (2010). The free-energy principle: a unified brain theory? Nat Rev Neurosci. **11**:127–138.

Friston KJ, Stephan KE. (2007). Free-energy and the brain. Synthese. **159**:417–458.

Hinton GE, Dayan P, Frey BJ, Neal RM. (1995). The "wake-sleep" algorithm for unsupervised neural networks. Science. **268**:1158–1161.

Hinton GE, Ghahramani Z. (1997). Generative models for discovering sparse distributed representations. Philos Trans R Soc Lond B Biol Sci. **352**:1177–1190.

Hinton GE, Salakhutdinov RR. (2006). Reducing the dimensionality of data with neural networks. Science. **313**:504–507.

Hinton GE, Zemel RS. (1994). Autoencoders, minimum description length and Helmholtz free energy. In: Advances in Neural Information Processing Systems 6 (NIPS 1993) (Cowan JD et al., eds), pp. 3–10.

Hubel DH, Wiesel TN. (1962). Receptive fields, binocular interaction and functional architecture in the cat's visual cortex. J Physiol. **160**:106–154.

Hyvärinen A, Hurri J, Väyrynen J. (2003). Bubbles: a unifying framework for low-level statistical properties of natural image sequences. J Opt Soc Am A. **20**:1237–1252.

Jardine N, Sibson R. (1968). A model for taxonomy. Math Biosci. **2**:465–482.

Jardine N, Sibson R. (1971). Mathematical Taxonomy. London: Wiley.

Linsker R. (1990). Perceptual neural organization: some approaches based on network models and information theory. Annu Rev Neurosci. **13**:257–281.

Ma WJ, Beck JM, Latham PE, Pouget A. (2006). Bayesian inference with probabilistic population codes. Nat Neurosci. **9**:1432–1438.

MacKay DM. (1956). The epistemological problem for automata. In: Automata Studies (Shannon CE, McCarthy J, eds), pp. 235–251 Princeton, NJ: Princeton University Press.

Marr D. (1969). A theory of cerebellar cortex. J Physiol. **202**:437–470.

Marr D. (1970). A theory for cerebral neocortex. Proc R Soc Lond B Biol Sci. **176**:161–234.

Marr D. (1971). Simple memory: a theory for archicortex. Philos Trans R Soc Lond B Biol Sci. **262**:23–81.

Marr D. (1982). Vision: A Computational Investigation into the Human Representation and Processing of Visual Information. San Francisco, CA: W. H. Freeman.

McClelland JL, McNaughton BL, O'Reilly RC. (1995). Why there are complementary learning systems in the hippocampus and neocortex: insights from the successes and failures of connectionist models of learning and memory. Psychol Rev. **102**:419–457.

McCulloch WS, Pitts W. (1943). A logical calculus of the ideas immanent in nervous activity. Bull Math Biophys. **5**:115–133.

McLachlan G, Peel D. (2004). Finite Mixture Models. New York: Wiley.

Michie D. (1968). Memo functions and machine learning. Nature. **218**:19–22.

Minsky M, Papert S. (1969). Perceptron: An Introduction to Computational Geometry. Cambridge, MA: MIT Press (expanded edition 1988).

Moffat A, Neal RM, Witten IH. (1998). Arithmetic coding revisited. ACM Trans Inf Syst (TOIS). **16**:256–294.

O'Reilly RC, Johnson MH. (1994). Object recognition and sensitive periods: A computational analysis of visual imprinting. Neural Comput. **6**:357–389.

Oja E. (2002). Unsupervised learning in neural computation. Theoret Comput Sci. **287**:187–207.

Olshausen BA, Field DJ. (1996). Emergence of simple-cell receptive field properties by learning a sparse code for natural images. Nature. **381**:607–609.

Oram MW, Földiák P, Perrett DI, Sengpiel F. (1998). The "Ideal Homunculus": decoding neural population signals. Trends Neurosci. **21**:259–265.

Poggio T. (2012). The Levels of Understanding framework, revised. Perception. **41**:1017–1023.

Pouget A, Dayan P, Zemel RS. (2003). Inference and computation with population codes. Annu Rev Neurosci. **26**:381–410.

Rao RP, Ballard DH. (1997). Dynamic model of visual recognition predicts neural response properties in the visual cortex. Neural Comput. **9**:721–763.

Rosenblatt F. (1962). Principles of Neurodynamics: Perceptrons and the Theory of Brain Mechanisms. Washington, DC: Spartan.

Shannon CE, Weaver W. (1949). The Mathematical Theory of Information. Urbana, IL: University of Illinois Press.

Sibson R. (1970). A model for taxonomy. II. Math Biosci. **6**:405–430.

Simoncelli EP, Freeman WT, Adelson EH, Heeger DJ. (1992). Shiftable multiscale transforms. IEEE Trans Inf Theory. **38**:587–607.

Sneve MH, Grydeland H, Nyberg L, Bowles B, Amlien IK, Langnes E, et al. (2015). Mechanisms underlying encoding of short-lived versus durable episodic memories. J Neurosci. **35**:5202–5212.

Sokal RR, Sneath PH. (1963). Numerical Taxonomy: The Principles and Practice of Numerical Classification. San Francisco, CA: W. H. Freeman.

Uttley A. (1955). The probability of neural connexions. Proc R Soc Lond B Biol Sci. **144**:229–240.

Uttley A. (1959). Conditional probability computing in a nervous system. In: Proceedings of the 17th Symposium on the Mechanisation of Thought Processes, vol. 1, pp. 119–148. London: HMSO.

Wallis G, Baddeley R. (1997). Optimal, unsupervised learning in invariant object recognition. Neural Comput. **9**:883–894.

Willshaw D, Hallam J, Gingell S, Lau S. (1997). Marr's theory of the neocortex as a self-organizing neural network. Neural Comput. **9**:911–936.

Zhaoping L. (2014). Understanding Vision: Theory, Models, and Data. Oxford: Oxford University Press.

Postlude

Chapter 10

David Marr, 1945–1980

Lucia M. Vaina

In the first section of this chapter, I follow David's early intellectual and scientific trajectory. I then describe his passions other than science: music and flying. The coherent thread running through these two sections and the later section, "The last challenge," is of David Marr as a young man who never gave up in the face of any challenge, no matter how big, how hard. He was so determined, so intense and full of passion that he rose victorious above every challenge and this made him really happy. One could see it in his unique smile, a mixture of softness, warmth, and pride in victory, and in the indescribable, also unique, twinkle in his eyes.

Beginnings

David Courtenay Marr was born on January 19, 1945 in Woodford in Essex, England. From 1958 to 1963 he attended Rugby School on a scholarship. Education at Rugby was broad, rigorous, and challenging; it aimed to maximize the students' learning potential and uncover their unique gifts. It was the best school for David's interests and abilities in mathematics, physics, and music (with the exception of the emphasis on sport!). After taking his O (Ordinary) level exams at the end of the first year, when he was only 14, he had two years for his A (Advanced) levels, a year for S (Scholarship) levels, and a final term for the university scholarship examination. After O levels, David chose to double major in mathematics and physics but, as required at Rugby, he also took several additional courses. Among them was a language requirement, and he chose Russian.

Peter Williams, David's best friend in those years, remembers that during the S levels and mathematics scholarship term, the two of them and William Y. Arms (later professor of computer science at Cornell University) would sit at the front of the otherwise empty Old Big School facing the blackboard and teacher, learning almost as much from each other while competing to find the shortest and best solution to mathematical problems. The syllabus was advanced and stimulating, but David's mind went beyond it. At David's suggestion, they read and discussed *The Living Brain* by Grey Walter (Walter, 1953) which vividly presented the evolution of the brain, the invention and development of the EEG, and the way in which the rhythmic patterns of someone's personality are revealed in specific "brain prints." It also shows how these electronic processes can throw light on brain functions such as memory, vision, and sleep. David spoke with great enthusiasm about the possibility of developing a "mathematical theory of the brain." And this enthusiasm was not a fleeting one.

After Rugby, David was awarded a scholarship to study mathematics at Trinity College, Cambridge, and started in October 1963. At Cambridge his results were outstanding. He took the final undergraduate mathematics exams after only two years, with his first class in finals ("Part II") giving him the title of "Wrangler." The rules for the BA degree required a third year's study, in which he passed Part III—essentially a master's degree—with distinction.

During this time his supervision partner was Denis Mollison, who became a close friend. Denis vividly remembers their first meeting in David's room in Whewell's Court across the road from the porters' lodge:

> His seriousness, love of exactness, and wide interests, and the laughter that bubbled up through the most serious discussions, were immensely appealing. As to seriousness, it was striking to meet someone who at the age of 18 had so clearly planned his future work: he knew already that his aim in life was to try to understand the brain; had decided that that required in-depth understanding of mathematics as well as physiology; and that he should learn the mathematics first as that was a young person's skill (email from Denis Mollison, 2015).

They were supervised by some of the most eminent, if intimidating, of the Trinity fellows. The most supportive was Peter Swinnerton-Dyer, who played an important part in David's life. He generously took his students on opera excursions, mainly to Covent Garden in London. Denis Mollison wrote to me, "I recall queuing overnight for Wagner's Ring Cycle—but he would fill his large car with us and treat us to a fine dinner afterwards, returning us all to Trinity around 2.00am." Denis further remembers David's sense of mischief: "For example, one time when he turned up for the daily sherry with Peter Swinnerton-Dyer on election day in 1966, he told him that he had just been out to cancel Peter's vote. The assumption was that Peter had voted Conservative but David voted for the Labour candidate, who did indeed win the seat from the Conservatives that day."

For part of his time at Cambridge David shared a suite of rooms with Tony Gardner-Medwin who was a research student of Giles Brindley, working on the cat visual pathway. David was attracted by Brindley's rigorous work and toward the end of the mathematics course he approached him and asked whether he could do theoretical research on the brain under his supervision. Brindley advised him to spend a full year studying what was known empirically about the brain and come back with a proposal for what he wanted to do.

In June 1966, after his success in the Part III Mathematics Tripos, David was awarded the CouttsTrotter Studentship by Trinity College, which allowed him a year's study, free from any examinations, in neurophysiology, neuroanatomy, experimental psychology, biochemistry, and other subjects related to brain science. He read avidly and attended courses in physiology, biochemistry, and psychology, all new subjects to him. His reading was in large part focused on neuroanatomy, in particular Ramón y Cajal's *L'histologie du système nerveux* (Ramón y Cajal, 1911) and the Eccles, Ito, and Szentágothai book *The Cerebellum as a Neuronal Machine* (Eccles et al., 1967). Both provided a solid ground for his thinking at that time, and significantly influenced the three papers discussed in this book.

David had many friends: some were musicians, some studied mathematics or science. To mark his twenty-first birthday in 1966, Denis Mollison gave him the 12 volumes of Proust's *Remembrance of Things Past* and many of his other friends signed the last volume. I have those volumes, and have corresponded via email with several of those who signed it. Paul Dean, a contributor to this book, was one of them. Denis Mollison and Tony Gardner-Medwin wrote to me giving their personal memories about David and Cambridge at that time, and Peter Rado (now deceased) provided a beautiful letter for a previous book on David (Vaina, 1991).

Having decided not to become a professional musician, David immersed himself with vigor in the quest to understand the brain's function from its detailed structure. Consistent with his early intuition at Rugby, he thought that mathematics provided the framework for relating the details of brain circuitry and neural events to their function. He was in an excellent place for pursuing this, as Trinity College was a strong magnet for both mathematicians and physiologists. During his studentship there, David benefited from lectures and interactions with eminent physiology fellows whose work remains of seminal importance to the study of neuroscience. Among these were Alan Hodgkin, who in 1963 (jointly with Andrew Huxley and John Eccles) was awarded the Nobel Prize in Physiology or Medicine for work on the ionic mechanisms of action potentials; William Rushton, whose work on color vision and the principle of univariance are central to the study of visual perception; Horace Barlow, who was among the first to ask what were the computational aims of the visual system, suggesting that one was the reduction of redundancy; and Giles Brindley, who, following Donald Hebb's hypothesis concerning learning, developed a formal theory of modifiable synapses and investigated how learning can be achieved by the brain. As will become clear, Giles Brindley had a great influence on David.

In the summer of 1967 David received a scholarship from Trinity College and the UK Medical Research Council (MRC), and began theoretical research under Giles Brindley. Brindley was known not to be a "hand-holder," which perfectly suited David; his research ideas were already clear, and all he wanted was to discuss them and have time to write them up. Brindley provided that opportunity.

In July 1968, he submitted a dissertation "The cortical analysis of sensory information. A theoretical investigation" (Marr, 1968), for which he was awarded the Prize Research Fellowship at Trinity. It was very unusual for scholars to receive these fellowships after just one year of research. In the introduction to the dissertation he gave a brief account for the basis of his research ideas.

> There are only three current ideas of substance about information processing in the nervous systems: these are first about reduction of redundancy in the signals carried by sensory pathways (Barlow, 1959/1961); second, the ideas associated with Hebb's book "The Organization of Behavior" (Hebb, 1949); and third, the more abstract approach of Prof. Zeeman (Zeeman, 1962), the tolerance spaces). The literature outside these groups of ideas is large and depressing: the subject has more than its fair share of lunatics. In particular, there is the field of artificial intelligence which has a volume of publications entirely inconsistent with the fact that no ideas have emerged in it for at least ten years; what is worse, those ideas from other fields that really are of some use are ignored.

David went on to discuss the ideas current in neurophysiology, finding Brindley's work on modifiable synapses (Brindley, 1967) to be particularly important. He was also excited by the then unpublished work of Brindley on neural nets, which he was shown during a discussion and thought to be of relevance to the work on modifiable synapses. He was also inspired by the studies of Jardine and Sibson (Jardine et al., 1967) on cluster analysis, thinking that "the topic was relevant to neurophysiology because classification is something that biological brains do. Since, as it appears, there is only one sensible way of classifying, biological brains must do it that way."

The chapters of the dissertation are the seeds for the three articles David published in the following three years and which are the focus of this book. In the fall of 1968, David moved to London and lived in Giles Brindley's house (Brindley was at Berkeley at that time), and in less than three months had rewritten the cerebellum chapter from his fellowship dissertation. It was published in the *Journal of Physiology* (Marr, 1969). As Brindley puts it "it was the first substantial theoretical paper that the journal had ever published" (Vaina, 1991). David remained in London for another 18 months after Brindley's return, at first full time, then part time while commuting from Cambridge. During this time he significantly expanded the fourth chapter of his dissertation on the classifying and memorizing functions of the cerebral cortex. In 1970 he published "A theory for the cerebral neocortex" (Marr, 1970) and in 1971 the "Simple memory: a theory for archicortex" (Marr, 1971). While in London and working at the Institute of Psychiatry, David met Dick Passingham, with whom he talked about work, and ideas. They enjoyed concerts together, and developed a close and warm friendship.

In London David worked with Stephen Blomfield, and they published a short paper in *Nature*, "How the cerebellum may be used" (Blomfield and Marr, 1970). David also collaborated with Denis Mollison and Stephen Blomfield on character recognition, but it is unclear why that work was never published or pursued further.

In 1971 David received an MA in mathematics and a PhD in neurophysiology from the University of Cambridge and accepted an appointment to the scientific staff of the MRC Laboratory of Molecular Biology in the Division of Cell Biology led by Francis Crick and Sydney Brenner. He gave several seminars based on his three papers. I have some detailed lecture notes which suggest that in 1971–1972 David talked more often on the neocortex paper than on the other two. The lecture notes were very structured. Setting up the principal landmarks of the talk, he introduced the theory by first describing in detail the motivation for it, then asking what the neocortex does, followed by dissecting the criteria for those functions, and finally presenting in detail the general scheme of the theory.

David read extensively on animal and human neuroanatomy and neuropsychology, and wrote many pages of reviews and notes for several related papers aimed at extending his published papers on the neocortex and archicortex. One draft, of about 40 handwritten pages, is called "A review of the anatomy and neuropsychology of the hippocampus and related structures." He read Douglas and Pribram (1969) very attentively and critically and toward the end of the draft he stated, "I applaud their work and in particular their opinion that neuropsychological thinking should be based on the results of experiment, not on the abstract generalizations of the learning theories. I hold that opinion with some passion." David also wrote that, "the purpose of this review is to achieve, in so far as is possible, a precise statement of the Douglas & Pribram theory and to indicate the regions in which it fails. This will make the motivation for my own theory clear." This draft is accompanied by detailed and critical handwritten notes on Douglas and Pribram (1966) and Douglas and Pribram (1969).

In this review, David also aimed to "discover what information is stored in the hippocampus, and how this stored information is used by the rest of the nervous system. For this it is necessary to study all the available information about the limbic system and related structures. The literature is large, diffuse, and of variable quality." The purpose of this long review was to distill from it that information which seemed to be firmly established. He considered this a necessary step before he could write the subsequent article, "How the hippocampus may be used," for which he produced a full (typed) draft, dated 1972, but the manuscript was never published. In the review of the amygdala and limbic system in general, he discussed the orienting reflex and the learning deficits produced by amygdalectomy. He also addressed problems with the current literature on the amygdala. The draft was much influenced by Broadbent's theory of information processing (Broadbent, 1971), and it discussed the kinds of information storage that appear to be necessary for an efficient attentional system.

A short, unfinished draft, entitled "Chapter Y: Evidence from experimental psychology about attention and memory" contains a table of contents and only a few pages: 1. Introduction; 2. Evidence from neuropsychology ("has to come to mean experiments that combine the technique of animal behavioral studies with those of neurosurgery: usually a brain lesion is made and an examination is made of the way in which the animal is subsequently handicapped. The logic of such experiments has to be rather carefully constructed, but with a decent amount of luck the technique can provide much important information"); 3. Evidence from clinical studies on man ("this falls into two parts, one is planned to focus on information obtained from humans with surgical lesions or other injuries; and two on information about Korsakoff's syndrome. Few definite conclusions can be made from these sources, but those that can be made are very firm"); 4. Evidence from experimental studies on man ("this is the area of experimental psychology that examines the kind of information processing of which humans are capable and is roughly defined as that area covered by Broadbent's book *Decision and Stress* (Broadbent, 1971) together with one or two closely related topics"); 5. Summary.

At the end he noted that the paper would focus on

> three rather separate areas of study from which useful and firm information can be obtained: the first is neuropsychology, and the second and third areas which are exclusively human—human clinical studies and experimental psychology. These three areas are briefly reviewed in the next three sections. Conclusions from them fall into three classes: those that are firmly established, those that seem likely to be true, but which cannot yet be regarded as firm, and those towards which the present work points. In the general summary that follows the review sections, I set out conclusions and their firmness, so that the reader may compare the established findings with the hypotheses that I have to make before developing the subsequent theory.

This chapter was left at only a few pages, but much of the planned content is discussed over many pages in another manuscript dated 1972, also unpublished, "Neuropsychology of the limbic system", part two of "A review of the anatomy and neuropsychology of the hippocampus and related structures." On these drafts he made the following short comment:

> Marr's hypothesis: both amygdala and hippocampus can control orienting reflex: amygdala control depends on the force of an affective quality associated with a stimulus; the hippocampus control depends on novelty. The amygdala is also involved with other innate attention related responses like fear reaction to stimuli.

Short handwritten drafts on each of the three areas defined in Chapter Y also exist, but they have not been completed.

In 1978, after David had been at MIT for a few years and was immersed in computational theories of vision, he added this handwritten comment at the end of his still unpublished manuscript of "How the hippocampus may be used":

> Very mechanism-oriented, but it nevertheless hints at some interesting ideas. On the whole, however, this is the least interesting of the early notes. Are there good, general addressing strategies? What is an affective quality—what's it for, and how should it (therefore) be organized?

The fundamental link between all David's work during his time in Cambridge, UK was expressed later in his vision book (Marr, 1982): "Truth, I believed, was basically neuronal, and the central aim of research was a thorough analysis of the structure of the nervous system." This early work was aimed at understanding structure in functional terms, and the mathematical framework allowed him to make predictions which, especially his paper on the theory of the cerebellum, have inspired many experimentalists over the years. It was this paper about which he wrote in his dissertation that the "theory was testable."

The three published papers that are the focus of this book and the unpublished drafts formed a continuum in David's mind, as he concluded in his 1968 dissertation. While the published papers belong to theoretical neurophysiology where "one is bound to push hard at the theoretical approach, for it is here that advances will come most quickly," he also wrote that

> there are other big problems about which one must start thinking and for which there is probably no conceptual background. These come under the broad heading of the nature of emotions, and the way they are related to cortical analysis. I think that one may hope to approach these problems through an understanding of the function of the cortex, by observing the effects upon it that various emotions have: you simply chose a suitable task, and watch the changes in the way it is done that accompany various emotional pressures (Classifying tasks would be most suitable). From this one would hope to deduce what is happening at the cellular level by correlating these changes with alterations in cluster density criteria. Once one knows both the way cortex works and the effect upon it which the various emotions produce, one has satisfied the prerequisites for a rigorous approach to behavior, and that must be our ultimate goal.

Crossing the Atlantic: from Cambridge to Cambridge

While David was with Sydney Brenner, he came into contact with Benjamin Kaminer, a close friend of Brenner and Seymour Papert from their student years in Johannesburg,

South Africa. Kaminer became chairman of the Department of Physiology at Boston University's School of Medicine, and Seymour Papert was at MIT, in the Artificial Intelligence Laboratory. They remained in touch with Brenner and met frequently when he came to work during the summer at the Woods Hole Marine Biological Laboratory. Ben Kaminer decided to organize a conference at Boston University to promote inter-disciplinary exchange and interaction between eminent people from different fields—molecular biology, neurobiology, neuroanatomy, mathematics, computer science, and theoretical physics—all of whom were interested in understanding the human brain. He discussed this proposal with Sydney Brenner, who told him that a good starting point for discussion would be recent papers about the organization of the cerebral cortex by a young scientist named David Marr who was working in his group.

In May 1972 Ben Kaminer therefore set up an interdisciplinary workshop centered around David's work. The group included computer scientists involved in designing net-works and models creating "artificial intelligence." In addition to David, among the main participants were neuroanatomists such as Walle Nauta (MIT) and Alan Peters (Boston University), Sydney Brenner, Francis Crick, and Stephen Blomfield (MRC, Cambridge, UK), Freeman Dyson (Institute of Advanced Studies, Princeton), Seymour Papert and Marvin Minsky (Artificial Intelligence Laboratory, MIT), Stephen Kuffler, David Hubel, Torsten Wiesel, and John Dowling (Harvard), and Horace Barlow (who at that time was at the University of California at Berkeley). Students from Harvard, MIT, and Boston University were also invited.

The meeting had only two formal lectures, one by David and the other by Seymour Papert. It was otherwise devoted to informal discussions, which were lively and provoca-tive. In his opening remarks David emphasized the application of an "inverse square law" to theoretical research, according to which its value varies inversely with the square of the generality, and stressed the importance of establishing top-down relationships firmly sup-ported by functional (computational) understanding together with bottom-up relation-ship grounded in understanding of the mechanisms. The rest of his talk discussed three critical questions: What does the brain do? What are the logical equivalents? What are the actual mechanisms? Papert's lecture addressed "artificial brains" and "perceptrons" and discussed a simple system involved in catching a piece of chalk.

The two talks elicited intense discussions, which continued during and after the week-end. Several participants were invited by Albert Szent-Györgi to his beach cottage at Woods Hole and David and others went on a boat trip to Martha's Vineyard. David spent much time with Minsky and Papert and, as Francis Crick notes, this boat trip was to be his road to Damascus! He was invited to come to the Artificial Intelligence Laboratory at MIT, and a verbal invitation was followed by a letter from Marvin Minsky and Seymour Papert, sent on November 21, 1972. "This is an official invitation to come for three months or 6 months as you wish, more if you like. *Stipend* $1,250 per month. *Obligation:* Do something great." He certainly did.

In March 1973 David came as a visiting scientist to the MIT Artificial Intelligence Laboratory. Prior to his arrival, he submitted a proposal for research to be conducted during his visit to the lab. The project was called "KLUMSY," and the purpose was "to investigate the problems that arise in the control of a simple sensorimotor system, like a robot arm and to study how such a system could acquire and use knowledge about itself and about the environment." The proposal was quite detailed and very broad, describing the potential world of the robot arms, the sensors to be used, and the problems that it would solve. David went on to outline how he would program KLUMSY, the database organization, the knowledge base, and the motor programs. To develop and program KLUMSY, David proposed to become fluent in MacLisp and in Conniver, both high-level programming languages developed at the MIT Artificial Intelligence Laboratory (Sussman and McDermott, 1972), running on the PDP-10, the main computer then used for artificial intelligence research at the laboratory. However, KLUMSY didn't make it.

After his arrival at the Artificial Intelligence Laboratory, David gave a series of lectures to students and researchers in artificial intelligence, and was amazed by how little they knew about the brain: "any aspect of brain functions, they had no idea what a synapse was and of what it did, and had very vague ideas what the brain did." Those who thought they knew something about the brain were influenced by Piaget's theories which Seymour Papert had brought back after working with Piaget for a few years in Switzerland. In the Artificial Intelligence Laboratory playroom, David talked about neuroanatomy, Cajal, Eccles, and neurophysiology, discussing these subjects broadly and at a high computational level. His main message was that artificial intelligence was the road for understanding the functions of the brain. However, he conveyed very clearly that understanding computers was entirely different from understanding computations carried out by the brain and its information processing tasks.

In the first couple of months at MIT, David got in touch with Jack Pettigrew, who was at Berkeley at the time with Horace Barlow, and visited him in May 1973. They had corresponded a few years before as both were interested in the neuronal circuit diagram incorporating modifiable synapses that had been introduced by Brindley a few years earlier. Jack Pettigrew recollects that "when David visited me at UC Berkeley our interactions mainly concerned the *personalities* of individual cortical neurons. He was interested to correlate these highly specific properties with those that he surmised might be found on the basis of information theory and the complex circuitry of cortical neurons known from anatomy." They wrote an Artificial Intelligence Laboratory Working Memo (Marr and Pettigrew, 1973), which was never published.

Pettigrew wrote "the unpublished paper that we wrote at that time reflects this approach: to try to estimate the tuning and range of trigger features in V1 from an information theoretical point of view." The experimental data they used in this working paper were from Jack Pettigrew's studies of the cat visual cortex. The visit and discussions with Pettigrew proved to be very important to the direction that David's work would take. "[Jack Pettigrew] is studying the development of the visual cortex, and has the most extraordinary results! The features coded for really do depend on what the kittens see. He was full of the results you mentioned, and especially those of Zeki. Apparently there is a stereo area, a movement area, as well as a colour one" (from a letter to Stephen Blomfield, in 1973).

In parallel, David read prodigiously in the field of artificial intelligence, from MIT Artificial Intelligence Laboratory papers and PhD theses, to many artificial intelligence papers on visual recognition. In the summer of 1973 he briefly worked with Carl Hewitt on the problem of the representation of knowledge about the three-dimensional world and scene recognition. This combined ideas about low-level visual processing, specifically the idea that there were several specialized visual areas, with more abstract notions about the representation of knowledge in intelligent systems which should be organized into quite large chunks, called frames, as proposed by Marvin Minsky around that time (Minsky, 1973/1974). They produced a 36-page document (Marr and Hewitt, 1973) entitled "Video Ergo Scio: An essay on some of the things that a vision system should deal with to achieve recognition." This draft described a simple experimental world of mechanical assemblies of various parts and shapes of different sizes made from a Fischertechnik construction kit. An outcome of this work was that David decided to focus on vision first, and tackle the more cognitive issues later.

Enthusiastic about Edwin Land's research, "the only scientist in the field actually concerned with handling real pictures, in his case, colour film," in September 1973, David wrote to Sydney Brenner " I see a bright future for vision in the next few years, and am anxious to stay in the subject, doing my own AI research as well as acting as interface with neurophysiology." A few weeks later he wrote to Giles Brindley that, because "the facilities and people are really impressive," he had decided to stay on for "a year or two" and work on vision, "hoping that insight into the functions you had to perform to recognize something, together with detailed neurophysiological knowledge and unexcitable disposition, would be capable of illuminating many questions that are surely not vulnerable to the microelectrode." The MIT Artificial Intelligence Laboratory was more than happy to extend his stay. In 1975 David decided that he would stay permanently at MIT, and he accepted a position as associate professor in the psychology department, ultimately receiving tenure and promotion to full professor in April 1980.

David's enthusiasm for research, his creativity, acute intuition, and infinite energy, were contagious, and soon after his arrival at MIT he had started a "vision group" of Artificial Intelligence Laboratory students working with him on their theses. The work went very well. After the initial paper, "The computation of lightness by the primate retina" inspired by Land and McCane's Retinex theory (Land and McCann, 1971), he went on to investigate early cortical processing of visual information and published a series of important papers (all discussed and cited in his Vision book, Marr, 1982) which he then extended through collaborations with his graduate students in the vision group and with Tommy Poggio, who at that time was at the Max Planck Institute für biologische Kybernetik in Tübingen, working on vision with Werner Reichardt.

David and Tommy visited each other often, since they realized very quickly after they met in 1973 that they were an extraordinarily matched pair. Tommy Poggio remembers the first time when he came to the Artificial Intelligence Laboratory specially to work with David: "I was understanding more and more David's work on vision. In retrospect it took a lot of time. Really new ways of thinking cannot be understood at once. A thousand different facets must be communicated with the magic of a language and the fascination of a style. David's papers on early vision all have these rare properties" (Vaina, 1991). What David and Tommy had in common was that both were working on vision, both had a powerful analytic background, and both were very knowledgeable and interested in neurophysiology and psychophysics. So it was easy to have a long and productive collaboration, and to become close friends.

They were the "dynamic duo", as the vision group referred to them, because of the energy and enthusiasm they spread around, which charged everyone and instilled an intense desire to excel in research. Together David, his students, and Tommy were seeking computational insights into the working of the visual system, and they put them to the test of implementation as computer models. Within only a few years they had published many groundbreaking papers on computational vision, discussed and extended in the vision book (Marr, 1982).

Among David's first students was Shimon Ullman, a perfect intellectual match for David. Shimon remembers that, "working with David was always challenging, exciting and rewarding." When later on I talked with David about his various students, he used exactly the same words to described the working relationship with Shimon, and added "he is very smart, smarter than me!" They became very close friends—a warm and lasting friendship.

David always thought big, and wanted to instill this type of thinking in his students as well. Ellen Hildreth, one of David's PhD students whom he warmly and caringly supported, recollects that

> it wasn't enough to study an aspect of stereo, a sub-problem of motion or a particular type of texture problem. You gritted your teeth, and went in to tackle the whole problem of stereo, motion or texture head on. He always preferred to present a whole theory of something, which might be a bit lacking in detail, than to present an explanation for any part of the problem ... . He trained his students to stand on their own two feet, and be their own people—sometimes playing the devil's advocate, just to get us to argue with him.

Ellen nicely describes David's generosity with ideas: he would solve a large part of the problem but insist that the student did it all alone. Ideas would come to him any time. In a note I asked her for in November 1980, and published much later (Vaina, 1991), Ellen wrote

> Sometimes David would call at 9:00 on a Sunday morning and would ask, 'I was just wondering if by any chance you might have planned to come into work today; I have a new idea you might like to try out'.

The 70's were a different era, if you wanted to use a computer you went into the lab, and the AI lab was busy round the clock with people working. So going in on a Sunday was not all that unexpected. As David's vision work was progressing, his emphasis was mainly on the theory of the process and possible algorithms, and much less on specific implementation. David was thinking deeply about how biological information processing must be understood before it can be said that one understood in completely. He thought of a fundamentally novel approach to biological information processing which required that any problem must be addressed at several different levels of abstraction. What exactly was the task executed by the system? On what properties of the world could a system performing this task be expected to rely? What methods could be shown to be effective in the performance of the task? Given a particular method, what were the algorithms suited to implementing it? Given a particular algorithm, what was the neural circuitry sufficient to carry it out?

These questions formed the core of his research philosophy, and he brainstormed about them in long discussions with Tommy Poggio in 1976. They wrote their first paper on this framework for a book published by the Neuroscience Research Program, founded at MIT by Frank Schmitt (Marr and Poggio, 1977) where they proposed four levels of understanding information processing problems. Later, in his vision book, David explicitly formulated this framework as three levels of explanation of information processing. At the highest level is a computational theory of how a task could be performed. The computational theory must specify what is being computed and why it is a useful thing to compute it. At the next level is the representation of the task and an algorithm (or a set of algorithms) for achieving that representation. At the third level lies the question of how the algorithm is actually implemented in the hardware of the brain. A key point which David emphasized in the book is that the three levels should be considered relatively independently.

Music—the clarinet

David's sister Rowena and Peter Williams, his best friend at Rugby, vividly remember David as an accomplished clarinetist even at school. David studied with Thea King in London, and in 1961 he obtained a place in Britain's National Youth Orchestra (NYO). He often performed in the NYO concerts, and it was there that he met Tony Pay, who studied clarinet at the Royal Academy of Music and later mathematics at Cambridge. Tony Pay pursued a musical career, in 1968 becoming the principal clarinetist in the Royal Philharmonic Orchestra. David and Tony became close friends.

In a note to himself, June 1977, David wrote about why he decided not to pursue a career in music.

> I always had to be the best at things (& I was always very competent) and I felt horribly if I wasn't. I remember vividly what a shock it was meeting Tony Pay: for the first time he was someone clearly better than me at something that I did. It caused incredibly traumatic feelings in me, awful insecurity, and I was quite unable to play well in that context, and I even left the National Youth Orchestra after a year because I could not face being so obviously second rate there. Yet the funny thing is that even now (years later) I believe that I wasn't, that I did have something special about my playing that perhaps even he didn't have.

Tony Pay wrote years later "music sprang from his heart, and though he possessed a formidable intellect, he never tried to reduce this side of his life to anything theoretically manageable or systematizable. His relationship with the instrument was a very physical one, and he obviously loved the act of performing" (Vaina, 1991).

David didn't give up music, he only chose not to pursue music as a career. He continued playing the clarinet, and indeed excelled at it. He had a unique way of interpreting the music that remained unforgettable for those who heard him play. He gave himself entirely to the music, living it deeply and fully, whether playing informally with his music friends in Cambridge, or performing Berlioz's *Beatrice and Benedict* overture with the orchestra. David loved the feel of playing, and the intellectual and emotional effort required to express music's meaning, "always with an open mind that admitted there might be alternative ways of interpreting a piece" (email from Denis Mollison, 2015). Peter Rado, another friend from Trinity, remembered a very special trip when David borrowed a Land Rover and they went to a Youth Music Festival in Bayreuth. "I vividly remember David prowling around with his clarinet, looking for a soprano ('any soprano') to sing with him Schubert's 'Shepherd on the Rocks'" (Vaina, 1991). In the summer of 1966, just before Peter was going on kidney dialysis and was going to lose his freedom, David and Denis Mollison took him rowing around Loch Morar, a wonderful freshwater loch in Scotland. This holiday was a gift to Peter, a gift of friendship and music, with David playing parts of the Mozart clarinet quintet—unforgettable by all who heard him play!

While he worked with Giles Brindley, who was a bassoonist, they read music and often played together. Their repertory contained the three Beethoven duets (WoO 27) and Poulenc's Sonata for Clarinet and Bassoon (FP 32a). David played often and everywhere. Everyone who heard him remembers the purity of the sound, the intensity and emotion. The stack of clarinet music scores from which David played is very tall, which testifies to his deep and lifelong relationship with the clarinet. It was in no way just a hobby. His listeners knew that, and immediately felt the intensity of his relationship with the instrument and its music. "His excellence as a clarinetist was, to begin with, an excellence of attitude and response. He was always committed to what he did," said Tony Pay (Vaina, 1991).

This remained so throughout his life, and he took the clarinet wherever he traveled. Tommy Poggio remembers him playing Beethoven's Clarinet trio in B-Flat Major -Opus 11 with two members of Max Planck Institute in Tübingen. "I never was so struck by music as I was that evening by David's clarinet. It was beautiful and perfect, so full of emotion as to be almost unbearable. The audience—it was quite clear afterwards—had a similar experience" (Vaina, 1991).

At home, in Cambridge, Massachusetts, standing tall, he often played in the quiet of the evenings, completely immersed, slowing and speeding tempos, stopping and restarting to emphasize a passage. He treated the music as if it happened spontaneously, for the first time. In his playing, the clarinet voices—the clarinet has more than one—rose straight to heaven fresh and with the utmost grace. His repertoire included Mozart, Brahms, Cavallini, Beethoven, Crussel, Hindemith, and the Schubert Octet, Opus 166, to list just a few.

His ethereally beautiful interpretation of the clarinet piece, "Abîme des oiseaux" (Abyss of the birds), the third movement of the clarinet solo from Messiaen's "Quartet for the End of Time" was unique. We both loved it. First sad, then joyous, then sad again, pure, gentle, and forceful, an intense prayer in the silence of the night, rising above and beyond the intellect into pure emotion and into the unknown, invisible, eternity. When he stopped, David sat silent for some time and then, on those occasions, he did not play anything else.

Flying

In a note to himself, David describes that even before starting in the program of study at Trinity in 1963, he lived through a difficult period, questioning himself about everything, feeling unsure and worried that he could achieve the great things that he had set out to do—in fact he doubted that he could do anything at all. This was a very hard period, but he didn't give up. Instead, he took on every challenge, and overcame every difficulty.

> I realized that I was afraid of heights and being in a plane seemed terrifying. I made myself do it. The reason why I was so happy afterwards is that I actually have won over myself as well as putting myself in the hands of nature, armed only with my skills. I must do this parachute bit too. I really think is worthwhile facing these things, it makes me more confident, so I don't have to go on proving myself

His pilot's log book records that he began taking flying instruction at the end of March 1963, and obtained a private pilot's license soon thereafter that qualified him to fly day and night. Flying became a passion: it was freedom, fun, adventure, imaginative! After moving to MIT, he went on to obtain a US private pilot's license. The entries in his pilot's log book were frequent, and the destinations many. The entry of June 6, 1976 describes flying with Tommy Poggio, his good friend and closest collaborator at that time, from Laconia, New Hampshire to the Lake Region and discussing their cooperative algorithm for computing stereo disparity, which was published later that year in *Science* (Marr and Poggio, 1976).

A particularly unforgettable day in the sky, again with Tommy, was June 27, 1976. The Tall Ships were coming into Newport on their way to New York and, David recorded in his log book that, "the day was beautiful and we set out to fly to Newport." It became an adventure that Tommy later described:

> In the afternoon the weather deteriorated quite suddenly. There was a storm and ghastly winds. Back to the airport, we thought for a while to leave the plane and go back to Boston in some other way. David phoned several times to inquire about the weather at Hanscom. It was clear so he decided to start. Airborne again, drops of rain slashed across the windscreen until we came from the low clouds out in the sun. It was eternally beautiful weather to which poets have accustomed us. But the feeling in a small plane without instruments is quite different. David, however, was relaxed. There was nothing to do but fly straight and wait for the clouds to dissolve.[1].

The last challenge

On December 2, 1977, after two weeks of being unwell with a fever, David was admitted for investigations to the Mount Auburn Hospital which is affiliated with MIT. He

---

[1] At my request Tommy wrote his memories of David, in late November 1980. They are published in the 1991 book (Vaina, 1991).

was diagnosed with acute myeloid leukemia and received remission induction therapy. After being released from the hospital, he decided to go England, to his parents' home in Cornwall to rest and recuperate. While there, he went for a consultation at Addenbrooke's Hospital in Cambridge, UK, where he received remission consolidation therapy before embarking on a maintenance program. David went on working and interacting with his students almost as if the illness that ultimately took his life didn't exist—all this despite treatments that were hard, with unpleasant side effects, and despite relapses and more chemotherapy. His courage and determination are impossible to describe.

In the summer of 1978 David was in remission and returned to MIT to continue hands-on collaborations with the members of his vision group, Keith Nishihara, Ellen Hildreth, Eric Grimson, Ken Stevens, Shimon Ullman, Whitman Richards, and Tommy Poggio who visited frequently from the Max Planck Institute in Tübingen. There were also others: younger students engaged in the MS or PhD programs.

Whitman Richards remembers vividly the uniqueness of Marr's vision group, where everyone's "energy level, excitement, and dedication was exceptional" and the activity was prodigious. In the three years following David's diagnosis with leukemia, the group produced 120 publications.

In 1979, whether undergoing treatment, or suffering strong side effects from the chemotherapy, or being in remission, David worked on his book "*Vision: a Computational Investigation into the Human Representation and Processing of Visual Information*" (Marr, 1982), which beautifully and eloquently presents the work of the group, and the philosophy of the approach. It was published posthumously by Freeman in 1982. Each chapter of the draft of the book, written by hand, was carefully organized in a dedicated binder. The book is a lucid presentation of the framework for vision research, and involves the construction of representations specific to David and the vision group's research. It proposes a general theory of the visual processing stages for the symbolic representations of the visual world that are created, maintained, and interpreted by the visual information processing. The stages progress from a description of the input image up to three-dimensional shape recognition.

As the writing was coming to an end, in April 1979, David and Tommy Poggio went to visit Francis Crick, during a longer period of remission. Crick had moved to the Salk Institute in La Jolla, California, and now worked on neuroscience. In the mornings David and Tommy worked together, then the three of them had lunch and talked for hours every day. In a note (Vaina, 1991) Crick recounts how educational these intense daily talks were for him. Characteristically, Crick challenged David's functional approach, while David, who thrived on challenge, fiercely argued every point. Fired with lots of energy, they engaged in a great contest of ideas and opinions. David was perfectly able to answer every provocation from Francis. The last chapter of the Vision book is written as a debate staged between them, inspired by those long April afternoons of conversations and challenges that remained as wonderful memories.

While the writing of most of the book went smoothly, the last chapter that simulated conversations with Francis Crick was much harder. David commented on this in several letters to me from Addenbrooke's Hospital, where he was being treated, or from his parents' home in Cornwall, where he was recovering. Because my US immigration application process was ongoing, I was unable to travel outside the country. For periods of time that felt infinitely long, we could only communicate by letters and phone when David was between treatments in Cornwall, at his parents' cottage. However, we made the best of the situation, and wrote long letters almost daily, sometimes several letters a day.

In one of these letters David wrote that it was hard writing the last chapter of the book, not just because it was intended as a clear message of his views on computational vision, but also because it was meant to explain to the reader how to think computationally. David wanted them to absorb *why and what* one must do to really understand visual information processing. In a letter he sent me on May 3, 1979, after he had again been admitted into the hospital for treatment, David wrote, "I thought of the book whose introduction I charted yesterday, and I felt it strong within me. I shall try very hard to make it a good book. I am sure that what it says is important: my task is to fulfill its potential."

Almost 35 years have passed since the publication of the Vision book, yet it remains stimulating to researchers in many fields, from brain and cognitive science to computer vision and philosophy. In addition to presenting focused problems in visual perception, David addressed the broader problems of the brain and how its visual functions can be studied and understood. The book is a living example of David's "thinking big."

It is also a powerful testament to David's will to rise to the last challenge. The book was published first in 1982 by W. H. Freeman, and then republished by MIT Press in 2010. In this last edition I asked his two best friends during his time at MIT, Shimon Ullman and Tommy Poggio, to write an introduction and an epilogue. Though the book is now more than 30 years old, over 3000 copies were sold during the first five years of this second edition.

By the summer of 1979 the research on vision was going well, several computational modules had been defined and algorithms implemented, and the vision group was hard at work. David was becoming interested in the development of possible hardware devices that might be capable of solving real-life problems. He wrote to me from Cornwall,

> I am trying not to think about going back there [Addenbrooke's Hospital]—it's depressing. And you how know I hate the drugs. A small victory yesterday though, I climbed up the path onto the cliff walk [in Cornwall], which I could not have done a week ago! I am starting to get back into shape. More good news, I got the design drawings for our vision chip! It should be tested now, I think, but I haven't heard anything. I wonder if it works. Christ there is such a future in that sort of technological development, and it's something that really can only be done at the AI Lab. I am sure Shimon and Tommy (when he comes to MIT) will push it.

He was very enthusiastic about this chip, so much so that after he returned at MIT in the fall of 1979, together with Shimon Ullman he went to DARPA in Washington DC to meet the sponsors of their research at the Artificial Intelligence Laboratory. Shimon remembers that at some point they were asked about their views regarding new directions the agency could take. "David snapped 'grow wires,' without offering any additional explanation. I could see the puzzlement in the other person's expression, but David saw no need to elaborate the issue further" (Vaina, 1991). He was extremely quick, he expected those around him to be equally quick, and he liked to tease.

A letter from the Federal Aviation Administration, dated November 2, 1978 informed David that he did not meet the medical standards of the Federal Aviation Regulations because of a disqualifying hematological condition, and that it was unlawful to exercise airman privileges unless he held an appropriate medical certificate allowing him to fly. There was nothing to do. But the Boston area scenery was still incredibly beautiful, whether walking in Great Meadows in Concord, or looking at the Boston skyline at sunset, enjoying the sun playing in the water at Walden Pond, or the dramatic sunset sky in Cambridge. David loved these views.

And suddenly, there was hope for the future! At Addenbrooke's a group of physicians lead by Abraham Karpas developed a vaccine against the type of leukemia David had, and he was one of the five patients selected to get it. The protocol included three doses, a few weeks apart. David had the first two in the spring of 1980, after which he came back to Cambridge, Mass., and things seem to go well. We were happily planning the next few years, celebrating life with friends, and felt hopeful. On May 15 he went back for the third dose of the vaccine, but the blood tests indicated that it had not helped. He relapsed and there were no additional promising treatments that could be offered there.

David returned immediately to Boston and in June 1980 he began a new and aggressive chemotherapy treatment at the Sydney Farber Cancer Institute (now known as the Dana Farber Cancer Institute) in Boston. The side effects were terrible, he became weak and could barely walk. I thought that if he could not walk, he would still be able to swim. I asked the hospital staff if we could have the afternoon off. They agreed, and I drove to Walden Pond, and slowly we walked into the water. It was almost sunset, and the sunlight reflected happily in David's eyes. "I swim! I can swim! I don't need to fly to see and feel beauty, this is all so beautiful. I love it," he said. After sunset we drove to the Willow Pond Kitchen, a small and simple restaurant nearby, and we each had a lobster and a beer. We returned to the hospital very late, it was almost 11 pm. We were victorious and happy, and it showed, so that when the worried hospital personnel saw us walking in, they greeted us with heartfelt warm smiles, but also with great relief. They understood.

By midsummer David was in remission, and this allowed us ten days at home. Out of the hospital! David seemed happy, we celebrated life over a bottle of champagne on our terrace together with Shimon Ullman. We were working on the last version of the article we wrote together (Marr and Vaina, 1982). It was a unique experience for me, at home, sitting at the desk side by side, discussing every sentence. Every word had to be absolutely right.

One beautiful breezy late afternoon, we were sitting on the terrace, the wind was gently moving the leaves, and the blue sky was turning into the dramatic sunset colors that David loved so much. We were creatively planning things to do or to work on, without ever letting the word "if" sneak in. Toward the evening, he went into the living room and picked up his clarinet and the score of the "Abîme des oiseaux." It is an extremely challenging piece, long held tones stretch ever so slowly and then stop abruptly, depicting the lone singing of the bird into the abyss of endless time, interlaced with chirps—fleeting moments of optimism. Davids interpretation of it was perfect, amazing, intense, and romantic.

But not then. He tried, tried again, and again. Quietly he put the clarinet away, and softly said that he could no longer feel the instrument. It was the neuropathy from the repeated courses of chemotherapy. Messiaen's quartet was composed in homage to the Angel of the Apocalypse, who raises his hand toward heaven saying: "There shall be no more time." The clarinet solo piece is "Time with its sadness, its weariness. The birds are the opposite of Time; they are our desire for light, for stars, for rainbows, and for jubilant songs" (Messiaen, 1941).

In the remaining time we had together, we listened to records or tapes of our favorite music. The clarinet was almost always present, and David listened with the same intensity and emotion he transmitted when playing. It was an afternoon in November 1980 when we were listening to Schubert's Octet in F major with Gervase de Peyer on the clarinet, and after the fifth movement David smiled softly "Serene and peaceful, let's stop here. He is good, but I am also really good" he said proudly and had that special, irresistible, twinkle in his eyes.

As much as I could, I was reading about innovations in treatment for David's type of leukemia. I discovered an article by a Japanese doctor, Mutsuyuki Kochi, and colleagues, which described good results with a treatment for leukemia they had developed. I managed to contact him by phone at his institute in Japan; he was kind and very positive, although it was really hard for us to understand each other in English. In October 1980 I received a letter from him saying that he would send a large amount of the medication and a detailed protocol on how to administer the drugs. The duration of the treatment was to be as long as possible. Tommy Poggio brought the medicines from Germany. (I cannot remember why they could not be sent here directly.) In the meantime David and I talked at length with the doctors at Dana Farber, but they were skeptical that it would work. David was very weak, was experiencing many strong side effects, and the conclusion of a long meeting with his doctors was that this exploratory treatment would not gain time and remission, but possibly have just the opposite effect. The treatment was not approved by the US Food and Drug Administration, but it wasn't that that stopped us from trying it: rather we listened to the opinion of his doctors, and considered David's medical condition at the time.

Every day I read his medical chart, and around mid-November the report from a bone-marrow test showed that he had no stem cells left, which meant that another remission was very unlikely. I am sure David knew it as well, but we never talked about it. There were so many wonderful things to talk about, to plan, as if our future together was still ours. Members of the vision group visited often and discussed research results, and David's feedback, as always, was quick, to the point, and incisive.

Sunday November 16, 1980, was an unusually beautiful sunny and warm day. In the early morning at the hospital we started planning the menu for our Christmas dinner: it was still a while away, but we always liked to plan everything in exquisite detail and refine the plans until the last minute. The dinner was going to start with champagne and special appetizers, followed by roast duck and orange sauce. The sun reflected in his eyes, he was luminous, full of life. Around 11 am the resident on duty, a young man full of pimples, came in. David closed the eyes and appeared immobile. The resident asked him questions, but he didn't respond. The resident asked louder, and then louder again. I thought this was another of David's mischiefs, as he liked to tease this particular resident. But this time it wasn't a prank.

David suddenly went into a coma that day, without any warning. He died at 3:45 am the next morning, November 17th. His doctor and two nurses, although not on duty that day, were there all the time. A few days later I arranged a short service in the Bigelow Chapel at the Mount Auburn Cemetery, where he was buried. At some point during the service the minister paused, we all remained in silence and listened to the "Abîme des oiseaux" clarinet solo from the beautiful recording of Gervase de Peyer. I chose this piece for its purity and intensity, and because it goes up and up, until it stops suddenly, and nothing follows. It was the "end of time." Also because it was a piece that David played so beautifully.

A few days later I received a letter from Dr. Emil Frei III, the physician in chief and director of the Sydney Farber Cancer Institute , who often came by to chat with David. He wrote: "I was privileged to know him well enough to feel the warmth of his friendship and the light of his intelligence, cheerfulness and courage, even in the face of a most difficult medical situation. More than any other patient I have known for a long time, he evoked the admiration and concern of the medical and nursing staff."

This book

David's thinking, like his emotions, was almost a physical presence, palpable in everything he did, whether it was science, music, flying, or just playing. It captured everyone around him. David was an intellectual leader, who possessed a harmonious blend of insight, mathematical rigor, and deep understanding of anatomy and neurobiology that characterize his research. He gave us a new intellectual landscape, which remains fertile more than 35 years after his death. This book, dedicated to his 70th birthday, demonstrates that. It is also living proof that David did win the *final challenge*, just as he surmounted all other challenges he encountered in his life.

Acknowledgments

David and I met on July 4, 1978 at the MIT Boat House where our lab (the MIT Artificial Intelligence Laboratory) was celebrating the Fourth of July. At Christmas 1979 we got engaged to marry and were married on May 10, 1980. Thus a large part of the period before the "Last Challenge" is constructed from what I learned from many of David's friends and colleagues and from his letters, notes, and manuscripts that I have at home. David Willshaw kindly contacted some of David's friends from the Trinity era, who then wrote to me and generously sent detailed recollections of the years they were together in Cambridge, UK. Denis Mollison and Tony Gardner-Medwin wrote extensively. David's

Rugby School friend, Peter Williams, also supplied a very informative piece. I contacted Jack Pettigrew to better understand the roots of their MIT Artificial Intelligence Laboratory working paper, and he sent me his recollections about interacting with David in the early 1970s, when David was moving from his earlier work discussed in this book to studying vision. In a previous book (Vaina, 1991) I have published recollections about David by friends and colleagues from both side of the Atlantic, and these also helped me in building this chapter. I am thankful to all. Also many thanks to Peter Dayan, David Willshaw, Denis Mollison, and Dick Passingham for critically reading and commenting on this chapter and to Cathy Collis and Chris Randles for carefully proofreading it for language, grammar, and punctuation.

All inaccuracies that the reader may identify in this chapter are my own.

References

Barlow H (1959). Sensory mechanisms, the reduction of redundancy, and intelligence; Proceedings of the 17th Symposium on the Mechanisation of Thought Processes, vol. **2**, pp. 537–574. London: HMSO.

Barlow H (1961). Possible principles underlying the transformations of sensory messages. In: Sensory Communication, pp. 217–234. Cambridge, MA: MIT Press.

Blomfield S, Marr D. (1970). How the cerebellum may be used. Nature. **227**:1224–1228.

Brindley G. (1967). The classification of modifiable synapses and their use in models for conditioning. Proc R Soc Lond B Biol Sci. **168**:361–376.

Broadbent D. (1971). Decision and Stress. London: Academic Press.

Ramón y Cajal S. (1911/1955). Histologie du système nerveux de l'homme et des vertébrés. Paris: A. Maloine/Madrid: Consejo Superior De Investigation Cientificas.

Douglas R, Pribram K. (1966). Learning and limbic lesions. Neuropsychologia. **4**:197–220.

Douglas R, Pribram K. (1969). Distraction and habituation in monkeys with limbic lesions. J Comp Physiol Psychol. **69**:473–480.

Eccles JC, Ito, M, Szentagothai, J. (1967). The Cerebellum as a Neuronal Machine. Berlin: Springer.

Hebb DO. (1949). The Organization of Behavior: A Neuropsychological Theory. New York: Wiley.

Jardine C, Jardine N, Sibson R. (1967). The structure and construction of taxonomic hierarchies. Math Biosci. **1**:173–179.

Land E, McCann J. (1971). Lightness and retinex theory. J Opt Soc Am. **61**:1–11.

Marr D. (1968). The cortical analysis of sensory information. A theoretical investigation. Trinity College, Cambridge, UK.

Marr D. (1969). A theory of cerebellar cortex. J Physiol. **202**:437–470.

Marr D. (1970). A theory for cerebral neocortex. Proc R Soc Lond B Biol Sci. **176**:161–234.

Marr D. (1971). Simple memory: a theory for archicortex. Philos Trans R Soc Lond B Biol Sci. **262**:23–81.

Marr D. (1982). Vision: A Computational Investigation into the Human Representation and Processing of Visual Information. San Francisco, CA: W. H. Freeman.

Marr D, Hewitt C. (1973). Video Ergo Scio: an essay on some things we like a vision system to know. In: Artificial Intelligence Laboratory Working Paper 60, Massachusetts Institute of Technology.

Marr D, Pettigrew J. (1973). Quantitative aspects of the computations performed by the visual cortex in the cat, with a note on a function of lateral inhibition. Artificial Intelligence Laboratory Working Paper 55, Massachusetts Institute of Technology.

Marr D, **Poggio T.** (1976). Cooperative computation of stereo disparity. Science. **194**:283–287.

Marr D, **Poggio T.** (1977). From understanding computation to understanding neural circuitry. Neurosciences Res Prog. Bull. **15**:470–488.

Marr D, **Vaina LM.** (1982). Representation and recognition of movements of shapes. Proc R Soc Lond B Biol Sci. **214**:501–524.

Messiaen O. (1941). Introduction. In: Quatuor pour la Fin du Temps. Paris: Editions Durand & Cie.

Minsky M (1973/1974) A framework for representing knowledge. In: Artificial Intelligence Laboratory Memo 306, Massachusetts Institute of Technology.

Sussman GJ, McDemott DV. (1972). From PLANNER to CONNIVER: a genetic approach. Proc AFIPS '72 (Fall, part II), pp. 1171–1179, New York: ACM.

Vaina LM. (1991). From the Retina to the Neocortex: Selected Papers of David Marr. Boston: Birkhauser.

Walter, W Grey. (1953). The Living Brain. London: Duckworth.

Zeeman E. (1962). The topology of the brain and visual perception. In: Topology of 3-Manifolds (**M. K. Fort**, ed), pp. 240–256. Englewood Cliffs, NJ: Prentice-Hall.

Index

Tables, figures, and boxes are indicated by an italic *t*, *f*, and *b* following the page/paragraph number.